ADHD in Adolescents

Alison Schonwald
Editor

ADHD in Adolescents

A Comprehensive Guide

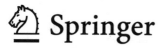 Springer

Editor
Alison Schonwald
Department of Pediatrics
Cambridge Health Alliance
Harvard Medical School
Touchstone Neurodevelopmental Center, LLC
Woburn, MA, USA

ISBN 978-3-030-62395-1   ISBN 978-3-030-62393-7   (eBook)
https://doi.org/10.1007/978-3-030-62393-7

This Springer imprint is published by the registered company Springer Nature Switzerland AG
The registered company address is: Gewerbestrasse 11, 6330 Cham, Switzerland

Introduction

The Value of a Diagnosis: Why Now?

When most people think of Attention-Deficit/Hyperactivity Disorder (ADHD), an overly active or inattentive grade-school student struggling to sit still or pay attention in class comes to mind. We might imagine an 8-year-old who is never still unless sitting in front of a screen, or a 10-year-old who is still losing everything, whose room and desk are a mess, whose teacher says, "He would do so much better in class if he could just pay attention." In fact, formal ADHD diagnostic criteria has long required ADHD symptoms to start in childhood, and according to the Diagnostic Statistical Manual of Mental Disorders – Fifth Edition (DSM-5), symptoms must be present before a child reaches 12 years of age [1].

So, why is this book about ADHD in *adolescents*? There are lots of reasons.

Let's think about what ADHD is: a neurobehavioral disorder occurring in anywhere from 7–10% of children and adolescents [2]. Many in this group don't outgrow the diagnosis: 45–85% diagnosed as children still have symptoms in adolescence, and 50–60% of that group show symptoms into adulthood [3]. Yet, we expect huge strides in maturity in the teen years, strides which depend on healthy underlying neurology. If we expect adolescents to drive a car, write term papers, babysit, join the army (and the list goes on), then we expect them to pay attention to their surroundings without distraction, inhibit their own interests and desires for a less preferred task at hand, plan for the immediate future, and again, the list goes on. Adolescents with ADHD may have a much harder time maturing into these skills, or demonstrating them consistently. Their underlying neurobiology is at the root of the problem, and the problem may not become fully apparent until facing this escalation in the expectations we have for them.

I've heard parents wonder,

"She has been on medication for ADHD for years. Shouldn't we have avoided some of these teen problems?"

"He isn't hyperactive like he was when his ADHD was first diagnosed. He shouldn't need medication now."

"She's made it this far without a diagnosis. Why does she need a diagnosis now?"

"He can't use this as a crutch, he just needs to figure it out."

"Diagnosing and treating her as a teenager is a mistake, life won't provide accommodations for her."

"We are teaching them not to use drugs, how can you put them on drugs?"

All are typical and reasonable thoughts and concerns, and may explain why you are picking this book up. Whether you are a parent with these questions, a clinician expected to reply to them, or a teacher spending much of your day with affected teens, this book should help.

Put simply, ADHD is important to identify and address in affected adolescents because it impacts them now, and can impact them in the future.

> Diagnosing and treating ADHD in teenagers is aimed at a single ultimate goal: **best outcomes now and later**.

"Outcomes" can mean different things for different people: best educational level reached? highest scores earned? best job kept? happiest relationships sustained? Regardless of the individual priorities, we know that, as a group, those with ADHD are more likely to have executive function problems, additional mental health diagnoses, substance use disorders, and lower professional attainment [4]. Yet, ADHD can be masked by other symptoms, diagnosed without standardized methods, and treated with ineffective options. Cultural differences in the perspective and language of health and developmental add another layer to consider. Unrecognized or misdiagnosed, the difficulties encountered by those with ADHD can negatively impact any and all life outcomes. Our goal is to offer every person their best opportunity to succeed, which means eliminating barriers they face. This book will help all readers understand, identify, and address the obstacles of ADHD so each affected person can thrive.

We do not focus on the unique strengths of each person. We don't have a chapter on the benefits of ADHD or the ways it improves lives. Yet, many incredibly successful adults have ADHD [5–7] and attribute their ability to lead, to excel, to think out of the box, and to come up with limitless ideas to their ADHD! ADHD is not a life sentence. While you celebrate and bolster the strengths in your child/student/patient, use this book to understand the complexity of ADHD in teens so your approach is as comprehensive and evidence-informed as possible.

Alison Schonwald
Department of Pediatrics, Cambridge Health Alliance
Harvard Medical School, Touchstone Neurodevelopmental Center, LLC,
Woburn, MA, USA

References

1. American Psychiatric Association. Diagnostic and Statistical Manual of Mental Disorders (DSM-5), 5th ed. Arlington: American Psychiatric Association, 2013.
2. Subcommittee on Attention-Deficit/Hyperactivity Disorder, Steering Committee on Quality Improvement and Management, Wolraich M, et al. ADHD: clinical practice guideline for the diagnosis, evaluation, and treatment of attention-deficit/hyperactivity disorder in children and adolescents. Pediatrics. 2011;128(5):1007–22. https://doi.org/10.1542/peds.2011-2654.
3. Roy A, Hechtman L, Arnold LE, et al. Childhood factors affecting persistence of ADHD in adulthood: results from the 16 year follow-up of the MTA study. [Poster presentation]. Annual Meeting of the American Psychiatric Association, 2016, May 14–18, Atlanta, GA, United States.
4. Biederman J, Petty CR, Fried R, et al. Educational and occupational underattainment in adults with attention-deficit/hyperactivity disorder: a controlled study. J Clin Psychiatry. 2008;69(8):1217–1222. https://doi.org/10.4088/jcp.v69n0803
5. Glazer J. ADHD Can Be a CEO's Superpower. [Huffington Post Blog]. 2015, September. Retrieved from https://www.huffingtonpost.ca/jessica-glazer/adhd-ceo-career_b_8124154.html
6. Kessler Z. I wouldn't give up my ADHD. ADDitude Magazine. 2018, November. Retrieved from https://www.additudemag.com/women-leaders-with-adhd/
7. Shoot B. The stars who aligned ADHD with their success. ADDitude Magazine. 2019, July. Retrieved from https://www.additudemag.com/successful-people-with-adhd-learning-disabilities/

Contents

Contributors

Jennifer Aites, MD Harvard Medical School, Division of Developmental Medicine, Boston Children's Hospital, Boston, MA, USA

Fern Baldwin, PhD Center for Autism and Related Disorders, Kennedy Krieger Institute, Baltimore, MD, USA

Rebecca Baum, MD The Olson Huff Center, Mission Children's Hospital, Asheville, NC, USA

Joshua Borus, MD, MPH Division of Adolescent/Young Adult Medicine, Boston Children's Hospital, Boston, MA, USA

Clement J. Bottino, MD, MPH Division of General Pediatrics, Boston Children's Hospital, Harvard Medical School, Boston, MA, USA

Jonas Bromberg, Psy.D. Boston Children's Hospital, Boston, MA, USA

Pediatric Physicians' Organization at Children's, Wellesley, MA, USA

Harvard Medical School, Boston, MA, USA

Olivia Carrick, MD Department of Psychiatry, Boston Children's Hospital, Harvard Medical School, Boston, MA, USA

Devon Carroll, APRN-BC Department of Psychiatry and Behavioral Sciences, Boston Children's Hospital, Boston, MA, USA

Natalie Cerda, MD, MPH Division of Developmental Medicine, Boston Children's Hospital, Boston, MA, USA

Nicholas Chadi, MD MPH Division of Adolescent Medicine, Department of Pediatrics, Sainte-Justine University Hospital Centre, Université de Montreal, Montreal, QC, Canada

Cassandra Conrad, MD Division of Developmental Medicine, Boston Children's Hospital, Boston, MA, USA

Danielle Doctor, MD Maine Medical Center, Portland, ME, USA

Katherine Driscoll, Ph.D. Division of Developmental Medicine, Boston Children's Hospital, Boston, MA, USA

Kida Ejesi, Ph.D. Developmental Medicine Center, Boston Children's Hospital, Boston, MA, USA

Leslie Green, MSW, LICSW Adolescent Substance Use and Addiction Program, Division of Developmental Medicine, Boston Children's Hospital, Boston, MA, USA

Jackie Hsieh, MD, MPH Harvard Medical School, Boston, MA, USA

Pediatrics at Newton Wellesley, Newton, MA, USA

Jennifer Johnson, MD Department of Pediatrics, Valley Children's Healthcare, Madera, CA, USA

Jill R. Kavanaugh, MLIS, AHIP Center on Media and Child Health (CMCH) and Clinic for Interactive Media and Internet Disorders (CIMAID), Boston Children's Hospital, Boston, MA, USA

Lauren Lindle, MD Developmental and Behavioral Pediatrician, Advocate Children's Hospital, Oak Lawn, IL, USA

Department of Clinical Sciences at Rosalind Franklin University of Medicine and Science, Oak Lawn, IL, USA

Kate Linnea, PhD Division of Developmental Medicine, Boston Children's Hospital, Boston, MA, USA

Carrie Mauras, PhD Department of Psychiatry, Cambridge Health Alliance, Touchstone Neurodevelopmental Center, Woburn, MA, USA

Anna Chaves McDonald, Ph.D. ASK Program, Primary Care Center, Boston Children's Hospital, Boston, MA, USA

Alison Rosenberg Mostyn, LICSW Boston Children's Hospital, Boston, MA, USA

Demetra Pappas, MD, MPH Harvard Medical School, Division of Developmental Medicine, Boston Children's Hospital, Boston, MA, USA

Joanna E. Perdomo, MD Division of General Pediatrics, Boston Children's Hospital, Harvard Medical School, Boston, MA, USA

Corinna Rea, MD, MPH Division of General Pediatrics, Boston Children's Hospital, Harvard Medical School, Boston, MA, USA

Michael Rich, MD, MPH Harvard Medical School, Boston, MA, USA

Center on Media and Child Health (CMCH) and Clinic for Interactive Media and Internet Disorders (CIMAID), Boston Children's Hospital, Boston, MA, USA

Harvard T.H. Chan School of Public Health, Boston, MA, USA

Sabrina Sargado, MD Division of Developmental Medicine, Boston Children's Hospital, Boston, MA, USA

Miriam Schizer, MD Adolescent Substance Use and Addiction Program, Division of Developmental Medicine, Department of Pediatrics, Boston Children's Hospital, Harvard Medical School, Boston, MA, USA

Dasha Solomon, PsyD Division of Developmental Medicine, Boston Children's Hospital, Boston, MA, USA

Anisha Srinivasan, MD, MPH Division of Developmental Medicine, University of Washington and Seattle Children's Hospital, Seattle, WA, USA

Michael Tsappis, MD Clinic for Interactive Media and Internet Disorders (CIMAID), Division of Adolescent Medicine and Department of Psychiatry, Boston Children's Hospital, Harvard Medical School, Boston, MA, USA

Rachel Tunick, Ph.D. Department of Psychiatry, Boston Children's Hospital, Harvard Medical School, Boston, MA, USA

Frinny Polanco Walters, MD Division of Adolescent/Young Adult Medicine, Boston Children's Hospital, Boston, MA, USA

Laura Weissman, MD Division of Developmental Medicine, Boston Children's Hospital, Boston, MA, USA

Liesl Windsor, MD Division of Developmental Medicine, Boston Children's Hospital, Boston, MA, USA

Jeffrey H. Yang, MD Department of Pediatrics, Valley Children's Healthcare, Madera, CA, USA

Samuel Zinner, MD Division of Developmental Medicine, University of Washington and Seattle Children's Hospital, Seattle, WA, USA

Part I
ADHD 101: The Basics

Chapter 1
Making the ADHD Diagnosis in Adolescents

Corinna Rea and Jackie Hsieh

Background

In the ever-changing world of adolescence, identifying Attention-deficit/hyperactivity disorder (ADHD) for the first time is tricky. Teenagers face an increasingly distracting world full of social stress and digital media. Society expects teens to take on more independent management of academic and work demands, all while noting that adolescents rarely get the sleep they need. Sustained attention and impulse control are required for safe driving, while new teen drivers must simultaneously screen out the often animated billboard advertisements marketing directly to them. We also expect them not to look at their smartphones, which feel like a third hand! Finally, the diagnostic terms change and leave open a range of interpretations for clinicians to unravel. How do we know whether inattentive, impulsive teens truly have an underlying disorder (ADHD) or are simply learning to manage the new demands of the world around them?

Case Example

Thomas is a 16-year-old who has always seemed intelligent but never put forth great effort in school. He did "fine" academically (Bs and an occasional C) and was not

C. Rea (✉)
Division of General Pediatrics, Boston Children's Hospital, Harvard Medical School, Boston, MA, USA
e-mail: Corinna.Rea@childrens.harvard.cdu

J. Hsieh
Harvard Medical School, Boston, MA, USA

Pediatrics at Newton Wellesley, Newton, MA, USA
e-mail: Jackie.Hsieh@childrens.harvard.edu

© Springer Nature Switzerland AG 2020
A. Schonwald (ed.), *ADHD in Adolescents*,
https://doi.org/10.1007/978-3-030-62393-7_1

in more trouble than other kids. He plays baseball and football and has a large social circle. Now in the middle of 10th grade, Thomas is earning Cs and Ds. He cannot stay on top of his work and has trouble keeping up with teachers who lecture (rather than engaging students in more active learning), despite studying and doing homework for hours at night. He thinks he might have ADHD.

Start with What You Know: ADHD Criteria and Presentations

Attention-deficit/hyperactivity disorder (ADHD) is diagnosed using standardized symptom criteria which are similar for all ages, from young children to centenarians. The American Psychiatric Association's *Diagnostic and Statistical Manual of Mental Disorders* (DSM-5) [1] outlines the type and number of symptoms (of inattention and/or hyperactivity/impulsivity) and several additional conditions required to diagnose ADHD. This provides a consistent framework for clinicians: more is required than a report of overactivity or poor attention for a diagnosis to be made.

But the diagnosis requires more than checking off enough symptoms on a checklist. For starters, the DSM-5 diagnostic criteria require several conditions to be met in addition to the symptoms presenting. Further, a diagnosis requires that reports from teachers and parents/guardians as well as a clinician's judgment after a comprehensive history and exam are interpreted to determine the diagnosis. The diagnosis ultimately is based on a clinician's judgment.

So, what do we do? How do clinicians decide? And how do we do this for adolescents?

Know the Diagnostic Choices

Diagnostic visits require that the clinician making the diagnosis knows the diagnostic choices, the known types of ADHD presentations. There are three common presentations of ADHD based on three combinations of symptoms. Each combination points toward a diagnosis, based on the individual's current symptoms. A given person with ADHD is diagnosed with only one presentation at a time, the presentation that best matches the current symptoms (Table 1.1).

Table 1.1 Three common presentations of ADHD

Three common presentations of ADHD	
1	Attention-deficit/hyperactivity disorder, combined presentation
2	Attention-deficit/hyperactivity disorder, predominantly inattentive presentation
3	Attention-deficit/hyperactivity disorder, predominantly hyperactive/impulsive presentation

The clinician making the diagnosis reviews information gathered and observed to determine what criteria are met (see Section "The Clinical Visit").

What Symptoms Does the Adolescent Have?

Symptoms of Inattention

1. Often fails to give close attention to details/makes careless mistakes on academic work
2. Often has trouble holding attention on tasks
3. Often does not seem to listen when spoken to directly or when having conversations
4. Often fails to follow through on instructions or tasks and deadlines
5. Often has trouble organizing tasks and activities, difficulty with time management
6. Often avoids tasks that require mental effort over a long period of time
7. Often loses valuable items such as cell phones, homework, books, keys, or clothes
8. Often is easily distracted by extraneous stimuli, such as unrelated thoughts
9. Often is forgetful in daily activities or regular duties (homework, keeping appointments)

Symptoms of Hyperactivity/Impulsivity

1. Often fidgets with or taps hands/feet
2. Often leaves seat when expected to remain in place
3. Often runs or climbs when it is inappropriate (teens/adults may feel restless)
4. Often unable to participate in leisure activities quietly
5. Often seems on the go or "driven by a motor" (teens/adults may be uncomfortable sitting still for extended time; may be experienced by others as restless of difficult to keep up with)
6. Often talks excessively
7. Often blurts out answers before questions are completed; finishes others' sentences
8. Often has trouble waiting for a turn (while waiting in line)
9. Often interrupts or intrudes on others (in conversations, uses others' things without asking; takes over what others are doing)

Gathering the symptoms comes from a comprehensive history and review of rating scales. See section "The Clinical Visit" to walk through those steps.

Are there enough symptoms to meet the diagnostic requirements? The number of symptoms required for each diagnosis is listed in the table below, distinguishing requirements for those younger than 17 from those who are older (Tables 1.2 and 1.3).

Table 1.2 ADHD symptom requirements for those under 17 years of age

Three common presentations of ADHD Diagnostic criteria: *up to age 17*	Minimum number of symptoms of inattention	Minimum number of symptoms of hyperactivity/impulsivity
Attention-deficit/hyperactivity disorder, combined presentation	6	6
Attention-deficit/hyperactivity disorder, predominantly inattentive presentation	6	0
Attention-deficit/hyperactivity disorder, predominantly hyperactive/impulsive presentation	0	6

Table 1.3 ADHD symptom requirements for those 17 year of age and older

Three common presentations of ADHD Diagnostic criteria: *17 years and older*	Minimum number of symptoms of inattention	Minimum number of symptoms of hyperactivity/impulsivity
Attention-deficit/hyperactivity disorder, combined presentation	5	5
Attention-deficit/hyperactivity disorder, predominantly inattentive presentation	5	0
Attention-deficit/hyperactivity disorder, predominantly hyperactive/impulsive presentation	0	5

Adolescents younger than 17 years old require six or more of the symptoms for diagnosis, while anyone 17 years and older requires only five or more of the symptoms.

Determine if the Additional Conditions Are Met

1. After reviewing the symptoms and determining whether there are sufficient symptoms to meet the symptom requirements for an ADHD diagnosis, several additional conditions must be met.
2. Symptoms must be present before age 12. Those with symptoms that start after the age of 12 do not qualify for any of these three ADHD diagnoses.
3. Symptoms must occur in two or more settings. For example, symptoms that are only present at home but not at school, or in public, or in any other observed setting do not meet criteria for any of these three disorders.
4. There should also be clear evidence that the symptoms interfere with and reduce the quality of social, school, or work functioning.
5. These symptoms are not better explained by another mental health or mood disorder [1].

Clinicians can also add a "specifier" or two to the diagnosis, giving it more detail. These specifiers are sometimes written in formal reports and other medical or psychological documentation.

- In partial remission (when full criteria were met in the past but not for the past 6 months but still cause impairment)
- Severity:
  - Mild (minimum number of required symptoms, cause minor impairment in function)
  - Moderate (in the middle of mild and severe)
  - Severe (many more symptoms present than needed to make the diagnosis and result in marked impairment in function)

When a person has impairing symptoms that do not meet the full criteria above, one of these two additional diagnoses may be appropriate.

What happens when the teen does not meet full criteria but no better explanation exists?

Lucky us! There are actually two more diagnostic options:

1. Other Specified Attention-Deficit/Hyperactivity Disorder
2. Unspecified Attention-Deficit/Hyperactivity Disorder

- When the clinician reports the specific reason that full criteria are not met, the diagnosis is "Other specified Attention-Deficit/Hyperactivity Disorder."
- When the clinician does not specify the reasons for failure to meet full diagnostic criteria, the diagnosis is "Unspecified Attention-Deficit/Hyperactivity Disorder."

Why? Why would such vague criteria be allowed? Sometimes we cannot get the history of the person from before age 12. Sometimes we have no history of symptoms before 12 at all, but we may intuit the person compensated so well in younger years that no symptoms were noted; high intelligence, solid work ethic, and an appealing personality can hide a young student's inattention or hyperactivity/impulsivity. Alternately, the environment could have prevented early ADHD symptoms from surfacing; for example, a student with inattention in a large class with relatively low work demands could "fly under the radar." Finally, a family/school so well matched (e.g., lots of activity, stimulation, structure, and individual attention) with the young child's needs might make ADHD symptoms irrelevant. Don't assume a clinician who gives these diagnoses is unsure or inaccurate; it might be the exact opposite situation.

The Confusion

The Name: Is It ADD or ADHD?

If this is so simple, why are so many people confused? It's all in a name. We often hear "She has ADD, she's not hyperactive," and medical records still pop up with "hyperkinesis." A brief history lesson will clear this right up [2].

While the first report of ADHD is as far back as 1798, over the years several diagnostic names were used for highly active, inattentive children. In the early 1900s, the "father of British pediatrics" Sir George Frederic Still described children with "an abnormal degree of passionateness" and "wanton mischievousness" with "exaggeration of excitability." Sound familiar? In the same era, early brain damage (e.g., from perinatal anoxia) with subsequent behavior or learning problems were described. After an encephalitis epidemic (1917–1928), surviving children often had what was called a "postencephalitic behavior disorder." They were described as hyperactive, distractible, and unmanageable in school. Their "hyperkinesis" led children to contact the environment continually, by touching, taking, and destroying. In the 1960s, "minimal brain dysfunction" was put forth as the most appropriate term by the Oxford International Study Group of Child Neurology. Referring to those with near average to above intelligence, affected children had various combinations of symptoms that included poor control of attention, impulse, or motor function. As awful as this name sounds, it was based on the understanding that children presenting with these problems had a true underlying organic problem. Some clinicians in current practice recall the days when "minimal brain dysfunction" was still diagnosed!

Recognizing that many children with this symptom constellation had no brain damage and that hyperactivity was the most marked symptom, others began using the term "hyperkinetic impulse disorder." The first formal diagnosis appeared in the 1968 *Diagnostic and Statistical Manual of Mental Disorders* (DSM-II) and was called "hyperkinetic reaction of childhood." Defined by only two descriptive sentences, the next DSM-III (1980) included three symptoms listed (hyperactivity, impulsivity, inattention) with numerical cutoffs and renamed the disorder attention deficit disorder (with or without hyperactivity). This is where the term ADD started, though it was on the books only from 1980 to 1987. A revised version was published in 1987 (DSM-IIIR) and renamed the disorder to our current attention-deficit/hyperactivity disorder. The DSM-IV (1994) kept the same name, along with three subtypes corresponding to the three presentations we have today. Current definitions listed above are from the DSM-5, published in 2013. The details of this are easy to read for those who want more detail at https://www.ncbi.nlm.nih.gov/pmc/articles/PMC3000907/.

The bottom line is that with increased understanding of the disorder, nomenclature and diagnostic criteria evolve. Belize used to be British Honduras, Croatia used to be Yugoslavia (and Croatia before that!). ♀ used to be Prince. Names change.

Why Does Everyone Say Something Different?

Sometimes families feel confused that one provider diagnosed ADHD combined type and another later diagnosed ADHD, predominantly inattentive type. Was the first provider wrong?

As you see from the history lesson above, the name for the disorder has changed over time. It is possible that the diagnostic terms changed over the course of a clinician's practice, such that they relook and rename a patient's presentations.

The diagnostic criteria certainly change. The DSM-5 was published in 2013 with fewer criteria required to make a diagnosis in those 17 and older, and also with modifications of criteria that are more appropriate for those beyond childhood. For example, the previous symptom "Often runs about or climbs in situations where it is inappropriate" is now followed by a note that "In adolescents or adults, may be limited to feeling restless" [1]. These changes not only make the diagnosis more fitting to those who are older but also contributed to an estimated 27% increase in the expected prevalence of ADHD among young adults, all based on the differences from the previous DSM-IV criteria [3]. Think of it this way: In 2012, a teen with a specific number and severity of symptoms might not have met criteria for ADHD, but the same person and same presentation then fit the (new) criteria in 2014.

Alternately, the presentation can change in the individual over the course of a life span, so that the person's diagnosis can change along with it. Symptoms, criteria, and diagnosis should be revisited with developmental maturity and changes in facing the increased demands of the world. For example, the young child with a combined presentation may transition to the predominantly inattentive presentation in adolescence.

The Clinical Visit

An adolescent should be evaluated for ADHD if they present with symptoms of inattention, hyperactivity, or impulsivity that interfere with function. The clinical evaluation includes a comprehensive medical, developmental, family, and social history as well as a clinical interview to determine the time of onset, course, duration, and impairment associated with symptoms [4]. In particular, the clinician should explore the presence of symptoms before age 12. The interview includes questions about the adolescent's functioning in school and other settings, and the clinician may find it helpful to review report cards and other school assessments [5]. Screening for comorbid psychiatric conditions is an important part of the diagnostic process [6–8], as well as inquiring about possible alternative causes for the symptoms such as substance abuse, anxiety, or digital media use [9–14].

If concerns about cognitive delays or learning disabilities surface (not understanding the work despite good effort, academic skills at a far lower level, "just seems younger"), neuropsychological testing may be appropriate [4, 15]. Finally, while most adolescents with ADHD have a normal physical examination, it is necessary nonetheless to identify other mimicking or masking conditions (hyperthyroidism, signs of suicidality such as self-harm, signs of substance use) and to document a baseline weight, height and blood pressure prior to considering treatment. The American Academy of Pediatrics recommends that the primary care clinician initiates the ADHD evaluation in most cases, but may refer children to a pediatric or mental health subspecialist in cases where the diagnosis is not clear or other comorbidities or concerns place it outside the scope of primary care [9].

Gathering Information About Adolescents

As with younger children, corroborative reports from people familiar with an adolescent's behavior and performance are imperative in making the diagnosis.

Most find it far more challenging to gather information for adolescents than for younger children [16]. Adolescents generally have multiple teachers at school who observe them in more limited circumstances. Similarly, parents may not see their children as much when they are older, or in as many contexts [9].

Unfortunately, limiting a history to the teen's own self-report is inadequate, as adolescents tend to minimize their own behavioral or academic difficulties [16–18]. It therefore remains optimal for clinicians to obtain information from multiple sources, including parents/caregivers, at least two teachers, as well as other people involved in the adolescent's life such as coaches or guidance counselors [19]. Recently, the development of apps and web-based portals such as myADHDportal. com serve to connect communities around an adolescent to improve the diagnostic accuracy, treatment efficacy, and treatment monitoring [20].

Identifying symptoms of ADHD in adolescents can itself be a challenge. Adolescents are less likely to exhibit hyperactivity in the same way as young children, and their impulsivity may seem like expected adolescent behavior [21]. They may quit jobs, end relationships, or exhibit emotional lability. They are also more likely to seek high reward activities such as using illicit substances, driving recklessly, or watching screens excessively [21]. Many adolescents have concurrent mental health and mood disorders that mask or enhance ADHD symptoms and need to be disentangled [21]. Some adolescents may also compensate for functional impairment with substance abuse [22].

To diagnose ADHD, clinicians look at the patient, thinking about symptoms and function over time and in the context of genetic predisposition, early childhood experiences, and evolving family, school, and community experience and function.

The clinician is "testing" to determine if there are sufficient symptoms to warrant a diagnosis and whether those symptoms are better explained otherwise. Rather than blood tests, clinicians use survey tools to ask about each and every ADHD symptom and about other disorders that could look similar. Rather than taking a picture of the brain with an MRI, the clinician gets a full picture of the teen's life by asking about school, mood, substance use, social context, and family status.

Think creatively when seeking symptoms from before age 12. Many adolescents with subtle symptoms may have been missed in childhood, especially those with above average cognitive abilities who were able to compensate for their symptoms, or those whose symptoms did not disrupt their functioning at school. Ask what school was like. Ask what report cards said. Does the teen recall how they felt in elementary school? Did the caregivers watch the teen play sports or give recitals or play on the playground? What did that look like? Listen for suggestive responses:

> He was sitting in left field playing with his toes.
> She was always the absent-minded student.
> She lost 10 red sweaters at camp one summer.

You might hear symptoms in the responses you get. Remember that girls are less likely to exhibit externalizing symptoms (outwardly aggressive or antisocial behavior) than boys and are often referred for evaluation later [23]. Girls' symptoms may very well be harder to see.

There are also aspects of adolescent medical care that make the diagnosis more challenging. Adolescents may be transitioning to adult care, where ADHD evaluation and treatment are less common. Some adult primary care physicians find that ADHD is outside the scope of their practice. Arguably the diagnosis is harder to make in the adult setting as original ADHD criteria are geared toward children [21]. Diagnosing and treating adolescents requires frequent follow-up visits, and compliance in young adults and adolescents can often be challenging.

Behavior Rating Scales

When considering a diagnosis of ADHD, parents/caregivers and other observers are usually asked to complete behavior rating scales. Rating scale data are then integrated with the information gathered from the clinical interview. Many behavior rating scales have been developed, including "narrowband scales" with questions limited to specific ADHD behaviors and "broadband scales" that cover a variety of symptoms, including those of ADHD but also other disorders like depression and anxiety. Once a concern arises that suggests ADHD, both narrow- and broadband scales are important. Use a broadband scale to identify alternative disorders or comorbid conditions to complete the initial assessment [24]. The validity of these tools depends on the age of the child, the person completing the scale, and the tool itself. Often the tools show signs of other conditions, either comorbid or mimicking.

Use narrowband scales to evaluate ADHD symptoms and then determine if the teen has sufficient symptoms and for which presentation.

An important limitation of survey use is that most studies of the tools are performed in specialty settings, meaning they are studied with a group of patients already identified as needing a highly trained specialist. Research findings on the accuracy of the scales reflect their accuracy when used with this specific population of patients referred, who may differ from a group of patients in the general population. Many children and adolescents are diagnosed with ADHD by their primary care providers, but we still use the scales with accuracy based on their use in a different population [25]. Note that this is standard practice; there isn't anything wrong with doing this. Families and providers simply recognize the need to interpret findings with some caution. Similarly, most ADHD measures were designed for elementary school-aged children; thus their applicability to adolescents is less clear [24]. Nevertheless, these scales are useful for gathering standardized information from multiple sources to help with diagnosis and tracking progress over time. Clinicians, caregivers, and teachers incorporate their findings into the current context of the adolescent.

A review of every ADHD rating scale is beyond the scope of this chapter, but some of the most commonly used tools are highlighted below.

1. *Vanderbilt Assessment Scales* (parent/teacher), aka "the Vanderbilt," are commonly used behavior rating scales. There are parent and teacher versions, both of which are based on the DSM-5 ADHD diagnostic criteria. The tools also include questions about several common comorbidities, such as oppositional defiant disorder (ODD)/conduct disorder, anxiety, and depression. Finally, there are questions about school performance and behaviors as well as social functioning. The Vanderbilt Assessment Scales have been validated in both community and referral settings [19, 26]. However, they are only designed for children aged 6–12, which limits their applicability in the adolescent population. Many clinicians still use this tool in the adolescent population due to its accessibility, ease of use, cost (it is free), and correlation with the DSM-5 criteria.
2. *The Swanson, Nolan, and Pelham Questionnaire* (SNAP): This is another commonly used tool that can be completed by both parents and teachers and corresponds to the DSM diagnostic criteria. There is a short version of the SNAP which is limited to symptoms related to ADHD and ODD, as well as a longer version with additional questions about ADHD and other disorders. This tool is designated for use in children age 6–18, but there is no specific adolescent version or adolescent normative data available, so again its use in the adolescent population may be limited [24, 27]. The tool is easy to use and free of charge.
3. *Conners 3rd Edition*: The Conners 3rd Edition [28] includes separate forms for parents and teachers of children age 6–18, as well as self-report forms for children age 8–18. There is a full-length version of each form which asks about

ADHD symptoms as well as common comorbid conditions, and also a short version which includes selected items from the longer form. The Conners 3rd Edition is not freely available, which may limit its use in some settings, but it is widely used nevertheless.

Case Revisited

Thomas presented at 16 years with dropping grades in 10th grade, wondering if he has ADHD. His clinician will need time to review Thomas's history of behavior and school function from elementary school. Interview, parent, and patient surveys should elicit symptoms of depression, anxiety, substance use, medical problems, or other factors that could explain his current symptoms. Thomas should identify adults who know him to complete surveys about his attention, hyperactivity, and impulsivity, which may also be completed by his parents and himself. In his case, report cards from mid-elementary school describe him as often inattentive but always mastering concepts and often completing classwork and homework with inattentive errors. Behavior programs sufficed in managing his classroom behavior. Parents report his room is messy and he loses things, but they have always provided reminders and prompts. No concerns for depression, anxiety, oppositional or defiant behavior, substance use, sleep problems, or medication side effects are identified. Attention Scales show sufficient symptoms to warrant a current diagnosis of ADHD, combined type.

Conclusions

Diagnosing the adolescent with ADHD is rarely straightforward. It can be hard to respect and empower teens while also requesting corroborating reports from parents, teachers, coaches, and others. Partnering with the teen where possible is key: identify shared goals and work together toward an accurate diagnosis and effective treatment.

Tips
- Think of the clinician as the test for ADHD. There is no routine need for blood tests, brain scans, neuropsychological testing, or fancy computer assessments when diagnosing most cases of ADHD.
- The hyperactivity of young children with ADHD tends to lessen over time, so that adolescents present with more restlessness and discomfort sitting for long periods.
- Other specified or unspecified ADHD diagnoses are just as real as the other ADHD diagnoses.

References

1. American Psychiatric Association. Diagnostic and statistical manual of mental disorders (DSM-5). 5th ed. Arlington: American Psychiatric Association; 2013.
2. Lange KW, Reichl S, Lange KM, Tucha L, Tucha O. The history of attention deficit hyperactivity disorder. Atten Defic Hyperact Disord. 2010;2(4):241–55. https://doi.org/10.1007/s12402-010-0045-8.
3. Matte B, Anselmi L, Salum GA, et al. ADHD in DSM-5: a field trial in a large, representative sample of 18- to 19-year-old adults. Psychol Med. 2014;45(2):361–73. https://doi.org/10.1017/S0033291714001470.
4. Pliszka S, AACAP Work Group on Quality Issues. Practice parameter for the assessment and treatment of children and adolescents with attention-deficit/hyperactivity disorder. J Am Acad Child Adolesc Psychiatry. 2007;46(7):894–921. https://doi.org/10.1097/chi.0b013e318054e724.
5. Thapar A, Cooper M. Attention deficit hyperactivity disorder. Lancet. 2016;387(10024):1240–50. https://doi.org/10.1016/S0140-6736(15)00238-X.
6. Fischer M, Barkley RA, Smallish L, Fletcher K. Young adult follow-up of hyperactive children: self-reported psychiatric disorders, comorbidity, and the role of childhood conduct problems and teen CD. J Abnorm Child Psychol. 2002;30(5):463–75. https://doi.org/10.1023/a:1019864813776.
7. Bird HR, Gould MS, Staghezza BM. Patterns of diagnostic comorbidity in a community sample of children aged 9 through 16 years. J Am Acad Child Adolesc Psychiatry. 1993;32(2):361–8. https://doi.org/10.1097/00004583-199303000-00018.
8. Connor DF, Edwards G, Fletcher KE, Baird J, Barkley RA, Steingard RJ. Correlates of comorbid psychopathology in children with ADHD. J Am Acad Child Adolesc Psychiatry. 2003;42(2):193–200. https://doi.org/10.1097/00004583-200302000-00013.
9. Wolraich ML, Hagan JF, Allan C; Subcommittee on Children and Adolescents with Attention-Deficit/Hyperactive Disorder, et al. Clinical practice guideline for the diagnosis, evaluation, and treatment of attention-deficit/hyperactivity disorder in children and adolescents. Pediatrics. 2019;144(4):e20192528.
10. Wilens TE, Martelon M, Joshi G, et al. Does ADHD predict substance-use disorders? A 10-year follow-up study of young adults with ADHD. J Am Acad Child Adolesc Psychiatry. 2011;50(6):543–53. https://doi.org/10.1016/j.jaac.2011.01.021.
11. Molina BSG, Pelham WE. Childhood predictors of adolescent substance use in a longitudinal study of children with ADHD. J Abnorm Psychol. 2003;112(3):497–507. https://doi.org/10.1037/0021-843x.112.3.497.
12. Mochrie KD, Whited MC, Cellucci T, Freeman T, Corson AT. ADHD, depression, and substance abuse risk among beginning college students. J Am Coll Heal. 2018:1–5. https://doi.org/10.1080/07448481.2018.1515754.
13. Sibley MH, Rohde LA, Swanson JM, et al. Late-onset ADHD reconsidered with comprehensive repeated assessments between ages 10 and 25. Am J Psychiatry. 2018;175(2):140–9. https://doi.org/10.1176/appi.ajp.2017.17030298.
14. Ra CK, Cho J, Stone MD, et al. Association of digital media use with subsequent symptoms of attention-deficit/hyperactivity disorder among adolescents. JAMA. 2018;320(3):255–63. https://doi.org/10.1001/jama.2018.8931.
15. Wolraich ML, Wibbelsman CJ, Brown TE, et al. Attention-deficit/hyperactivity disorder among adolescents: a review of the diagnosis, treatment, and clinical implications. Pediatrics. 2005;115(6):1734–46. https://doi.org/10.1542/peds.2004-1959.
16. Smith BH, Pelham WE Jr, Gnagy E, Molina B, Evans S. The reliability, validity, and unique contributions of self-report by adolescents receiving treatment for attention-deficit/hyperactivity disorder. J Consult Clin Psychol. 68(3):489–99. https://doi.org/10.1037/0022-006X.68.3.489.

17. Loeber R, Green SM, Lahey BB, Stouthamer-Loeber M. Differences and similarities between children, mothers, and teachers as informants on disruptive child behavior. J Abnorm Child Psychol. 1991;19(1):75–95. https://doi.org/10.1007/BF00910566.
18. Kramer TL, Phillips SD, Hargis MB, Miller TL, Burns BJ, Robbins JM. Disagreement between parent and adolescent reports of functional impairment. J Child Psychol Psychiatry. 2004;45(2):248–259. http://www.ncbi.nlm.nih.gov/pubmed/14982239. Accessed December
19. Wolraich ML, Bard DE, Neas B, Doffing M, Beck L. The psychometric properties of the Vanderbilt attention-deficit hyperactivity disorder diagnostic teacher rating scale in a community population. J Dev Behav Pediatr. 2013;34(2):83–93. https://doi.org/10.1097/DBP.0b013e31827d55c3.
20. Epstein JN, Kelleher KJ, Baum R, et al. Impact of a web-portal intervention on community ADHD care and outcomes. Pediatrics. 2016;138(2):e20154240. https://doi.org/10.1542/peds.2015-4240.
21. Brahmbhatt K, Hilty DM, Hah M, Han J, Angkustsiri K, Schweitzer JB. Diagnosis and treatment of attention deficit hyperactivity disorder during adolescence in the primary care setting: a concise review. J Adolesc Health. 2016;59(2):135–43. https://doi.org/10.1016/j.jadohealth.2016.03.025.
22. Molina BS, Hinshaw SP, Eugene Arnold L, et al. Adolescent substance use in the multimodal treatment study of attention-deficit/hyperactivity disorder (ADHD) (MTA) as a function of childhood ADHD, random assignment to childhood treatments, and subsequent medication. J Am Acad Child Adolesc Psychiatry. 2013;52(3):250–63. https://doi.org/10.1016/j.jaac.2012.12.014.Adolescent.
23. Gaub M, Carlson CL. Gender differences in ADHD: a meta-analysis and critical review. J Am Acad Child Adolesc Psychiatry. 1997;36:1036–45. https://doi.org/10.1097/00004583-199708000-00011.
24. Collett BR, Ohan JL, Myers KM. Ten-year review of rating scales. V: scales assessing attention-deficit/hyperactivity disorder. J Am Acad Child Adolesc Psychiatry. 2003;42(9):1015–37. https://doi.org/10.1097/01.CHI.0000070245.24125.B6.
25. Kemper AR, Maslow GR, Hill S, et al. Attention deficit hyperactivity disorder: diagnosis and treatment in children and adolescents; 2018. https://doi.org/10.23970/AHRQEPCCER203.
26. Wolraich ML, Lambert W, Doffing MA, Bickman L, Simmons T, Worley K. Psychometric properties of the Vanderbilt ADHD diagnostic parent rating scale in a referred population. J Pediatr Psychol. 2003;28(8):559–67. https://doi.org/10.1093/jpepsy/jsg046.
27. Bussing R, Fernandez M, Harwood M, et al. Parent and teacher SNAP-IV ratings of attention deficit hyperactivity disorder symptoms: psychometric properties and normative ratings from a school district sample. Assessment. 2008;15(3):317–28. https://doi.org/10.1177/1073191107313888.
28. Kao GS, Thomas HM. Test review: C. Keith Conners, Conners 3rd Edition Toronto, Ontario, Canada: multi-health systems, 2008. J Psychoeduc Assess. 2010;28(6):598–602. https://doi.org/10.1177/0734282909360011.

Chapter 2
Medical Evaluation for ADHD Symptoms in Adolescents

Cassandra Conrad and Jennifer Aites

Case Example

Britney is a 15-year-old, healthy girl, who starts struggling in 9th grade classes. She has been without any learning, developmental, or medical concerns until now. She tells her parents that she cannot pay attention in class and that she cannot follow what is being taught. She was a solid, hardworking student prior to this year. Parents scheduled a pediatric visit to figure out what's going on with her.

Background

This book has contributions from developmental behavioral pediatricians, pediatric psychologists, a psychiatric nurse practitioner, a social worker, and general pediatricians. While we present evidence-based practices, your clinician may view the same evidence from a different perspective. Chapter 1 focused on making the diagnosis: anyone making the diagnosis should complete a detailed history, review current and historical functioning in the home and community settings (which often requires attention rating scales completed by teachers or others), as well as review the diagnostic criteria in the *Diagnostic and Statistical Manual of Mental Disorders, 5th Edition* (DSM-5) [1]. Here we review the medical evaluation appropriate when a patient presents with the question of ADHD.

C. Conrad (✉)
Division of Developmental Medicine, Boston Children's Hospital, Boston, MA, USA
e-mail: Cassandra.conrad@childrens.harvard.edu

J. Aites
Harvard Medical School, Division of Developmental Medicine, Boston Children's Hospital, Boston, MA, USA
e-mail: Jennifer.aites@childrens.harvard.edu

© Springer Nature Switzerland AG 2020
A. Schonwald (ed.), *ADHD in Adolescents*,
https://doi.org/10.1007/978-3-030-62393-7_2

The Medical Evaluation and the Medical Evaluator

How do the fields differ in providing ADHD care? It's not entirely clear. National societies of pediatrics and psychiatry have has its own ADHD diagnosis and treatment guideline for its field [2, 3]. These guidelines are certainly more similar than different. Published research studies describe different patterns for prescribing ADHD medication across the disciplines, but not for diagnosing ADHD [4]. In our experience, practice patterns differ not only among clinicians but also within a discipline: some pediatricians are more comfortable diagnosing older or younger children than others. Some psychiatrists provide therapy along with medication, and some neurologists look harder for medical disorders before diagnosing and treating. More evident differences come when looking at regional patterns, reflecting access to specialists, educational services, and cultural preferences. Information in this book generally adheres to the AAP guidelines.

Across specialties, clinicians recognize that other conditions, mostly other emotional, behavioral, or neurodevelopmental disorders, as well as response to environmental stress, may mimic ADHD or co-occur with ADHD (Table 2.1). Chapters later in this book go into more detail about the specifics of each "mimicker."

The remainder of this chapter will review when additional medical evaluation may be necessary to differentiate the diagnosis of ADHD from other physical or medical conditions mirroring ADHD symptoms or co-occurring with ADHD symptoms. Physical or medical conditions that may mirror or co-occur with ADHD are listed in Table 2.2 [1, 5–10].

> Your clinician may recommend a different evaluation from what you see below. Ask why! There may be a very good reason, and you are sure to have an informative discussion.

Table 2.1 Disorders and contexts that create symptoms similar to ADHD

ADHD mimickers [1, 5–8]		
Emotional/behavioral disorders [1, 6, 7]	Psychosocial factors [6–9]	Neurodevelopmental disorders [1, 5–7, 9, 10]
Anxiety	Socioeconomic stressors	Learning disorders
Depression	Maltreatment/abuse	Intellectual disability
Oppositional defiant disorder/ conduct disorder	Bullying	Autism spectrum disorder
Mood disorders	Conflicts between child and parents, other family members, friends, or teachers	Speech and language disorders
Obsessive-compulsive disorder		Tic disorders
Post-traumatic stress disorder	Unsuccessful parenting or classroom management techniques	Stereotyped movement disorder
Adjustment disorders		

Table 2.2 Physical and medical conditions mimicking/co-occurring with ADHD

Hearing impairment	Fetal alcohol syndrome
Visual impairment	Brain injury
Seizure disorders	Genetic disorders (such as 22q11 deletion syndrome, neurofibromatosis, or fragile x syndrome)
Disordered sleep	
Narcolepsy	
Substance use	Metabolic disorders (such as phenylketonuria)
Thyroid disorders	Complications of central nervous system infection
Lead toxicity	Medication side effects (such as bronchodilators, thyroid replacement medications, corticosteroids, or neuroleptics)
Malnutrition	

History and Physical Examination

The medical evaluation begins within a comprehensive history as well as physical examination. The history should include a timeline of the presenting symptoms, current functioning across settings, educational history, birth history, developmental history, medical history, mental health history, and family and social histories [3, 10]. During a portion of the history, the adolescent should be interviewed alone, as they may not be comfortable discussing certain topics in front of parents or caregivers, including mistreatment, anxiety or depressive symptoms, substance use, and sexuality [3].

The physical examination should include a neurologic examination (checking that the nerves are working, from the eyes to the ankles), as well as hearing and vision screenings [6, 7]. Psychologists and social workers do not complete physical examinations and may defer to the primary care provider. Hearing and vision screen may be completed in a primary care office or referred elsewhere. Administration of a mental status examination can be helpful to elicit behavioral or emotional disorders [3]. A mental status examination assesses appearance, behavior, speech, mood, affect, thought process, thought content, cognition, insight, and judgment.

Neuroimaging Studies

Neurological studies and neuroimaging studies are not indicated in the medical workup of ADHD, unless concerns are elicited from the history and physical for another condition or disorder that presents with symptoms that overlap with ADHD and is diagnosed with imaging. In general, as there is no biological marker of ADHD, neurological and neuroimaging studies are nondiagnostic, and they cannot predict treatment response in ADHD [3, 12]. Furthermore, using neuroimaging studies that involve exposure to radioactivity or intravenous radioactive nucleotides to assess for ADHD is not recommended, given both safety concerns and a lack of evidence showing utility of the studies [3]. Neurological studies and neuroimaging studies used to research (not diagnose, just research) ADHD include magnetic resonance imaging (MRI), functional MRI (fMRI), single photon emission computed tomography (SPECT), positron emission tomography (PET), electroencephalogram (EEG), event-related potential (ERP), and computed tomography (CT or CAT) scan. Some studies have shown that as a population, children with ADHD have slow wave changes on their EEG, reduced brain volume, and possibly a delay in maturation of their brain, but these findings are nondiagnostic, and there can be overlap with other neurological or psychiatric disorders [1, 12]. Having one of these findings does not equate to a diagnosis of ADHD, nor does it explain how ADHD developed. Absence of one of these findings does not mean ADHD is an inaccurate diagnosis. Research shows there is much overlap between findings in brain structure and function between those with ADHD and those in the general population without ADHD [9].

> While ADHD research using these modalities has helped the medical field learn more about the disorder, including brain pathophysiology, these findings are not helpful in making the initial diagnosis of ADHD.

Seizures

Seizures in children and adolescents may present with primarily inattentive moments [7]. Staring may be a common symptom seen in both seizures and ADHD, and it is important to elicit information about staring; is it interrupted with physical contact? How often does the staring occur? Does it occur in a variety of settings [11]? Absence seizures present as moments of blank staring with cessation of talking, any time of day and in all contexts. Lasting 10–20 seconds, absence seizures may appear as a lapse of attention, accompanied by eye fluttering, chewing, or other motor movements. During the absence seizure, the staring behavior cannot be interrupted. Subsequently, the child does not recall being unavailable but resumes their baseline level of alertness. While children with ADHD may commonly stare, staring episodes can be interrupted, particularly with touch. One study comparing patients with ADHD to those with absence seizures found that inattention, unfinished homework, and reduced task persistence were seen significantly more in ADHD than in those with absence seizures. In contrast, these behaviors were found to occur in low frequency in those with absence seizures [11]. Neither EEG nor referral to a neurologist is routinely required for medical diagnosis of ADHD, unless history or physical examination is concerning for a seizure disorder or other unusual neurologic findings.

Sleep

The relationship between sleep, symptoms of inattention, and the diagnosis of ADHD is complex. Many sleep disorders, insufficient sleep, and snoring can significantly affect attention and may present with symptoms of inattention [7, 13]. Sleep disorders to consider include sleep apnea, narcolepsy, and periodic leg movements. Prior to making the diagnosis of ADHD, sleep disorders should be ruled out as a solitary cause of ADHD-like symptoms. A comprehensive sleep history should be obtained during the medical history component of an ADHD evaluation. Information about the number of hours of sleep, number and duration of nighttime awakenings, snoring, symptoms of apnea, movements during sleep, and daytime sleepiness should be obtained. In addition to sleep problems leading to symptoms that may mimic ADHD, those with ADHD can have comorbid sleep problems exacerbating symptoms of ADHD [13, 14]. If the medical history is suggestive of a sleep disorder, subjective and objective measures are needed to better assess for a sleep disorder [13]. Subjective measures might include self-completed or parent-completed sleep diary. Objective measures are polysomnography (sleep study), actigraphy (movement monitor), multiple sleep latency test, or serum ferritin levels [13, 14].

Hearing and Vision

Hearing and vision screenings should be part of the physical examination when considering ADHD. Each can present with symptoms of apparent inattention as well. If screenings performed or the elicited history are concerning for hearing loss and/or vision impairment, referral for audiologic evaluation or ophthalmologic evaluation should be made.

> Vision and hearing deficits are both common and can first develop or be recognized in teens.

Thyroid Disorders

Thyroid disease, including both hypothyroidism and hyperthyroidism, can present in adolescence and can lead to ADHD-like symptoms of inattention or hyperactivity, respectively [7]. Typically, with hypothyroidism or hyperthyroidism, there are additional associated signs and symptoms that help to differentiate them from a diagnosis of ADHD. These signs and symptoms may include agitation or irritability, emotional instability, decreased energy, impaired memory, goiter, or decreased growth velocity [3, 15, 16].

Routine screening for thyroid function tests is not recommended in the ADHD evaluation. In previous studies of children referred for an ADHD evaluation without other associated symptoms of thyroid dysfunction, thyroid function studies were normal [3, 15, 16].

Toxins

Children and adolescents exposed to toxins may present with symptoms of ADHD. Toxin exposure can occur prenatally or during childhood and adolescence. Toxins that are known to present with attentional symptoms include alcohol, lead, specific prescribed medication, and illicit substances [7]. Fetal alcohol syndrome often presents with symptoms of ADHD. Children with fetal alcohol syndrome have a higher incidence of ADHD compared to the general population [3]. The diagnosis of fetal alcohol syndrome is a clinical one that can be determined by history and physical examination findings; no medical testing is necessary to establish the diagnosis.

Lead exposure both prenatally and during childhood and adolescence is associated with an increased risk of ADHD. If the adolescent being evaluated has possible exposure to lead in their environment, such as living in an older home or in a home with old plumbing, performance of a serum lead level should be considered [3]. In general, lead exposure at any point presents with a number of impairments other than ADHD, and unless other symptoms are elicited during the evaluation of ADHD (headaches, belly pain, joint and muscle pain, memory difficulty), screening of serum lead levels should not be part of the medical evaluation for ADHD [3, 17].

Medications that can induce ADHD-like symptoms include bronchodilators (such as albuterol), corticosteroids, isoniazid, neuroleptics, and replacement thyroid hormones [1, 5]. The patient's medical history should include a medication reconciliation to reveal any medications potentially contributing to the symptoms. Finally, use of illicit substances may present with ADHD-like symptoms. In adolescents, substance use may present with symptoms of declining school performance, inattention, or distractibility [5, 7]. Substance use should be reviewed during a comprehensive history; as discussed above, an adolescent is more likely to disclose substance use when interviewed separately from the family. Treatment of substance use disorders should occur before a new diagnosis of ADHD is made, to determine what symptoms are present in the absence of illicit substances [5].

Genetic and Metabolic Disorders

Many genetic and metabolic disorders present with symptoms of ADHD [7]. However, additional symptoms are present as well. Examples are neurofibromatosis, fragile X syndrome, 22q11 deletion syndrome, and phenylketonuria [5–7, 9]. History and physical examination are the first step in the medical evaluation of a possible metabolic or genetic condition. Details suggesting genetic disorder include early and ongoing developmental or cognitive delays, involvement of other systems in the body, and specific facial features. Metabolic disorders are suggested by periods of developmental regression, failure to thrive, unusual odors, and difficulty tolerating otherwise minor illnesses. In the event that the medical history is suggestive, genetic or metabolic testing can be considered. While an underlying genetic disorder might account for the ADHD symptoms, remember that a comorbid diagnosis of ADHD can still be made if symptoms are present, are impairing, and are not commensurate with the patient's developmental level [1].

Nutritional Deficiency

Some research has suggested that iron deficiency and/or low ferritin levels may lead to symptoms of ADHD [18]. If the patient's history reveals selective eating or possible malnutrition, or if the physical examination is concerning for iron deficiency or anemia (pale, fast heart rate), laboratory work looking for iron deficiency or low ferritin levels may be considered. However, additional research is needed to fully understand the association between iron deficiency and ADHD [18].

Case Revisited

Britney's primary care provider completes a comprehensive history. She finds that Britney has indeed been healthy without exposure to toxins, medications, and trauma. She has no signs or symptoms of depression or anxiety, has an active social life, and looks forward to getting her driver's license next year. She sleeps well, 7 hours/night during the week and 12 hours at a stretch on weekends. Britney sees the blackboard well from the back of the class and is not aware of hearing issues; she passes office screening. She understands the academic material but loses track of what the class is doing. Her mother has seen Britney stop mid-sentence and stare off, unresponsive when her mother says her name or touches her arm. Her physical exam is entirely normal.

Britney undergoes an EEG for the specific concerns of absence seizures and then has a follow-up neurology visit to interpret and manage the abnormal findings of her EEG. Once she is treated for her absence seizures, Britney resumes her solid school performance. No ADHD diagnosis is warranted.

Conclusions

The medical evaluation for ADHD symptoms in adolescents warrants consideration of a vast differential diagnosis, explored through comprehensive history and physical examination. In order to diagnose ADHD, a history of symptoms should be present prior to the age of 12; new onset of ADHD symptoms in adolescence should be considered carefully. The importance of a comprehensive history and physical cannot be overstated. ADHD is a clinical diagnosis; laboratory, neurological, or neuroimaging tests are typically not indicated, unless concerning findings are elicited on history or physical.

Tips
- Different clinicians might have different approaches to the evaluation of ADHD.
- The diagnosis of ADHD in teens requires a lengthy conversation to review the history and ongoing symptoms, including a private and confidential conversation between the patient and clinician (no parents present). Plan the time accordingly!
- Most adolescents diagnosed with ADHD don't require medical testing with blood tests, CT scans, or MRIs.

References

1. American Psychiatric Association. Diagnostic and statistical manual of mental disorders (DSM-5). 5th ed. Arlington: American Psychiatric Association; 2013.
2. Wolraich ML, Hagan JF, Allan C; Subcommittee on Children and Adolescents with Attention-Deficit/Hyperactive Disorder, et al. Clinical practice guideline for the diagnosis, evaluation, and treatment of attention-deficit/hyperactivity disorder in children and adolescents. Pediatrics. 2019;144(4):e20192528.
3. Pliszka S, AACAP Work Group on Quality Issues. Practice parameter for the assessment and treatment of children and adolescents with attention-deficit/hyperactivity disorder. J Am Acad Child Adolesc Psychiatry. 2007;46(7):894–921. https://doi.org/10.1097/chi.0b013e318054e724.
4. Anderson LE, Chen ML, Perrin JM, Van Cleave J. Outpatient visits and medication prescribing for US children with mental health conditions. Pediatrics. 2015;136(5):e1178–85. https://doi.org/10.1542/peds.2015-0807.
5. French WP. Assessment and treatment of attention-deficit/hyperactivity disorder: part 2. Pediatr Ann. 2015;44(4):160–8. https://doi.org/10.3928/00904481-20150410-11.
6. Felt BT, Biermann B, Christner JG, Kochhar P, Van Harrison R. Diagnosis and management of ADHD in children. Am Fam Physician. 2014;90(7):456–64.
7. Feldman HM. Developmental-behavioral pediatrics. 4th ed. Philadelphia: Elsevier; 2009.
8. Brahmbhatt K, Hilty DM, Hah M, Han J, Angkustsiri K, Schweitzer JB. Diagnosis and treatment of attention deficit hyperactivity disorder during adolescence in the primary care setting: a concise review. J Adolesc Health. 2016;59(2):135–43. https://doi.org/10.1016/j.jadohealth.2016.03.025.
9. Feldman HM, Reiff MI. Clinical practice. Attention deficit-hyperactivity disorder in children and adolescents. N Engl J Med. 2014;370(9):838–46. https://doi.org/10.1056/NEJMcp1307215.
10. Efron D, Hazell P, Anderson V. Update on attention deficit hyperactivity disorder. J Paediatr Child Health. 2011;47(10):682–9. https://doi.org/10.1111/j.1440-1754.2010.01928.x.
11. Williams J, Griebel ML, Sharp GB, Lange B, Phillips T, Delosreyes E, Bates S, Schulz EG, Simpson P. Differentiating between seizures and attention deficit hyperactivity disor-

der (ADHD) in a pediatric population. Clin Pediatr (Phila). 2002;41(8):565–8. https://doi. org/10.1177/000992280204100802.
12. Bush G. Neuroimaging of attention deficit hyperactivity disorder: can new imaging findings be integrated in clinical practice? Child Adolesc Psychiatr Clin N Am. 2008;17(2):385–404, x. https://doi.org/10.1016/j.chc.2007.11.002.
13. Hvolby A. Associations of sleep disturbance with ADHD: implications for treatment. Atten Defic Hyperact Disord. 2015;7(1):1–18. https://doi.org/10.1007/s12402-014-0151-0.
14. Singh K, Zimmerman AW. Sleep in autism spectrum disorder and attention deficit hyper- activity disorder. Semin Pediatr Neurol. 2015;22(2):113–25. https://doi.org/10.1016/j. spen.2015.03.006.
15. Stein MA, Weiss RE. Thyroid function tests and neurocognitive functioning in children referred for attention deficit/hyperactivity disorder. Psychoneuroendocrinology. 2003;28(3):304–16. https://doi.org/10.1016/s0306-4530(02)00024-0.
16. Toren P, Karasik A, Eldar S, Wolmer L, Shimon I, Weitz R, Inbar D, Koren S, Pariente C, Reiss A, Weizman R, Laor N. Thyroid function in attention deficit and hyperactivity disorder. J Psychiatr Res. 1997;31(3):359–63. https://doi.org/10.1016/s0022-3956(96)00061-1.
17. Lidsky TI, Schneider JS. Lead neurotoxicity in children: basic mechanisms and clinical cor- relates. Brain. 2003;126(Pt 1):5–19. https://doi.org/10.1093/brain/awg014.
18. Percinel I, Yazici KU, Ustundag B. Iron deficiency parameters in children and adolescents with attention-deficit/hyperactivity disorder. Child Psychiatry Hum Dev. 2016;47(2):259–69. https://doi.org/10.1007/s10578-015-0562-y.

Chapter 3
Treating Adolescent ADHD with Medication

Danielle Doctor

Case Example

Clara is a 16-year-old who has generally done well academically. She has always been a hard worker, socially successful, and involved in sports. In 10th grade, she shares that she has always felt it was hard to focus. Now with so much more work, it's a bigger problem. She either has to stay up until 2 a.m. to complete her work or turn in incomplete efforts. She believes she has ADHD and that medication would help.

Background

Medication for the treatment of ADHD can be divided into two main categories: stimulants and non-stimulants. Stimulants are considered first-line therapy in the treatment of adolescents. Before initiating therapy, a physical exam and personal and family history should be performed with specific focus on the cardiovascular system. Vital signs as well as height and weight should be recorded. All teens should be screened for substance use, as part of the ADHD diagnostic process, before medication is prescribed and regularly thereafter.

To decide what medication to initiate, the questions below (Table 3.1) can yield important information:

D. Doctor (✉)
Maine Medical Center, Portland, ME, USA
e-mail: ddoctor@mmc.org

© Springer Nature Switzerland AG 2020
A. Schonwald (ed.), *ADHD in Adolescents*,
https://doi.org/10.1007/978-3-030-62393-7_3

Table 3.1 Questions to ask before choosing a medication

1	Are there certain times of day symptoms are the most disruptive?
2	What time in the morning can the patient take the medicine?
3	Can you swallow a pill?
4	Are there baseline troubles that we don't want to worsen with potential side effects of medication? Reduced appetite? Poor weight gain? Sleeplessness? Anxiety? Other psychiatric comorbidities?
5	Any relevant family history? ADHD medications that worked well or didn't work well?
6	Family history of cardiac rhythm disturbance? Sudden unexplained death in a healthy individual under 40? Individual history of chest pain, fainting, and heart problem?

Table 3.2 Methylphenidate-based medications

Generic	Brand name	Doses (duration)
Methylphenidate	Ritalin	5, 10, 20 mg (3–4 h)
	Methylphenidate Chewable	2.5, 5, 10 mg (3–5 h)
	Methylphenidate Solution	5 mg/5 mL, 10 mg/5 mL (3–5 h)
	Metadate ER	10, 20 mg (6–8 h)
	Metadate CD	10, 20, 30, 40, 50, 60 mg (8–12 h)
	Cotempla XR-ODT	8.6, 17.3, 25.9 mg (up to 12 h)
	Aptensio XR	10, 20, 30, 40, 50, 60 mg (up to 12 h)
	Adhansia XR	25, 35, 45, 55, 70, 85 mg (up to 16 h)
	Jornay	20, 40, 60, 80, 100 mg (delayed release)
	Quillivant XR	5 mg/mL (up to 12 h)
	QuilliChew ER	20, 30, 40 mg (6–8 h)
Methylphenidate SR	Ritalin SR	20 mg (6–8 h)
Methylphenidate OROS	Concerta	18, 27, 36, 54 mg (10–12 h)
Dexmethylphenidate	Focalin	2.5, 5, 10 mg (5–6 h)
	Focalin XR	5, 10, 15, 20 (10–12 h)
Methylphenidate LA	Ritalin LA	10, 20, 30, 40 mg (8–12 h)
	Daytrana	10, 15, 20, 30 mg (9–12 h)

Parent and patient preferences are important to discuss, so that decision making is shared and adherence is optimized.

Stimulants

For many adolescents, stimulants will be the first medication tried. There are two classes of stimulants: methylphenidates (Table 3.2) and amphetamines (Table 3.3). The response rate, as measured in reduction in hyperactivity or increase in attention, has been reported around 70% for first stimulant use and up to 80% when more than once stimulant is tried [1, 2]. Under these two classes, there are a variety of formulations to choose from to best fit the lifestyle and needs of the patient. The exact mechanism of action of stimulants in ADHD is unknown. It is hypothesized that an increase in dopamine and norepinephrine in pyramidal neurons in the prefrontal cortex enhances signal strength while decreasing the amount of noise, thereby reducing core symptoms of ADHD [3].

Table 3.3 Amphetamine-based medications

Generic	Brand name	Doses (durations)
Dextroamphetamine	Dexedrine®	5 mg (4–6 h)
Dextroamphetamine SR	Dexedrine Spansule®	5, 10, 15 mg (6–8 h)
Mixed Amphetamine Salts	Adderall®	5, 10, 20, 30 (4–6 h)
	Adderall XR®	5, 10, 15, 20, 25, 30 mg (8–12 h)
	Mydayis®	12.5, 25, 37.5, 50 mg (up to 16 h)
d- and l-amphetamine sulfates	Adzenys ER®	1.25 mg/mL
	Adzenys XR®	3.1, 6.3, 9.4, 12.5, 15.7, 18.8 mg (up to 12 h)
	Dyanavel XR®	2.5 mg/mL (up to 13 h)
	Evekeo®	5, 10 mg (4–6 h)
d-amphetamine sulfate	Zenzedi®	2.5, 5, 7.5, 10, 15, 20, 30 mg (4–6 mg)
	Procentra®	5 mg/5 mL (4–6 h)
Lisdexamfetamine dimesylate	Vyvanse® Vyvanse Chewable®	10, 20, 30, 40, 50, 60, 70 (up to 10 h) 10, 20, 30, 40, 50, 60

Amphetamine-Based Medications

Administration

In general, long-acting formulations tend to be more convenient; for children over the age of 6, long-acting options are often the first treatment. Effects of stimulant medication can be seen within 20 min of administration of first dose. Dosing should be titrated up every 3–7 days until maximum effect is observed, and the medication is tolerated with minimum side effects. Common side effects include insomnia, decreased appetite, and mood lability (particularly in younger patients). Psychosis and cardiac complications are rare; however, taking a comprehensive cardiac history is imperative.

Both classes of stimulants appear to be equally efficacious in studies and therefore either can be tried first.

Non-stimulants

The overall response to non-stimulants is around 50% [4]. They are typically tried after stimulants were found to be ineffective or side effects were not tolerable. Side effects tend to be less severe than with stimulant use, the most prominent being sedation and nausea.

Non-stimulants can be used as adjunctive therapy to stimulants, in cases where comorbidities prevent treatment with a stimulant, or based on patient and family preferences.

Atomoxetine

Atomoxetine (Table 3.3) is noradrenergic reuptake inhibitor which is thought to act in ADHD by selectively increasing levels of norepinephrine in the synapses of the prefrontal cortex [5]. It can be considered for first-line therapy in patients with active substance use disorder, anxiety, or tic disorders. The full effect of the medication is usually not seen until week 6 of treatment, so it is important to give adequate time for trialing the medication [6]. Serious but rare complications include an increase in suicidal thinking, liver injury, cardiovascular effects, and priapism. More common side effects are weight loss, sedation, abdominal pain, headaches, and irritability.

Alpha-2 Adrenergic Agonists

Clonidine and guanfacine are alpha-2 adrenergic agonists which come in both short-acting and extended release formulas (Table 3.4). The exact mechanism of action is unclear, but they are believed to work in ADHD via the modulation of dopamine and noradrenaline transmission through the synapse [7]. Initial effects may take up to 2 weeks to be seen. Side effects include sedation, depression, headache, irritability, hypotension, and bradycardia. Both require tapering with discontinuation to prevent rebound hypertension.

Table 3.4 Non-stimulant medications for ADHD

Generic	Brand name	Doses (durations)
Atomoxetine	Strattera	10, 18, 25, 40, 60, 80, 100 mg caps (24 h)
Clonidine	Catapres	0.1, 0.2 mg (4–6 h)
Clonidine long acting	Kapvay	0.1, 0.2 mg (12 h)
Guanfacine	Tenex	1 mg (6–8 h)
Guanfacine extended release	Intuniv	1, 2, 3, 4 mg (8 h)

Considerations in Treatment

Method of Administration

There are many other options for medication delivery other than tablets which can aid in medication compliance if a patient is pill adverse or cannot swallow a pill. Many come in both short-acting and extended release forms. A more detailed look at all the available options can be found at the ADHD Medication Guide listed below under resources. Other forms include:

- Liquids
- Orally disintegrating tablets
- Chewable tablets
- Capsules
- Transdermal patch

Sleep

Sleep disturbances have been found in 25–55% of individuals with ADHD [8]. These disturbances can be distressing to parents and worsen ADHD symptoms. Compounding sleep concerns further, insomnia is also a common side effect of stimulants. There is a difference between having trouble falling asleep and having trouble staying asleep. If having trouble falling asleep, the stimulant may be taken earlier or changed to a shorter-acting form. Other options include lowering the dose and/or adding a non-stimulant ADHD medication. If the trouble is in staying asleep, be sure to discuss sleep hygiene. Using medications for sleep such as melatonin and clonidine has shown improvements in sleep-onset latency and total sleep duration but should be used as a last choice after other options have been pursued [9].

Appetite

Appetite suppression is one of the most common side effects of stimulants and can become a problem for growth and development. These medications should be taken with or after a meal when possible. Diminished appetite is best met with nutrient dense foods at meals. High-fat foods, however, can affect drug metabolism resulting in delayed onset and increased peak concentrations [10]. Weekend and summer drug holidays may be considered when growth trajectories cross two percentile lines [11]. Switching medication to atomoxetine may also be considered, given its lesser effect on appetite.

Anxiety

The comorbidity rate of anxiety disorders and ADHD is approximately 25% [12]. There is an overlap in symptoms characterizing each disorder; therefore effective treatment of ADHD with stimulants may also reduce symptoms of anxiety [13]. However, a possible side effect of stimulants is anxiety. It is important to take a detailed history and helpful to screen with a validated questionnaire for anxiety-related disorders; the SCARED questionnaire is commonly used, easy to deliver and score, and free for use [14]. Using atomoxetine as therapy when comorbid anxiety is present at baseline may be considered. Studies have found improvement in both anxiety and ADHD symptoms with the use of atomoxetine [15]. The addition of an antidepressant when symptoms are moderate or severe may be needed as well as psychotherapy.

Tic Disorders

Tic disorders are a common comorbidity occurring in about 20% of those with ADHD. ADHD usually precedes the emergence of tics by 2–3 years. Therefore, tics may emerge or worsen during stimulant treatment; however, stimulants are not associated with an increased rate, severity, or persistence of tic disorders. There is no evidence of increased risk of new-onset tics with stimulant medication in children with ADHD without preexisting tics [16]. Although quality of evidence is low, a review of eight studies found use of methylphenidate, clonidine, guanfacine, desipramine, and atomoxetine to reduce symptoms of ADHD in children with tics, while high-dose dextroamphetamine may worsen tics. In individual cases when stimulants are found to worsen tics, alpha agonists and atomoxetine can be used or added to ADHD treatment [17].

Substance Use

The rate of ADHD in patients with substance use disorders is around 25%, a rate considerably higher than the general population [18]. Cigarette use has been shown to start earlier and be more severe in those with ADHD. However, there is a 1.9-fold reduction in the risk of substance use disorders in youths treated with stimulants [19]. In the cases of comorbid substance use, once-daily extended-release formulations allow for easier monitoring. It is important to coordinate with co-treaters and to consider less abusable medications such as lisdexamfetamine, atomoxetine, or guanfacine.

Monitoring

> With both stimulant and non-stimulant treatment, monitoring and follow-up is imperative and can range from every 3 to 6 months depending on the patient.

Parent and teacher scales should be administered frequently during dose titration to assess changes in core symptoms and efficacy of treatment. Height, weight, and vitals should be monitored due to common side effects affecting appetite, growth, blood pressure, and heart rate.

Treatment Not Working?

If only some improvement in symptoms results from medication, it is possible the patient needs a higher dose. Dose adjustments are frequently needed as treatment progresses. If a maximum dose is reached, or side effects are not well tolerated, adding a second medication may be warranted.

If not seeing any improvement in symptoms, some further questioning may help. Is the patient actually taking the medication? There could be many reasons for medication nonadherence including method of administration, social stigma, patient denial, or diversion of medication. If the medication is taken as directed, a trial of a different medication may be effective. Reconsidering the diagnosis is always helpful, along with thoughtful exploration of evolving comorbidities.

Case Revisited

Clara does not fit the typical profile of a teen with ADHD, as symptoms of ADHD should emerge more clearly before 12 years of age. First, other explanations for her lack of focus and increased struggle completing her work should be explored (Depression? Sleep disorder? Social stressors? Executive function needs? Substance use?). If she does meet sufficient criteria to warrant a diagnosis, and no other explanation is found, she may have ADHD, inattentive subtype. In fact, some with inattentive ADHD who always worked hard and were well behaved might have been missed in the earlier years (especially girls). On the other hand, through thorough history, we should find some symptoms noticed by others of inattention at an early age. Further, suspicion for misuse is reasonable in an adolescent first presenting with inattention. Clara can be given suggestions for optimizing her homework environment at home and for accessing support to improve her organization skills.

Neuropsychological testing can confirm evidence of inattention. Should medication be pursued, a trial of stimulant or non-stimulant should be discussed.

Conclusions

Medication is the single most effective treatment for ADHD, but no single prescription works best for every person. As a result, a stepwise approach can be helpful in choosing the right medication plan. Use of adjunctive medications can help make treatment both more tolerable and more effective. The process requires shared decision-making including both parent and child for successful treatment while also keeping in mind access and adherence. Treatment must be tailored to the family, and best care includes frequent monitoring. Medication often plays an important role in treatment for the adolescent with ADHD, but the complexity of this developmental stage often requires far more than a prescription to optimize outcomes.

Tips
- Use free resources!
  Table chart including visuals of medications: http://www.adhdmedication-guide.com/
  Teaching a child how to swallow a pill:
  http://www.pillswallowing.com
- Medication can be first started in a teen for ADHD, but there should be a story of earlier symptoms and an explanation for why they weren't treated.
- Choose an ADHD medication based on how it differs from the others, in duration, formulation, side effects, and risk profile.

References

1. Elia J, Ambrosini PJ, Rapoport JL. Treatment of attention-deficit-hyperactivity disorder. N Engl J Med. 1999;340(10):780–8. https://doi.org/10.1056/NEJM199903113401007.
2. Arnold LE. Methylphenidate vs. amphetamine: comparative review. J Atten Disord. 2000;3:200–11. https://doi.org/10.1177/108705470000300403.
3. Stahl SM. Mechanism of action of stimulants in attention-deficit/hyperactivity disorder. J Clin Psychiatry. 2010;71(1):12–3. https://doi.org/10.4088/JCP.09bs05890pur.
4. Wigal SB, Chae S, Patel A, Steinberg-Epstein R. Advances in the treatment of attention-deficit/hyperactivity disorder: a guide for pediatric neurologists. Semin Pediatr Neurol. 2010;17(4):230–6. https://doi.org/10.1016/j.spen.2010.10.005.
5. Garnock-Jones KP, Keating GM. Atomoxetine: a review of its use in attention-deficit hyperactivity disorder in children and adolescents. Paediatr Drugs. 2009;11(3):203–26. https://doi.org/10.2165/00148581-200911030-00005.

6. Michelson D, Faries D, Wernicke J, et al. Atomoxetine in the treatment of children and adolescents with attention-deficit/hyperactivity disorder: a randomized, placebo-controlled, dose-response study. Pediatrics. 2001;108(5):E83. https://doi.org/10.1542/peds.108.5.e83.
7. Arnsten AF. Toward a new understanding of attention-deficit hyperactivity disorder pathophysiology: an important role for prefrontal cortex dysfunction. CNS Drugs. 2009;23(Suppl 1):33–41. https://doi.org/10.2165/00023210-200923000-00005.
8. Corkum P, Tannock R, Moldofsky H. Sleep disturbances in children with attention-deficit/hyperactivity disorder. J Am Acad Child Adolesc Psychiatry. 1998;37(6):637–46. https://doi.org/10.1097/00004583-199806000-00014.
9. Anand S, Tong H, Besag FMC, Chan EW, Cortese S, Wong ICK. Safety, tolerability and efficacy of drugs for treating behavioural insomnia in children with attention-deficit/hyperactivity disorder: a systematic review with methodological quality assessment. Paediatr Drugs. 2017;19(3):235–50. https://doi.org/10.1007/s40272-017-0224-6.
10. Wender EH. Managing stimulant medication for attention-deficit/hyperactivity disorder [published correction appears in Pediatr Rev. 2001 Sep;22(9):292]. Pediatr Rev. 2001;22(6):183–90. https://doi.org/10.1542/pir.22-6-183.
11. Pliszka S, AACAP Work Group on Quality Issues. Practice parameter for the assessment and treatment of children and adolescents with attention-deficit/hyperactivity disorder. J Am Acad Child Adolesc Psychiatry. 2007;46(7):894–921. https://doi.org/10.1097/chi.0b013e318054e724.
12. Biederman J, Newcorn J, Sprich S. Comorbidity of attention deficit hyperactivity disorder with conduct, depressive, anxiety, and other disorders. Am J Psychiatry. 1991;148(5):564–77. https://doi.org/10.1176/ajp.148.5.564.
13. Abikoff H, McGough J, Vitiello B, et al. Sequential pharmacotherapy for children with comorbid attention-deficit/hyperactivity and anxiety disorders. J Am Acad Child Adolesc Psychiatry. 2005;44(5):418–27. https://doi.org/10.1097/01.chi.0000155320.52322.37.
14. Birmaher B, Khetarpal S, Brent D, et al. The screen for child anxiety related emotional disorders (SCARED): scale construction and psychometric characteristics. J Am Acad Child Adolesc Psychiatry. 1997;36(4):545–53. https://doi.org/10.1097/00004583-199704000-00018.
15. Geller D, Donnelly C, Lopez F, et al. Atomoxetine treatment for pediatric patients with attention-deficit/hyperactivity disorder with comorbid anxiety disorder. J Am Acad Child Adolesc Psychiatry. 2007;46(9):1119–27. https://doi.org/10.1097/chi.0b013e3180ca8385.
16. Roessner V, Robatzek M, Knapp G, Banaschewski T, Rothenberger A. First-onset tics in patients with attention-deficit-hyperactivity disorder: impact of stimulants. Dev Med Child Neurol. 2006;48(7):616–21. https://doi.org/10.1017/S0012162206001290.
17. Osland ST, Steeves TD, Pringsheim T. Pharmacological treatment for attention deficit hyperactivity disorder (ADHD) in children with comorbid tic disorders. Cochrane Database Syst Rev. 2018;6(6):CD007990. Published 2018 Jun 26. https://doi.org/10.1002/14651858.CD007990.pub3.
18. Charach A, Yeung E, Climans T, Lillie E. Childhood attention-deficit/hyperactivity disorder and future substance use disorders: comparative meta-analyses. J Am Acad Child Adolesc Psychiatry. 2011;50(1):9–21. https://doi.org/10.1016/j.jaac.2010.09.019.
19. Wilens TE, Faraone SV, Biederman J, Gunawardene S. Does stimulant therapy of attention-deficit/hyperactivity disorder beget later substance abuse? A meta-analytic review of the literature. Pediatrics. 2003;111(1):179–85. https://doi.org/10.1542/peds.111.1.179.

Chapter 4
Behavioral and Therapeutic Treatment of ADHD in Adolescents

Liesl Windsor and Demetra Pappas

Case Example

Adina is an 11th grader with ADHD. She has never been an outstanding student; instead she shines as a musician. She works "hard enough" to earn passing grades and hopes to pursue her musical career after high school. Adina sometimes takes stimulant medication, particularly when cramming for exams and taking them. Otherwise, she feels most creative without medication. Taking her first business class, she sees how important these skills will be for her career; Adina would like to do better in this class, but the volume and nature of long-term projects and assignments overwhelm her.

Background

Although the use of medication and school supports are the most frequently implemented approaches in the treatment of ADHD, behavioral and therapeutic interventions also have important roles when caring for individuals with ADHD. The Multimodal Treatment Study of ADHD (MTA) was a multisite clinical trial spanning 14 months [1]. The study included 579 children randomly designated to receive routine community care or one of three treatments: medication management, intensive behavioral treatment, or the combination of both medication and behavioral

L. Windsor (✉)
Division of Developmental Medicine, Boston Children's Hospital, Boston, MA, USA
e-mail: Liesl.windsor@childrens.harvard.edu

D. Pappas
Harvard Medical School, Division of Developmental Medicine, Boston Children's Hospital, Boston, MA, USA
e-mail: demetra.pappas@childrens.harvard.edu

© Springer Nature Switzerland AG 2020
A. Schonwald (ed.), *ADHD in Adolescents*,
https://doi.org/10.1007/978-3-030-62393-7_4

therapy. Although the MTA study only included children between the ages of 7.0 and 9.9 years, it is still the largest clinical ADHD trial to date. As such, the findings of this study have been considered applicable to various pediatric patient populations and have informed the standard of care for management of ADHD [2].

Adolescents represent a distinct subset of pediatric patients. The complexity of relationships with parents, teachers, and peers increases dramatically during the teenage years. As parental supervision decreases and opportunities for autonomy increase, the possibility for treatment refusal grows. Middle and high school students face increased academic demands, and those with ADHD may struggle with assignment submission, attendance problems, and completion of high school [3]. The requirement for teens to prepare for college and employment can place additional stress on youth with ADHD in whom executive functioning is already compromised. Furthermore, children with ADHD are at a significantly increased risk of developing additional conditions including oppositional defiant disorder, conduct disorder, depression, anxiety, learning disabilities, and substance use and abuse. These conditions may be further exacerbated by the increased social, emotional, and academic pressures that teens are facing as well [4]. These challenges highlight the importance of additional treatment modalities that may address vital areas not fully managed by medication alone. Figure 4.1 displays the range of behavioral treatment available, each explained more fully below (Fig. 4.1).

Therapeutic Options

Given the unique nature of challenges facing teens in general and particularly those with ADHD, most who are affected would benefit from some type of psychosocial support.

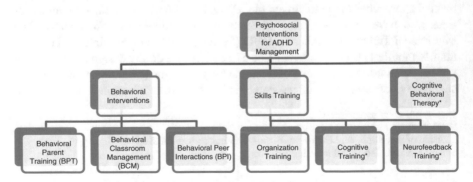

Fig. 4.1 Overview of well-established psychosocial interventions. (Asterisks indicate interventions that are still experimental [cognitive training], possibly efficacious [neurofeedback], and not considered evidence-based for ADHD treatment alone [CBT])

These approaches vary in core practices, target group, therapeutic goals, and setting. They are not universally applicable to all adolescents, and there is some variability in evidence-based efficacy among the therapeutic options. Overall, consistency is vitally important, and adolescents respond best when supports are provided in a variety of settings. Interventions should be considered carefully, on an individual basis, to formulate a treatment plan that is feasible and appropriate for each teenager and their family.

Behavioral Interventions

Behavioral interventions refer to a set of management practices applied to a person's environment that are intended to change that person's behavior. This approach relies on the principles of contingency management with a goal of increasing the frequency of positive behavior and reducing the occurrence of undesirable behavior. Target behavior may occur at home, at school, and/or among peers. Both positive (reward systems) and negative consequences can be used (Table 4.1), though positive methods typically are more powerful in changing behavior.

Behavior management is most effective when applied consistently across contexts. Practically, these techniques can be employed in a number of ways. In order to ensure efficacy, training programs have been developed to equip parents and teachers to craft an environment that is conducive to the success of the teenager. The most commonly used approaches to this intervention are behavioral parent training (BPT), behavioral classroom management (BCM), and behavioral peer interventions (BPI) [6].

Behavioral Parent Training

Behavioral parent training (BPT) is geared toward teaching parents how to set clear expectations for their teenagers. Many structured programs exist, all employing similar foundational principles with some variation in the hands-on application of

Table 4.1 Behavioral intervention tools

Method	Example behavior	Example consequence
Positive reinforcement of desirable behavior	Maintain grades of Bs or higher	Allowed to drive
	Turn in all homework assignments on time	Extra allowance
Removal of privileges as a consequence of undesirable behavior	One or more grades drops below Bs	Earlier curfew
	Skip any single class unexcused	Loss of cell phone

those tenets. Each is designed to support and empower parents of children with ADHD to facilitate the success of the child. Parents are coached on practical ways in which they can create an organized home environment. Parents are also taught to use positive feedback to encourage desired behavior and ways in which to institute consequences for negative behavior routinely. Some of these tools may already be used in the home, but training sessions help parents implement them accurately and consistently.

For parents of adolescents, BPT is modified to take into consideration the developmental stage of the teenager. Although the framework of principles largely remains the same, the actual application should look different from that used for younger children. Positive reinforcement may involve access to electronics, a vehicle, or event tickets. Consequences for undesirable actions may be denial of access to electronics or friends (grounding) or tasking the adolescent with more chores to complete at home. Additionally, parents and teens should meet with a psychologist/facilitator to learn how to approach difficult situations and find resolutions that are agreeable to both parents and teens. Parents are taught how to bargain for improvements in specific behaviors in exchange for feasible rewards that are desirable to the adolescent. Involving teenagers in the decision-making process is vital in motivating them to change their behavior [7].

> When parents implement behavior management at home, parent report of behavior generally improves with the intervention.

However, it is difficult to ascertain whether the improvement reported is due to the parent having a better understanding and ability to manage difficult behavior or if it is due to actual improved behavior on the part of the child. However, reports show that the relationship between parent and child improves overall.

Several existing programs are available to help parents optimize their approach to managing behavior at home. Although the methods may differ, parents and clinicians should ensure that any BPT program being considered includes the following components [8]:

- Parents are taught practical ways to implement positive reinforcement, structure, and consistent discipline.
- Parents learn positive ways to interact and communicate with their child.
- Activities are assigned for parents to work on with their child at home.
- Meetings are scheduled regularly with the family to monitor progress and provide ongoing support.
- Opportunities for reassessment and adjustment of strategies are included as deemed necessary.

Table 4.2 Examples of classroom interventions for teachers

1	Use nonverbal cues to redirect an affected student's attention
2	Maintain appropriate pacing to match a student's attention
3	Provide clear expectations for projects and assignments
4	Distribute outlines for note-taking
5	Teach note-taking skills explicitly
6	Highlight salient information with emphatic tone or labels ("This is important!")
7	Assign seats so the student with ADHD is away from distractions
8	Assign group project partners so students with ADHD learn from organized peers

Behavioral Classroom Management

ADHD is a neurobiological disorder, and adolescents with this diagnosis cannot be expected to overcome their difficulties through sheer effort alone. School-based educational accommodations, often stipulated by a 504 Plan or Individualized Education Program (IEP), allow adolescents with ADHD to access the curriculum more effectively. Behavioral classroom management entails crafting an educational environment that encourages positive behavior from students. Many of the same methods employed in BPT can be modified and applied to the classroom setting. Table 4.2 lists examples of classroom interventions for teachers (Table 4.2).

Behavioral Peer Interventions

In addition to their challenges with relating to adults, adolescents with ADHD often have a hard time fostering relationships with their peers [9]. Behavioral peer interventions employ contingency management strategies (e.g., token economy) to reinforce desired social behaviors (i.e., communication, participation, and collaboration). This particular intervention is typically implemented in various social situations, and the goal is to improve social proficiency in children with ADHD [10]. Interventions such as the Summer Treatment Program (STP) create opportunities for children to engage appropriately with peers in recreational settings [4]. Data suggests that these strategies improve peer acceptance and social skills [6].

Skills Training [11]

Skills training pertains to a group of techniques focused on equipping teens with the tools needed to function optimally in everyday life. This treatment tactic seeks to address the challenges with organization and executive functioning deficits commonly experienced by children with ADHD. Executive functioning refers to working memory, inhibitory control, and mental flexibility [12]. Children and adolescents are expected to develop the ability to recall important information on demand and switch from one task to another efficiently while tuning out extraneous environmental stimuli. Implementing treatment modalities focusing on augmenting organizational skills and executive functioning in youth has real-life benefits as adolescents navigate their teenage years and transition into adulthood.

Organization Training

The term "organizational skills" refers to the ability to manage assignments, belongings, and time [13]. The demands on these skills increase as children get older. Children with ADHD often misplace their homework and school materials. They may have difficulty submitting projects in a timely fashion and adequately preparing for exams. In general, organizational skills programs use token economies and reward systems to encourage adoption of specific target organizational goals (e.g., assignment tracking, time management, and physical organization of materials) in participants. Parents and teachers are then taught how to reinforce the reward system so the responsibility is shifted from the program facilitator to the caregivers and school staff over time. Studies indicate that although teacher ratings of organizational skills may not be significantly impacted by these interventions, parent ratings and academic performance do improve after students receive direct skills training [13].

Other ways to impart organizational skills include the use of an executive functioning coach and, more recently, the use of digital games for the purpose of teaching organizational skills [14]. Parent and teacher ratings of time management indicate that these games can result in mild to moderate treatment benefits in participants.

Cognitive Training

Cognitive training is another area of interest which is currently being studied. Cognitive training entails exercises geared toward improving working memory, inhibition, cognitive flexibility, and/or overall attention.

1. Computerized training programs: These can be played by the individual for a designated period of time. Some evidence suggests an improvement in working memory with this approach, although to date there has been no significant observable difference in caregiver- or teacher-reported hyperactivity, inattentiveness, or academic achievement.
2. Programs that confront participants with increasingly complex auditory and visual stimuli: These improve learners' attention and inhibition skills by requir-

ing them to identify specific signals among multiple distractions [11]. Facilitators then give the participants practical tips on how the skills learned can be applied to daily context. This approach has shown some promise, demonstrating a significant effect on portions of neuropsychological testing as well as caregiver-rated (but not teacher-rated) ADHD symptoms and executive functioning.

Neurofeedback Training

Neurofeedback training is based on the premise that those with ADHD have different patterns of brain wave activity in comparison with their unaffected peers. Neurofeedback training uses EEG sensors to provide participants with visual and auditory cues of changes in their brain waves. Participants are then taught how to monitor and suppress the waves associated with inattentiveness. This change in brain wave activity is believed to cause changes in behavior [15].

> While there is some evidence suggesting that neurofeedback may be effective in decreasing symptoms of ADHD, it has not been widely studied, and further investigation is necessary.

Cognitive Behavioral Therapy

Cognitive behavioral therapy (CBT) is a form of psychological treatment which directly focuses on the individual and is geared toward helping them recognize negative mindsets and deliberately apply practiced techniques to change those mindsets [5]. CBT is an effective tool for treating depression and anxiety disorders, as well as alcohol and drug use problems [16]. CBT has not been shown to be efficacious in the management of ADHD. However, it may provide some relief for comorbid conditions which are more likely to manifest in children and adolescents with ADHD [1]. As such, although CBT should not be routinely recommended for teens with ADHD alone, clinicians must screen these adolescents for symptoms of coexisting mental health conditions that may warrant a referral for CBT. Each child must be properly evaluated, and CBT is recommended when appropriate.

Physical Activity

The American Academy of Pediatrics recommends 60 min/day of physical activity for children. Exercise is not considered an evidence-based treatment option for ADHD, but there is some evidence to suggest that exercise may have positive effects on oppositional defiant symptoms, mood, and peer interactions in those with ADHD [11]. However, it has not yet been established that these effects are statistically significant. As such, while physical activity may improve motor ability, physical fitness, attentiveness, and social behavior [17], more investigation is required to characterize the ideal approach and target population.

Challenges

Although the first-line treatment for ADHD in adolescents is a combination of medication and psychosocial therapy, there is a significant disparity between the percentages of children receiving each of these treatment modalities [18]. Children and adolescents with ADHD are far more likely to receive medication therapy than they are to have been exposed to any of the aforementioned therapeutic options. Some of the reasons for this disparity may include lack of understanding of the importance of psychosocial interventions, difficulty finding and accessing appropriate therapists, and financial and time constraints.

Additionally, there have been a number of studies showing the efficacy of psychosocial interventions in the pediatric population, but only a relatively small amount of data exists pertaining specifically to individual 12–18-year-olds. There is some preliminary support for the use of psychosocial interventions in youth; however, more research is needed in this cohort to determine the true impact of behavioral and therapeutic management on this unique subgroup of pediatric patients.

Case Revisited

Adina's story suggests that she is having trouble with the organization and management of her business class workload. After determining whether inattention/impulsivity is interfering with her success (suggesting medication could be appropriate) and exploring whether an additional co-occurring mental health disorder has developed (such as anxiety or depression), Adina may benefit from organization training to directly improve her skills in managing the long-term projects and assignments that overwhelm her. Several resources may also be useful for Adina, whose motivation and insight predict her willingness and interest in mature self-improvement.

Conclusions

Medication is rarely enough to treat the adolescent with ADHD. In fact, successful interventions may include a broad range of methods to help the teen with ADHD succeed, often added to medication for a combined approach. Some methods shape behavior with motivation and reinforcement; other methods help the teen build their own skills to better manage ongoing challenges. Finding the right behavioral and therapeutic strategies is similar to finding the right medication: the first try is often not the last, and what works at one point in time might need adjustment later.

Tips
- Adolescents should always be involved when behavioral and therapeutic interventions are chosen. Buy-in is key!
- More than one type of behavioral intervention can be used at the same time.
- Lots of existing resources are helpful; use our list below.

Resources for Parents, Educators, and Clinicians Caring for Adolescents with ADHD

Books

- *A Bird's-Eye View of Life with ADD and ADHD: Advice from Young Survivors*
- Alex Zeigler, Chris A. Zeigler Dendy
- *Applying to College for Students with ADD or LD: A Guide to Keep You (and Your Parents) Sane, Satisfied and Organized Through the Admission Process*
- Blythe Grossberg
- *Teenagers with ADD and ADHD: A Guide for Parents and Professionals*
- Chris Dendy
- *Putting on the Brakes: Young People's Guide to Understanding Attention Deficit Hyperactivity Disorder*
- Patricia Quinn, Judith Stern
- *Taking Charge of ADHD: The Complete, Authoritative Guide for Parents*
- Russell A. Barkley
- *Your Defiant Teen: 10 Steps to Resolve Conflict and Rebuild Your Relationship*

- Russell A. Barkley, Arthur L. Robin

Websites

- Children and Adults with Attention-Deficit/Hyperactivity Disorder (CHADD)
- https://chadd.org/
- National Institute for Children's Health Quality
- https://www.nichq.org/resource/caring-children-adhd-resource-toolkit-clinicians
- National Institute of Mental Health

- https://www.nimh.nih.gov/health/topics/attention-deficit-hyperactivity-disorder-adhd/index.shtml
- American Academy of Child and Adolescent Psychiatry
- https://www.aacap.org/AACAP/Families_and_Youth/Facts_for_Families/FFF-Guide/Children-Who-Cant-Pay-Attention-Attention-Deficit-Hyperactivity-Disorder-006.aspx
- US Department of Education

  - Building the Legacy: IDEA 2004
    https://sites.ed.gov/idea/
  - Identifying and Treating Attention Deficit Hyperactivity Disorder: A Resource for School and Home
    https://www2.ed.gov/rschstat/research/pubs/adhd/adhd-identifying-2008.pdf
  - Teaching Children with Attention Deficit Hyperactivity Disorder: Instructional Strategies and Practices
    https://www2.ed.gov/rschstat/research/pubs/adhd/adhd-teaching-2008.pdf
  - Students with Disabilities Preparing for Postsecondary Education: Know Your Rights and Responsibilities
    https://www2.ed.gov/about/offices/list/ocr/transition.html
  - Protecting Students with Disabilities: Frequently Asked Questions About Section 504 and the Education of Children with Disabilities
    https://www2.ed.gov/about/offices/list/ocr/504faq.html

- Centers for Disease Control and Prevention
  https://www.cdc.gov/ncbddd/adhd/index.html

References

1. Jensen PS. A 14-month randomized clinical trial of treatment strategies for attention-deficit/hyperactivity disorder. Arch Gen Psychiatry. 1999;56:1073.
2. Subcommittee on Attention-Deficit/Hyperactivity Disorder, Steering Committee on Quality Improvement and Management, Wolraich M, et al. ADHD: clinical practice guideline for the diagnosis, evaluation, and treatment of attention-deficit/hyperactivity disorder in children and adolescents. Pediatrics. 2011;128(5):1007–22.
3. Kent K, Pelham W, Molina B, et al. The academic experience of male high school students with ADHD. J Abnorm Child Psychol. 2010;39:451–62.
4. Fabiano G, Schatz N, Pelham W. Summer treatment programs for youth with ADHD. Child Adolesc Psychiatr Clin N Am. 2014;23:757–73.
5. Chan E, Fogler J, Hammerness P. Treatment of attention-deficit/hyperactivity disorder in adolescents. JAMA. 2016;315:1997.
6. Evans S, Owens J, Bunford N. Evidence-based psychosocial treatments for children and adolescents with attention-deficit/hyperactivity disorder. J Clin Child Adolesc Psychol. 2014;43(4):527–51.
7. Children and Adults with Attention-Deficit/Hyperactivity Disorder (CHADD). Parent training and education. 2020. Retrieved from https://chadd.org/for-parents/parent-training-and-education/

8. Centers for Disease Control and Prevention. Parent training in behavior management for ADHD. 2019. Retrieved from https://www.cdc.gov/ncbddd/adhd/behavior-therapy.html
9. Hoza B. Peer functioning in children with ADHD. Ambul Pediatr. 2007;7(1 Suppl):101–6.
10. Lerner M, Mikami A, McLeod B. The alliance in a friendship coaching intervention for parents of children with ADHD. Behav Ther. 2011;42(3):449–61.
11. Evans S, Owens J, Wymbs B, Ray A. Evidence-based psychosocial treatments for children and adolescents with attention deficit/hyperactivity disorder. J Clin Child Adolesc Psychol. 2018;47(2):157–98.
12. Harvard University Center on the Developing Child. Executive function: skills for life and learning. Retrieved from https://developingchild.harvard.edu/resources/inbrief-executive-function-skills-for-life-and-learning/
13. Langberg J, Epstein J, Girio-Herrera E, et al. Materials organization, planning, and homework completion in middle-school students with ADHD: impact on academic performance. School Psychol Rev. 2011;3:93–101.
14. Bikic A, Leckman JF, Christensen TØ, et al. Attention and executive functions computer training for attention-deficit/hyperactivity disorder (ADHD): results from a randomized, controlled trial. Eur Child Adolesc Psychiatry. 2018;27(12):1563–74.
15. Steiner N, Frenette E, Rene K, et al. In-school neurofeedback training for ADHD: sustained improvements from a randomized control trial. Pediatrics. 2014;133(3):483–92.
16. American Psychological Association. What is cognitive behavioral therapy? 2020. Retrieved from https://www.apa.org/ptsd-guideline/patients-and-families/cognitive-behavioral.aspx
17. Jeyanthi S, Arumugam N, Parasher R. Effect of physical exercises on attention, motor skill and physical fitness in children with attention deficit hyperactivity disorder: a systematic review. Atten Defic Hyperact Disord. 2019;11(2):125–37.
18. Danielson M, Visser S, Chronis-Tuscano A, et al. A national description of treatment among United States children and adolescents with attention-deficit/hyperactivity disorder. J Pediatr. 2018;192:240–246.e1.

Chapter 5
Complementary and Alternative Treatment of ADHD in Adolescents

Jennifer Johnson and Jeffrey H. Yang

Case Example

A 17-year-old with attention deficit hyperactivity disorder (ADHD) has become vegan and, in doing so, wonders if there are more natural ways to treat her disorder than the prescription medication she has taken (successfully and without side effects) for several years. She and her parents begin to look into options and find much written about different supplements on the Internet. She and her family share interest in changing her treatment from her stimulant to a combination supplement marketed specifically to treat ADHD.

Background

Complementary and alternative medicine (CAM) approaches include a wide variety of interventions, ranging from substances ingested by the patient (e.g., diets, nutrients, "detoxifying" substances) to actions or activities performed by or on the patient (e.g., yoga, exercise, biofeedback, sensory therapy). Many find these options appealing, expecting positive results without negative consequences. In fact, some CAM interventions are promising, but some are potentially harmful. Understanding the risks and benefits of any treatment plan is paramount but tricky in a world of limitless Internet "information." Explanations below address many of the more common CAM treatments, with a chart for easy reference (Table 5.1).

J. Johnson (✉) · J. H. Yang
Department of Pediatrics, Valley Children's Healthcare, Madera, CA, USA
e-mail: JJohnson8@valleychildrens.org

© Springer Nature Switzerland AG 2020
A. Schonwald (ed.), *ADHD in Adolescents*,
https://doi.org/10.1007/978-3-030-62393-7_5

Therapy	Recommendation				Effect size			SECS criteria*			Concerns about current evidence				Comment
	For general health	For ADHD	Not recommended	Unclear	small	moderate	large	Safe	Easy to use	Cost (Not expensive or time-consuming)	Anecdotal	No control group comparison	Likely confounders	Small/exclusive population	
Health nutritional habits	X	X						X	X	X					
Feingold diet			X		X			X		X				X	
AFC elimination diet	X				X			X	X	X					
Gluten-free diet			X†							X	X			X	Recommended only in wheat allergy or celiac disease
Sugar elimination diet	X							X		X	X				
Few-foods diet			X†		X					X				X	May be used briefly as a diagnostic tool
Omega-3 fatty acids or fish oil	X	X			X†	X†		X	X	X		X			Small effect for impulsivity; moderate for oppositional behavior & emotional lability
Omega-6 fatty acids			X					X	X	X		X			
Amino acids			X						X	X		X			Encourage high-quality proteins in diet instead
Carnitine			X†					X	X	X		X		X	May be acceptable in those with Fragile X syndrome
SAMe				X				X†	X	X		X			May not be safe for those on serotonin medications, with bipolar disorder, or immuno-compromised
Gly-conutrients				X				X	X	X		X		X	
DMAE		X			X			X	X	X		X			
DMAA			X						X			X			Unsafe; known significant side effects
Multivitamin	X	X			X			X	X	X		X			
Megadose vitamins			X						X			X			
Vitamin D			X†					X	X	X		X		X	For low vitamin D
Vitamin Bs				X					X	X		X			

Table 5.1 Summary table of complementary and alternative treatments
*Sensibility (in SECS criteria) not included as it is, by definition, subjective and dependent on individual values
†See comments

													Notes
Vitamin C				x				x	x		x			
Iron				x†	x			x†	x	x		x		x	For low ferritin
Magnesium				x†				x†	x	x		x		x	For low magnesium
Zinc				x†				x†	x	x		x		x	For low zinc
Gingkobiloba				x					x	x		x			
Pycnogenol				x					x	x		x			
TCM herbal supplements				x		x†			x	x		x		x	Very limited data; many components may have psychostimulant properties
Valerian			x						x	x		x			
Kava kava			x						x	x		x			
Chamomile			x						x	x		x			
Rhodiola Rosea				x				x	x	x		x		x	
St. John's Wort			x						x	x		x			
Fungal treatments			x						x						
Melatonin	x†							x	x	x		x			For sleep problems
Caffeine			x						x†	x†		x			In small doses
Marijuana/THC			x									x			
CBD oil			x†	x†					x			x†			OTC preparations not recommended due to inconsistent quality; Epidiole and prescription preparations have inadequate data, except for in epilepsy
Proprietary formulations			x						x		x	x	x	x	
Exercise	x	x				x		x	x	x					
Neuro-feedback		x					x	x			x		x	x	
Mindfulness/Meditation				x	x			x	x	x				x	
Yoga				x		X (as adjunct)		x	x	x				x	
Martial Arts				x				x	x					x	
Chiropractic manipulation				x				x			x		x	x	
Acupuncture				x				x			x			x	
CogMed or working memory training				x				x						x	

Table 5.1 (continued)

rTMS			X			X						X		
Anthroposophic therapies			X			X†					X		X	Depends on intervention used
Occupational therapy supports	X					X†	X†			X	X		X	Depends on intervention used
Sensory integration			X			X								May be helpful for sensory problems with goal of improving function
Chelation		X												

Table 5.1 (continued)

Nutritional Interventions

The last few decades have seen an increased interest in the impact of nutrition and diet on behavior. There is emerging evidence suggesting a significant relationship between quality of diet and mental health [1]. Thus, families of children with ADHD are often interested in manipulation of nutrition and diet as a way of changing behavior, including the core symptoms of ADHD. Evidence for these interventions remains very limited but generally falls into three categories [2]:

1. Healthy nutritional habits
2. Elimination diets
3. Specific nutrient supplementation

Nutritional Habits

The presence of an ADHD diagnosis has been associated with several "unhealthy" dietary habits, including skipping breakfast, preference for fast foods, and frequent candy/soft drink intake (i.e., higher intakes of total fat, saturated fat, refined sugars, and sodium) [1–3]. Non-medicated children with ADHD are at an increased risk of obesity compared to the general population [1, 3]. That being said, children with ADHD often struggle with self-regulation, making it unclear whether these associations result from the diets themselves or from poor regulation of food intake secondary to ADHD symptoms. However, some limited evidence does suggest that a balanced diet rich in fish, vegetables, fruit, legumes, and whole grain foods (i.e., pescetarian or pesco-vegetarian diet that includes eggs and dairy) can improve attention in addition to its benefits on general health and well-being [2, 3]. When implementing a dietary change, it is also important to consider the impact on parent-child interactions. The potential benefits from the diet must be balanced with the stress of enforcing it [4].

Elimination Diets

Feingold/Kaiser Permanente Diet and Artificial Food Coloring Elimination

In 1973, Dr. Benjamin Feingold proposed that certain food additives, including salicylates, artificial food colorings, and artificial flavorings, led to hyperactivity and learning problems [5]. The resulting diet seeks to eliminate artificial flavors and dyes in addition to sausage, hot dogs, lunch meat, grapes, and apples [3]. Despite the initial claim that more than 50% of children responded to the diet, meta-analyses have shown only very small improvements on parent rating scales, regardless of whether the child was initially rated as hyperactive [5]. Despite the fact that these studies were all performed with children whose parents believed the child's symptoms to be responsive to diet, only 11–33% showed improvement with the diet implementation [5]. This improvement was not demonstrated on observer or teacher rating scales [5].

Rather than focusing on salicylate elimination, a related diet focuses on eliminating artificial food coloring (AFC) alone from children's diets. In preschool-age and young school-age children with both children and parents blinded to the administration, small but significant increases in hyperactivity scores were observed when AFCs were provided, regardless of whether a child met criteria for ADHD [4, 5]. This suggests that the potential benefits to AFC elimination may apply to all children regardless of ADHD diagnosis [4, 5]. These studies led to increased restrictions on AFCs in the European Union [5]. AFC elimination has an estimated average effect size of 0.28 (small) in children with hyperactivity; in comparison, average effect size of stimulant medications is 0.8 (large) [6]. Thus, the magnitude of improvement resulting from stimulant use is far greater than it is when eliminating AFCs. It is estimated that approximately 8% of children with ADHD have symptoms related to AFCs, but most studies showing effect have dealt with young children rather than adolescents [6, 7]. Although *not recommended as a primary treatment for ADHD*, it would be reasonable to eliminate AFCs from children's diets to the best extent possible given that AFCs do not add nutritional value [6].

Gluten-Free Diet

Gluten has been a part of the human diet for at least 10,000 years and leads to well-known adverse reactions in individuals with wheat allergy and celiac disease, such as abdominal pain, vomiting, weight loss, and chronic diarrhea. In hopes of mitigating such symptoms and associated behavioral problems, many families have adopted gluten elimination or gluten-free diets (GFD) [2]. *GFD may improve symptoms in documented cases of wheat allergy and celiac disease but does not target ADHD symptoms directly.* Supervision by a qualified health professional is important because this diet may not promote healthy eating habits. GFD is more likely to be deficient in fiber, B vitamins, iron, zinc, and folic acid and to contain higher proportions of simple sugars and fats [2].

Sugar Elimination

Sugar intake has long been blamed for hyperactivity; however, no studies have supported this claim [6]. Although sugar-free diets have not been shown to decrease symptoms, it has been shown that parents are more likely to rate their child as hyperactive when the parent believes the child has ingested sugar [6]. Given the increase in childhood obesity and obesity-related conditions, *it may be reasonable to limit the amount of sugar intake, but this would not be expected to affect a child's core ADHD symptoms.*

Allergen-Free/Few Foods Diets

The most extreme dietary restriction utilized by some for ADHD management is known as an oligoantigenic or "few foods" diet. All foods with allergenic potential, such as milk, eggs, chocolate, wheat, citrus, and nuts, are removed from the child's diet and then reintroduced into the diet one at a time (one per week) to document any potential changes in the child's behavior upon reintroduction of the food [3]. Most studies have struggled to reduce bias in their design due to the difficulties of establishing a blinded condition and because participants tend to have a pre-existing interest in dietary management [7]. Additionally, some of the reported effects are likely secondary to increased structure within the home prompted by strict dietary regulations [7]. A meta-analysis found that up to 30% of children with hyperactivity may respond to some version of an elimination diet with an effect size of 0.29 (small), but no pattern was seen in the foods correlated with symptoms [6]. However, elimination diets have also been noted to have the potential for harm due to a lack of nutritional balance. *A few foods diet is generally not recommended as a primary treatment for ADHD.* It may be useful for a brief period of time to determine whether a child is behaviorally sensitive to an individual food [7]. Rating scales from parents and teachers in the weeks before and after instituting the diet can be helpful in tracking symptoms more systematically. If a few foods diet is pursued, a daily multivitamin may be recommended as well as consultation with a dietician [6]. It is not recommended to continue a few foods diet beyond 2 weeks if no benefit from the diet is perceived by that time [6].

Supplements

Omega-3 Fatty Acids

Omega-3 fatty acids, found in fish oil, have been shown to positively affect neuron growth and play a role in dopamine regulation [8]. Lower levels have been measured in children with ADHD, particularly in males [8], compared to same aged peers. Studies of omega-3 fatty acid supplementation suggest an effect size of 0.31

(small to moderate) for oppositional behavior and emotional lability. There may also be some short-term reduction of impulsivity with associated improvements in reading and spelling [2, 3, 6, 9]. Although parent rating scales have shown significant improvement for inattention and hyperactivity, similar improvements have not been shown on teacher rating scales in most studies [9].

Effects of fish oil supplementation have only been demonstrated over a 3- to 6-month period, suggesting that they may not be a great choice for acute treatment of the primary symptoms of ADHD [6]. One study demonstrated that concurrent fish oil supplementation was associated with lower doses of methylphenidate and less appetite suppression in children with ADHD [10]. Thus, there may be a role for fish oil as an adjunctive therapy to standard medication treatment.

Omega-6 fatty acids are found in plant oils and, unlike omega-3's, have not been shown to have any benefits on behaviors or mood. Fish oil supplements vary in their ratio of omega-3 to omega-6 fatty acids. Therefore, results of fish oil supplementation may vary widely depending on their content and quality. Increased fish intake itself (as opposed to fish oil supplements) has also not shown any benefit for ADHD symptoms [1].

If utilized, supplementation should occur with at least 600 mg of mercury-free or USP grade omega-3 fatty acids per day for at least 3 months (some studies recommend 1–2 g and at least 500 mg of EPA) [3, 4, 9]. No major side effects have been demonstrated with use. It is unknown if those with seafood allergies may safely take fish oil supplements. Given the small to moderate effect sizes demonstrated in studies as well as their beneficial effect on triglyceride levels, *omega-3 fatty acids are reasonable to use as an adjunctive treatment for ADHD*.

Amino Acids

Children with ADHD may have lower levels of some amino acids. Some demonstrate nitrogen wasting, and many exhibit problems with nutrition and growth [4]. It has been suggested that supplementing amino acids can make up for these deficits and improve behavioral symptoms. However, data regarding the impact of amino acid supplementation is inconsistent. Positive studies have shown only small, short-term benefits for these supplements and a litany of reported risks [6]. Specifically, tyrosine and phenylalanine supplementations have shown no effect on ADHD symptoms [7]. One study using tryptophan supplementation showed an improvement on parent rating scales but not on teacher ratings [7]. Therefore, *amino acid supplementation is not recommended for primary or adjunctive therapy* [6]. Instead, a safer and more reasonable alternative may be to find ways of encouraging children to consume more high-quality proteins [4].

- *Carnitine* is derived from amino acids in the body and is involved in fatty acid transport and energy production [4, 7]. It has been shown to *reduce ADHD symptoms in children with fragile X syndrome but not in children with ADHD alone* [7]. Some evidence seems to suggest that the increase in energy production may worsen hyperactivity and impulsivity in those predisposed [4]. Thus, carnitine supplementation may have inconsistent results at best and be counterproductive at worst.

- *S-adenosyl-L-methionine (SAMe)* is produced in the body from the amino acid methionine and assists in cell regulation [11]. Although it has shown some promise in the treatment of depression, it has *not been studied for ADHD* [11]. SAMe should not be used in those with bipolar disorder due to a risk of worsening manic episodes, those who are on serotonin-containing medications due to the risk of inducing serotonin syndrome, or those who are immunocompromised due to the possible enhancement of *P. carinii*, a microorganism responsible for severe infections [11].

- *Glyconutrients, DMAE, and DMAA* Organic compounds, such as glyconutrients and dimethylaminoethanol (DMAE), are involved in cell communication and functioning [6]. Glyconutrients have recently been studied for ADHD treatment, but all studies to date have been poorly designed and inconclusive [4, 6]. In contrast, studies using DMAE have shown a weak but significant effect on ADHD symptoms with no serious safety concerns [4]. The Food and Drug Administration has classified it as "possibly effective" [4]. It is important to note that DMAE may be confused with 1,3-dimethylamylamine (DMAA), an amphetamine derivative sometimes found in weight loss and sports performance supplements despite its ban in dietary supplements in 2013 [11]. DMAA has no supporting evidence and many safety concerns, including elevated blood pressure, shortness of breath, and heart attack, particularly if coupled with caffeine use [11]. For this reason, *DMAA should be expressly recommended against.*

Vitamins and Minerals

Studies in the United Kingdom have shown improvement in attention and concentration with multivitamin supplementation to meet recommended daily allowances (RDA), indicating that a *daily multivitamin may be beneficial* [6]. In contrast, megavitamin therapy (vitamins given at large doses, often many times greater than RDA) has not been shown to be beneficial and also presents major safety concerns [6]. In fact, one study using megavitamin therapy showed worsening of ADHD symptoms in 25% of children as well as an elevation in liver enzymes in half of those receiving the megadoses [3, 7].

Vitamin D

Vitamin D is integral to many functions in the body, including regulation of calcium and phosphate, bone growth and remodeling, cell growth modulation, inflammation reduction, and immune function [11]. Correlational data suggests that low levels of vitamin D in children may be associated with increased risk of ADHD diagnosis, whereas higher levels of maternal vitamin D in the neonatal period may be associated with lower ADHD symptoms in toddlers [1]. However, the majority of intervention studies have not shown vitamin D supplementation to improve ADHD symptoms [12]. A few notable studies in subjects with comorbid vitamin D deficiency showed subsequent improvement in evening symptoms [11]. However, they were not able to distinguish between the direct effect of vitamin D on ADHD symptoms and the benefit of resolving vitamin D deficiency. Given the risk for heart and kidney damage if given in excess and the lack of clear benefit on ADHD symptoms, *vitamin D should not be supplemented without a documented low serum vitamin D level* [11].

Vitamin B

Several of the B vitamins – including vitamin B6 (pyridoxine), B9 (folate), and B12 (cobalamin) – have roles in neurotransmitter production and fatty acid metabolism. Deficiencies have been proposed as contributing to ADHD [7]. Low levels of B2, B6, B9, and B12 have been found to correlate with ADHD diagnosis, with B2 and B6 correlating with severity of symptoms [1]. However, *no studies have been identified looking at vitamin B supplementation for ADHD symptoms.*

Vitamin C

Vitamin C has also been proposed for supplementation given its antioxidant effects as well as its role in iron absorption [7], but *no studies were found on its use for treatment of ADHD.*

Iron

Iron plays a role in fatty acid metabolism as well as dopamine synthesis and transport [7, 8]. Iron deficiency is a known cause of cognitive impairment and is also associated with restless leg syndrome, which shares many symptoms with ADHD [7]. Low ferritin (iron store) levels have been correlated with hyperactivity, impulsivity, inattention, and higher levels of amphetamine medications required to control symptoms [3]. It is important to note that these symptoms can also appear with sleep deprivation or poor quality sleep, as seen with restless leg syndrome. Iron supplementation in low-resource, overseas populations has been shown to moderately reduce ADHD symptoms; however, no major studies have been performed in high-resource populations, such as the United States. Thus, it remains unclear whether the benefits are related to treatment of ADHD or nutritional deficiency [6]. In a small-scale US study, iron supplementation in children with low ferritin improved ADHD symptoms.

However, the study did not control for sleep quality; the improvement may have been secondary to improved sleep quality due to the reduction of restless leg syndrome that was also seen [8]. Iron often induces constipation and, if given in excess, can lead to hemochromatosis [4]. It would be reasonable to assess ferritin levels in those children who are at risk for nutritional deficiencies or who exhibit symptoms of restless leg syndrome and to correct any deficiencies discovered. *Evidence, therefore, does not support iron supplementation as a primary treatment for ADHD.*

Magnesium

Studies on magnesium have been performed in Eastern Europe and other regions of the world where nutritional deficiencies are prevalent. These showed moderate decreases in ADHD symptoms, but no large-scale studies have been performed in the United States or the United Kingdom [6]. Magnesium levels of children with ADHD in the United States have been within normal ranges in a number of studies [4]. Animal studies with magnesium supplementation have shown a U-shaped response curve for behavior, indicating that *supplementation in children who are not nutritionally deficient may worsen symptoms* [6]. Additionally, magnesium often results in diarrhea, and doses over 10 mg/kg/day or 200 mg/day have been shown to be toxic and may result in death [4].

Zinc

Zinc helps to regulate dopamine and norepinephrine (two key neurotransmitters in ADHD) and plays a key role in melatonin production (important in sleep regulation) [4, 8]. Although zinc has been shown to be an effective supplement in overseas studies of children with presumed nutritional deficiency, studies in the United States have not shown any benefit of zinc supplementation alone [6]. However, low zinc levels have been shown to correlate with inattention, and one study reported lower required doses of amphetamine medication with zinc supplementation [3, 8, 10]. High levels of zinc supplementation (greater than 15 mg/day) may interfere with iron and copper absorption; so, it *should not be used as a treatment for ADHD symptoms without documented low blood levels of zinc* [4].

Herbs

Herbs are defined as parts of plants that have pharmacological activity [4]. Since herbs are not regulated by the FDA, the quality and concentrations are inconsistent [4]. As with all pharmacologic agents, they have the propensity to interact with other herbs and medications, sometimes to a greater degree since herbs can have multiple active components. Furthermore, they may be contaminated with toxins, such as lead, particularly in herbs imported from Asia [4]. As with any supplement or over-the-counter medication, it is extremely important to notify the child's doctor of use.

Ginkgo biloba Extract

Ginkgo biloba extract, taken from the maidenhair or ginkgo tree, has been shown to increase blood flow to the brain while also inhibiting platelet activation [4]. Studies on *Ginkgo biloba* in the general, adult population have shown improved attention, memory, processing speed, and executive function, but studies in teenagers with ADHD have been very small, pilot studies [8]. One study showed some benefits on both parent and teacher rating scales, but there is *not yet enough data on efficacy or side effects in children to recommend its use* [12]. Side effects may include nausea, headaches, and rashes as well as subdural or eye bleeding more rarely [4, 8]. It should be avoided in anyone taking aspirin, warfarin, or heparin, and it must be held for 2 weeks prior to surgery [8].

Pycnogenol (Pine Bark Extract)

Pycnogenol, an extract taken from maritime pine bark, is thought to work by improving blood flow, particularly to the brain [11]. Little research to date has been performed using Pycnogenol; its effects are inconclusive [4]. One trial has shown positive results on ADHD symptoms, including improved attention, decreased hyperactivity, and improved visual-motor coordination [4, 6]. However, *safety has not been adequately studied at this time.*

Traditional Chinese Medicine Herbal Supplements

Ningdong and duodongning are supplements consisting of multiple herbs and ground animal products that are typically used for their calming properties and recently used as a treatment for ADHD and Tourette's syndrome. Ningdong's main noted side effect is drowsiness and increased sleep, while duodongning may decrease appetite. Although one small-scale study for each supplement showed improvement in ADHD symptoms similar to stimulant medication based on parent and teacher report, *little information is yet available about the efficacy and safety of these supplements* [10, 12]. Similarly, Yizhi mixture and Jingling liquid, made from a number of herbs, have each shown improvement in ADHD symptoms when given as an adjunct to stimulant medication, but they have not been looked at with larger studies, and little information on their safety is available at this time [10].

Valerian Root

Valerian root, taken from a perennial, flowering plant and previously used as a treatment for insomnia, has *not been shown to have any positive effect in ADHD* [4, 6]. Its use has been associated with heart problems, headaches, and restlessness. It is not recommended for children or for ADHD treatment [4].

Kava kava

Kava kava supplements, taken from the root of the kava shrub, have *not demonstrated any positive effect for ADHD symptoms* and are associated with a number of side effects, including high cholesterol, liver damage, heart problems, weight loss, and blood in urine [4, 11]. Its use is not recommended.

Chamomile

Chamomile, a daisy-like flower, is often administered in tea form by combining dried chamomile flowers with water and has long been used for its calming properties. There is *no data supporting chamomile's use for ADHD* symptoms in children or adults [4]. It may produce bleeding, vomiting, and hypersensitivity reactions [4]. Therefore, it is *not recommended* for use in children, regardless of the presence or absence of ADHD.

Rhodiola Rosea

Rhodiola, taken from a dried flowering plant, is proposed to act through elevations in dopamine, serotonin, and norepinephrine levels [8]. Studies of this herb have not focused on those with ADHD, but *several studies have shown a benefit for attention, memory, and accuracy as well as mood* [8]. Because it has a mild antiplatelet effect, Rhodiola *may cause increased bruising as well as induce dizziness and dry mouth* [8, 11]. If utilized, it may be provided in doses ranging from 50 to 500 mg/day in children [8].

St. John's Wort

St. John's wort, taken from a flowering plant, has traditionally been used to relieve symptoms of depression and has been found to inhibit the reuptake of dopamine, serotonin, and norepinephrine [13]. Although one study showed improvement in

ADHD rating scales with St. John's wort supplementation in children with ADHD, several other studies have shown no improvement [4, 6, 10]. Additionally, St. John's wort can elicit sun sensitivity and increase anxiety [11]. Most notably, it interferes with many prescription medications, including antidepressants, birth control medications, and warfarin, and it can induce serotonin syndrome, particularly when coupled with psychiatric medications [4]. Therefore, it is *not recommended for ADHD treatment*.

Fungal Treatment

There is currently *no evidence* for oral fungal medications having use in ADHD treatment; however, it has several associated risks, including affecting liver, kidney, and heart function [4].

Melatonin

Sleep problems affect 25–55% of children with ADHD and may be attributable to poor sleep hygiene, stimulant side effects, sleep-onset insomnia, restless leg syndrome, or comorbid psychiatric conditions such as anxiety [8]. Melatonin is a neurohormone secreted by the pineal gland that regulates our sleep-wake cycle [8]. Although melatonin has *not been shown to target core ADHD symptoms*, it is often beneficial for children with chronic sleep problems, which may indirectly improve their concentration and hyperactivity [6]. It may be given in doses of 1–6 mg 30 min prior to desired sleep onset and has not been associated with any major side effects [8]. As melatonin does play a minor role in reproductive functioning, it may theoretically induce amenorrhea in large doses, which is readily reversible with cessation of the supplement [14]. Though studies on melatonin's effect on long-term hormonal impact have yet to be performed, it is generally believed to be safe for long-term use.

Caffeine

Caffeine functions as a weak stimulant and thus has been proposed as a home remedy for children with ADHD. However, studies have shown small or no benefit and, in some cases, worsening of attention and activity level [6]. It is associated with tachycardia and palpitations at high doses [6]. Its use is *not recommended as a treatment for ADHD*.

Marijuana/Cannabidiol (CBD) Oil

With the recent explosion in "medical marijuana" use, many families have begun to express an interest in marijuana use or CBD oil for ADHD symptoms. Marijuana contains two primary chemicals: delta-9-tetrahydrocannabinol (THC) and cannabidiol (CBD). THC is a mind-altering substance associated with the "high" experienced from marijuana. CBD, on the other hand, is not associated with intoxication effects. A form of CBD oil is approved by the Food and Drug Administration for use in two rare and severe seizure disorders that are difficult to control with typical seizure medications, but no studies to date have been published focusing on CBD oil as a treatment for ADHD [11]. As with other herbs and supplements, CBD oil preparations are not currently monitored for purity or safety; therefore, it is unknown how much THC is contained in these preparations. One study of CBD products ordered online found that approximately 70% of products were inaccurately labeled, including 21% that contained THC [15]. THC has been known to cause clouding of thinking, hallucinations, anxiety, and psychosis over short periods of time as well as long-term changes in the brain that may result in lowered IQ, impairment of learning and memory, and worsening of psychiatric conditions, such as anxiety, depression, and schizophrenia [11]. In addition to changes in the brain, marijuana and THC have been linked to increased lung infections, increased chance of heart attack, and severe nausea and vomiting requiring hospitalization [11]. As data on the safety, efficacy, and reliability of CBD oil is scarce at this time, it *should not be recommended for symptoms of ADHD.*

Proprietary Formulations

Many products are marketed as specialized formulations for ADHD symptoms. Most appear to contain a mixture of various herbs, vitamins, and other dietary supplements, but labels are often unclear, limited, or absent. These products should be used with extreme caution given the lack of independent research, FDA oversight, clear labeling, and data regarding consistent and safe dosing [6].

Mind-Body Therapies

Increasingly, there is an understanding of how our physical and mental states may influence each other, impacting our feelings, emotions, and behavior. Children with ADHD are often physically dysregulated and frequently appear to others as having a poor connection between their thoughts and actions. There is some data suggesting that these children can have decreased parasympathetic nervous system activity, which, in turn, is associated with poor emotional regulation [8]. Families may turn to mind-body therapies to help children with ADHD learn to calm their bodies, increase parasympathetic activity, and calm their minds.

Exercise

Exercise has been shown to produce an increase in dopamine, norepinephrine, and serotonin release as well as an increase in cerebral blood flow, presumably helping to stimulate the prefrontal cortex, the primary area affected by ADHD [16, 17]. Several studies have demonstrated an improvement in executive functioning following aerobic exercise, particularly when exercise incorporates strategic thinking, anticipation, and cooperation [18]. Exercise has also been shown to improve reading comprehension and mathematics performance in the short term [18]. In meta-analyses of the effect of exercise programs in children with ADHD, aerobic exercise was associated with improvements in impulsivity, anxiety, inattention, social disorders, self-esteem, cognitive speed, classroom behavior, and executive functioning that persist for days to weeks [16, 18]. Given the wide range of health benefits associated, *regular exercise of at least 30 min/day for 3–5 days a week should be encouraged in all children*, including those with ADHD.

Neurofeedback

Neurofeedback uses real-time displays of brain activity in an attempt to teach participants to better regulate their attention and focus. The goal of neurofeedback is to decrease theta wave activity in the brain, which is associated with hyperactivity, impulsivity, and inattention and is the type of brain activity seen during daydreaming states [6]. In addition, neurofeedback seeks to simultaneously increase beta wave activity in the brain, which is seen during periods of concentration and active engagement in activities [6]. Typically, neurofeedback consists of one to three sessions per week administered over 2–12 months [8]. A meta-analysis of trials in the 1990s and 2000s showed an effect size of 0.69; however, the studies were limited by a lack of follow-up after treatments, unstandardized methods, and a lack of control groups [6]. One study demonstrated statistically significant effect sizes ranging from 0.4 to 0.6 on both teacher and parent rating scales of inattention and impulsivity with continued improvement still seen 6 months after the intervention [8]. Although neurofeedback shows promise for the treatment of ADHD, given that the treatment is time-intensive, expensive, not typically covered by insurance, and less effective than stimulant medication, there *is inadequate data to recommend neurofeedback as a primary treatment at this time.*

Mindfulness/Meditation

Mindfulness-based practices focus on regulation of attention [19]. These strategies can be utilized as young as 7 years old [19]. In adults, mindfulness-based programs targeting stress reduction have demonstrated increased gray matter development, associated with memory, learning, and emotional regulation [8]. Although no large-scale studies have been conducted on teenagers using mindfulness training, several small studies with both teenage and adult participants showed improvements in ADHD symptoms, anxiety, depression, and tasks involving attentional conflict, which was similar to results of mindfulness-based practices in younger children [19]. Additionally, mindful parenting programs have been created with the goals of reducing parental stress, decreasing reactivity, and improving executive functioning, particularly in parents who also demonstrate symptoms of ADHD [19]. Mindfulness parenting programs have demonstrated *some benefit by lowering parental symptoms of inattention and hyperactivity while decreasing parental stress and overreactivity* [19]. These programs are thought to benefit kids as parents improve their abilities to respond productively to their child's behaviors while also modeling appropriate ways of self-regulating [17]. Mindfulness or meditation practices that actively focus on increasing attention and awareness appear to have an advantage over those that encourage people to let their mind wander freely, as latter practices have been shown to decrease blood flow to the frontal lobe and increase theta wave activity [17].

Yoga

Yoga integrates postures, breathing techniques, and meditation practices with the goal of regulating the body and attention [17]. Yoga has been shown to increase vagal tone and to increase alpha waves in the frontal lobe, which promotes relaxation [20]. *In studies of teenagers with and without ADHD, yoga has been associated with decreased impulsivity and anxiety as well as improved mood and decreased opposi-tionality* [7, 20]. One study utilizing yoga as an adjunct to medication for 34 weeks showed effect sizes of 0.6–0.97 on ADHD symptoms compared to a control group playing active games [20]. However, information about the true potential of yoga remains limited as the studies to date have been small and without control groups [6, 8].

Martial Arts

Martial arts have long been a recommended activity for children with ADHD given their emphasis on self-control and concentration [17]. Karate has been shown in one study to *improve attention on tasks* with an effect size of 0.88 [17]. Tai chi empha-sizes controlled breathing and attention to body movement and balance [17].

Although few studies have been done, one study in adolescents utilizing tai chi showed *decreased hyperactivity, improved attention, and decreased negative emotions and anxiety* [17]. These studies have all been performed on a small scale, limiting our ability to draw many conclusions.

Chiropractic Manipulation

Chiropractic care seeks to manipulate the musculoskeletal system in hopes of improving neurological functioning [13]. Little has been published on the subject of chiropractic manipulation for children with ADHD. Although at least one case study reported benefits, the studies have been limited by small sample sizes (one to seven children), lack of controls, and concurrent treatment with fish oil or other supplements [6]. The reports may also contain biases given that all authors of these studies are chiropractors reporting on their own patients; so there is a lack of comparison groups and blinding [6]. At this time, there is *inadequate data to draw conclusions regarding the use of chiropractic manipulation.*

Acupuncture

Acupuncture is a traditional Chinese medicine practice that involves the insertion of needles into designated acupoints with the goal of manipulating the flow of *qi* (life energy) [13]. Electroacupuncture provides additional stimulation to acupoints through the use of a pulsating electrical current attached to the inserted needles [13]. Very few studies of acupuncture have focused on treatment of ADHD in children, though both electroacupuncture and traditional practices have been used [6]. Although one study showed some functional improvement, *no studies have shown significant improvement in ADHD symptoms on standardized evaluation* forms or an advantage when compared to traditional treatments in children [12]. If acupuncture is used, it is important to check the provider's credentials and/or state registration due to the risk of infections, organ puncture, or nerve damage if administered incorrectly [11].

Cogmed/Brain Training Programs

The Cogmed program is a computer-based program focused on improving working memory that consists of 25 training sessions over 5 weeks [6]. Studies have been conducted in adolescents and have shown an improvement in primary memory (not secondary memory as is impaired in ADHD) without improvement in frontal lobe function [6]. Although parents reported improved attention, no improvement has been seen on teacher rating scales, and parents were not blinded to the intervention

[6]. Similar results have been demonstrated for other brain training programs [12]. Although brain training programs demonstrate improvement in the direct skills practiced, these skills do not appear to generalize to other tasks or show any effect on academic or cognitive functioning. Overall, there is *no evidence of benefit for ADHD symptoms resulting from these programs.*

rTMS

Repetitive transcranial magnetic stimulation (rTMS) is a relatively new intervention utilizing weak electrical current to stimulate the prefrontal cortex [21]. In TMS, a focal magnetic field is created that induces small electrical currents of varying amounts of strength, frequency, and interval as well as interval rest without stimulation. Placing the TMS magnet over the targeted brain region alters the firing patterns of the brain region underneath. Several studies demonstrated safety of the intervention and sufficient benefits for ADHD symptoms that the FDA approved use of TMS for ADHD in children 7–12 years of age [22, 23]. One small study of adolescents did not show improvement in this age group [24]; *more research is needed before TMS should be recommended for adolescents with ADHD.*

Anthroposophic Therapies

In anthroposophic therapy, ADHD is viewed as an equilibrium imbalance [6]. Therapy focuses on rhythm and movement through exercise, art, and rhythmic massage as well as supplements [6]. Several studies have shown some benefit, but these are complicated by participants self-selecting to this therapy, a lack of control groups, and a lack of consistent intervention strategies given the wide variety of anthroposophic therapies available [6, 13].

Occupational Therapy Approaches

Occupational therapy supports have become increasingly utilized for children with ADHD. Some common occupational strategies include flexible seating, chair bands, sensory integration therapy, weighted vests or lap pads, fidget toys (e.g., fidget spinners), and use of an interactive metronome. In several studies in elementary-age children, weighted vests of 10% of children's body weight were shown to improve in-seat behavior, processing speed, executive functioning, and attention with decreased fidgeting [25]. Similarly, the use of stability balls in classrooms has been shown to improve attention and on-task behavior as well as decrease hyperactivity [26]. Interactive metronome training, while effective for visual motor control, has not shown benefit for any of the core symptoms of ADHD [26].

One occupational therapy training program, the Cognitive-Functional (Cog-Fun) program, has shown some promise in young school-age children [26]. The Cog-Fun program is a parent and child training program that takes place over 12 weeks during 1 h/week sessions led by an occupational therapist. This program focuses on introducing cognitive strategies through the use of games and play activities to improve executive functioning [26]. Two small-scale studies with control groups have shown improvement in executive functioning with use of this program [26]. Several play-based occupational therapy programs, such as Theraplay, have also shown some improvement in ADHD symptoms as well as interpersonal relationships and communication [26]. The positive results of these programs likely stem from their similarities to behavioral parent training, but these approaches may be too simplistic for typically-developing adolescents.

Children with ADHD are often reported to have sensory-seeking or avoiding behaviors that induce many families to seek out sensory integration therapy. Sensory integration therapy is administered by occupational therapists and seeks to acclimate children to sensations by repeated and structured exposure. Although no studies have been identified looking at the effect of sensory integration therapy on ADHD symptoms, it may be utilized in specific cases where sensory aversions are impairing a child's ability to function well in their environment. If used, it is important that goals are specifically designed around improving a child's overall function and ability to engage in the activities and demands of daily life, rather than simply mitigating symptoms. Sample goals include tolerating a noisy environment *in order to remain in a regular classroom environment*, using a fidget toy/cushion *because it helps them focus and complete their work on time*, or expanding a very restricted diet *to improve nutrition*.

Chelation

Chelation is the use of an organic or inorganic compound to bind metal ions in the body so that the metal loses its physiological activity or toxic effect. It is used to treat children with documented heavy metal toxicity, such as lead levels over 25 µg/dL. In the case of lead toxicity, impulsivity and inattention are part of the toxidrome and, thus, may improve with treatment. However, chelation is dangerous for those with normal lead/heavy metal levels and may result in such effects as seizures, brain damage, heart arrhythmias, respiratory failure, liver or kidney damage, severe allergic reactions, increased bleeding risk and infections, or death [4]. *Its use should be restricted only to cases of heavy metal toxicity and under conditions of close medical monitoring.*

Case Revisited

While a more natural intervention may be desired, it is important to review the current treatment carefully, as subtle problems may contribute to the desire to switch. In the scenario described, the adolescent and her family should be asked – with authentic curiosity – their thoughts, concerns, and priorities. Many products are marketed as specialized formulations for ADHD symptoms. Most appear to contain a mixture of various herbs, vitamins, and other dietary supplements, but labels are often unclear, limited, or absent. Providing nonjudgmental factual information will be important, and they should be informed that such products should be used with extreme caution given the lack of independent research, FDA oversight, clear labeling, and data regarding consistent and safe dosing. Working together to find effective treatments that align with her beliefs and values should continue as the next step.

Conclusions

The world of CAM is ever changing, often confusing, and difficult to navigate. Though there are many promising therapies, data are often sparse and/or confounded, and there can be much variability among commercial products. A good rule of thumb for parents and clinicians to apply when determining whether a complementary and alternative medicine approach is appropriate for a child is the *SECS criteria: safety, ease, cost*, and *sensibility* given the evidence available [10].

Although it is often tempting for families and clinicians to institute multiple treatments at the same time in hopes that one will be effective, this should be avoided. Treatments may influence or interfere with each other's effect, and it becomes difficult to judge the impact of each treatment. Furthermore, the uncertainty and logistical complexity of adjusting multiple treatments simultaneously may add strain on the family that can also decrease potential effectiveness of the treatments [10]. Therefore, only one new therapy or medication should be adjusted at a time in order to better understand its impact on the child. Use of behavioral rating scales, such as Vanderbilt ADHD or Clinical Attention Problem Scale (CAPS) forms, from both caregivers and teachers, is recommended prior to the initiation and at follow-up of new treatments in order to more accurately gage child response.

Clinicians must be willing to ask families about their CAM practices in a nonjudgmental way in order to encourage them to divulge use. They must also be willing to help families explore the safety and efficacy of these practices. Families interested in the use of CAM should be encouraged to discuss practices and supplements of interest with their child's doctor. For up-to-date information on use of supplements and therapies, the National Institutes of Health's (NIH's) National Center for Complementary and Integrative Health website (https://nccih.nih.gov/) is an excellent resource for all interested parties.

Tips
- Only one new therapy or medication should be started and adjusted at a time in order to better understand its impact on the child.
- Think SECS when considering CAM treatment: safety, ease, cost, and sensibility.
- When weighing risks and benefits of CAM treatment, consider cost, time commitment, and whether the CAM treatment interferes with other important activities or opportunities.

References

1. Lange KW. Dietary factors in the etiology and therapy of attention deficit/hyperactivity disorder. Curr Opin Clin Nutr Metab Care. 2017;20(6):464–9. https://doi.org/10.1097/MCO.0000000000000415.
2. Cruchet S, Lucero Y, Cornejo V. Truths, myths and needs of special diets: attention-deficit/hyperactivity disorder, autism, non-celiac gluten sensitivity, and vegetarianism. Ann Nutr Metab. 2016;68(Suppl 1):43–50. https://doi.org/10.1159/000445393.
3. Millichap JG, Yee MM. The diet factor in attention-deficit/hyperactivity disorder. Pediatrics. 2012;129(2):330–7. https://doi.org/10.1542/peds.2011-2199.
4. Arnold LE, Hurt E, Lofthouse N. Attention-deficit/hyperactivity disorder: dietary and nutritional treatments. Child Adolesc Psychiatr Clin N Am. 2013;22(3):381–402, v. https://doi.org/10.1016/j.chc.2013.03.001.
5. Arnold LE, Lofthouse N, Hurt E. Artificial food colors and attention-deficit/hyperactivity symptoms: conclusions to dye for. Neurotherapeutics. 2012;9(3):599–609. https://doi.org/10.1007/s13311-012-0133-x.
6. Bader A, Adesman A. Complementary and alternative therapies for children and adolescents with ADHD. Curr Opin Pediatr. 2012;24(6):760–9. https://doi.org/10.1097/MOP.0b013e32835a1a5f.
7. Heilskov Rytter MJ, Andersen LB, Houmann T, et al. Diet in the treatment of ADHD in children - a systematic review of the literature. Nord J Psychiatry. 2015;69(1):1–18. https://doi.org/10.3109/08039488.2014.921933.
8. Sharma A, Gerbarg PL, Brown RP. Non-pharmacological treatments for ADHD in youth. Adolesc Psychiatry (Hilversum). 2015;5(2):84–95. https://doi.org/10.2174/2210676605021504301549 37.
9. Chang JP, Su KP, Mondelli V, et al. Omega-3 polyunsaturated fatty acids in youths with attention deficit hyperactivity disorder: a systematic review and meta-analysis of clinical trials and biological studies. Neuropsychopharmacology. 2018;43(3):534–45. https://doi.org/10.1038/npp.2017.160.
10. Hurt EA, Arnold LE. An integrated dietary/nutritional approach to ADHD. Child Adolesc Psychiatr Clin N Am. 2014;23(4):955–64. https://doi.org/10.1016/j.chc.2014.06.002.
11. National Center for Complementary and Integrative Health. National Center for Complementary and Integrative Health [Internet]. Bethesda: National Center for Complementary and Integrative Health; 2018 [updated 2018 Nov 9; cited 2019 Jan 12]. Retrieved from https://nccih.nih.gov/
12. Goode AP, Coeytaux RR, Maslow GR, Davis N, Hill S, Namdari B, et al. Nonpharmacologic treatments for attention-deficit/hyperactivity disorder: a systematic review. Pediatrics. 2018;141(6). https://doi.org/10.1542/peds.2018-0094.

13. Skokauskas N, McNicholas F, Masaud T, et al. Complementary medicine for children and young people who have attention deficit hyperactivity disorder. Curr Opin Psychiatry. 2011;24(4):291–300. https://doi.org/10.1097/YCO.0b013e32834776bd.
14. Masters A, Pandi-Perumal SR, Seixas A, et al. Melatonin, the hormone of darkness: from sleep promotion to ebola treatment. Brain Disord Ther. 2014;4(1). https://doi.org/10.4172/2168-975X.1000151.
15. Bonn-Miller MO, Loflin MJE, Thomas BF, Marcu JP, Hyke T, Vandrey R. Labeling accuracy of cannabidiol extracts sold online. JAMA. 2017;318(17):1708–9. https://doi.org/10.1001/jama.2017.11909.
16. Cerrillo-Urbina AJ, Garcia-Hermoso A, Sanchez-Lopez M, et al. The effects of physical exercise in children with attention deficit hyperactivity disorder: a systematic review and meta-analysis of randomized control trials. Child Care Health Dev. 2015;41(6):779–88. https://doi.org/10.1111/cch.12255.
17. Herbert A, Esparham A. Mind-body therapy for children with attention-deficit/hyperactivity disorder. Children (Basel). 2017;4(5). https://doi.org/10.3390/children4050031.
18. Den Heijer AE, Groen Y, Tucha L, et al. Sweat it out? The effects of physical exercise on cognition and behavior in children and adults with ADHD: a systematic literature review. J Neural Transm (Vienna). 2017;124(Suppl 1):3–26. https://doi.org/10.1007/s00702-016-1593-7.
19. Cassone AR. Mindfulness training as an adjunct to evidence-based treatment for ADHD within families. J Atten Disord. 2015;19(2):147–57. https://doi.org/10.1177/1087054713488438.
20. Balasubramaniam M, Telles S, Doraiswamy PM. Yoga on our minds: a systematic review of yoga for neuropsychiatric disorders. Front Psych. 2012;3:117. https://doi.org/10.3389/fpsyt.2012.00117.
21. Becker JE, Shultz EKB, Maley CT. Transcranial magnetic stimulation in conditions other than major depressive disorder. Child Adolesc Psychiatr Clin N Am. 2019;28(1):45–52. https://doi.org/10.1016/j.chc.2018.08.001.
22. Palm U, Segmiller FM, Epple AN, et al. Transcranial direct current stimulation in children and adolescents: a comprehensive review. J Neural Transm (Vienna). 2016;123(10):1219–34. https://doi.org/10.1007/s00702-016-1572-z.
23. U.S. Food and Drug Administration. FDA permits marketing of first medical device for treatment of ADHD [Press release]. 2019. Retrieved from https://www.fda.gov/news-events/press-announcements/fda-permits-marketing-first-medical-device-treatment-adhd
24. Weaver L, Rostain AL, Mace W, et al. Transcranial Magnetic Stimulation (TMS) in the treatment of attention deficit/hyperactivity disorder in adolescents and young adults: a pilot study. J ECT. 2012;28(2):98–103. https://doi.org/10.1097/YCT.0b013e31824532c8.
25. Bodison SC, Parham LD. Specific sensory techniques and sensory environmental modifications for children and youth with sensory integration difficulties: a systematic review. Am J Occup Ther. 2018;72(1):7201190040p1–p11. https://doi.org/10.5014/ajot.2018.029413.
26. Nielsen SK, Kelsch K, Miller K. Occupational therapy interventions for children with attention deficit hyperactivity disorder: a systematic review. Occup Ther Ment Health. 2017;33(1):70–80. https://doi.org/10.1080/0164212X.2016.1211060.

Chapter 6
Neuropsychological Testing for Adolescents with ADHD

Fern Baldwin and Kate Linnea

Introduction

Attention-deficit/hyperactivity disorder (ADHD) is the most common of several conditions that fall under the umbrella term neurodevelopmental disorder or an atypical development of the central nervous system (CNS) that becomes apparent in early childhood [1, 2]. Despite being categorized as a brain disorder, ADHD is defined behaviorally. As reviewed in Chap. 2, ADHD has no distinctive biomarker, meaning there is no blood test, brain scan, or other conclusive measure to determine this diagnosis. Instead, ADHD is diagnosed based on a child's developmental and clinical history, informal and standardized reports of behavior, clinician observations, and, sometimes, neuropsychological testing. An assessment of ADHD should ideally use a multimodal and multidisciplinary approach [3] and include information obtained from several sources to assess symptoms across settings, a comprehensive history to determine age of onset and duration of symptoms, assessment of functional impairment, and evaluation for possible coexisting conditions. Currently, many children and adolescents are diagnosed with ADHD by a primary care provider [4]; however, appointment time limitations interfere with consistent adherence to the diagnostic criteria outlined by the *Diagnostic and Statistical Manual of Mental Disorders, 5th Edition* (DSM-5) [5]. A brief visit with a primary care pediatrician is not the ideal setting for diagnostic conceptualization of a teenager with a new ADHD concern [6]. Comprehensive neuropsychological evaluations are

F. Baldwin (✉)
Center for Autism and Related Disorders, Kennedy Krieger Institute, Baltimore, MD, USA
e-mail: BaldwinF@kennedykrieger.org

K. Linnea
Division of Developmental Medicine, Boston Children's Hospital, Boston, MA, USA
e-mail: Kate.linnea@childrens.harvard.edu

© Springer Nature Switzerland AG 2020
A. Schonwald (ed.), *ADHD in Adolescents*,
https://doi.org/10.1007/978-3-030-62393-7_6

lengthy and more thorough and include formal testing, yet there is ongoing debate as to the added value of neuropsychological assessment in the diagnostic and treatment process in youth with ADHD. But in many regions, parents of children with inattention or school difficulties are automatically advised to "get a neuropsych eval." This chapter reviews what that means. We also cover who, when, and why a neuropsychological evaluation is indicated for an adolescent with ADHD symptoms. Finally, clinicians are directed to specific sections of this chapter, while parents and teachers may prefer to focus on boxed tips, search specific sections, or *find a specific test* to better understand its function [1–6].

Case Example

A 16-year-old boy with dyslexia is having increased academic difficulty in 9th grade. His grades are dropping, and he is not able to complete papers and long-term assignments by the deadline. He was diagnosed with "mild" Attention-deficit/ hyperactivity disorder (ADHD) and dyslexia at 9 years of age. Medication was never prescribed. Until this year, he has earned Bs and Cs while playing sports and receiving Individualized Education Program (IEP) services, including reading intervention. No substance use, depression, or anxiety is suspected. The high school recommends a full neuropsychological evaluation, but the family does not understand why he needs more testing.

Background

To understand the neuropsychological evaluation process of ADHD, specifically in teenagers, we first need to appreciate what a neuropsychological evaluation will— and will not—clarify. Most neuropsychological evaluations include several components: a comprehensive history of the teen (usually provided by the primary caregiver), behavioral observations, performance-based measures, standardized questionnaires (parent-, teacher-, and/or self-report), and individualized recommendations. The process of gathering a comprehensive history is reviewed in a previous chapter. The remaining components (performance-based measures, standardized questionnaires, behavioral observations, and individualized recommendations) are described below, as are the ways in which the information yielded contributes to the conceptualization of the adolescent, including whether or not they present with ADHD.

Performance-Based Measures

Performance-based measures are tests administered to a child and scored based on the responses. Results from these tests are typically interpreted in comparison to other individuals in the same age range as the test taker, resulting in standardized/norm-referenced scores that take a variety of forms. While there are numerous measures to assess these areas across the lifespan, some of the common tests used in pediatric and adolescent practice will be described so that a neuropsychological evaluation report is more accessible to every reader. Each assessment measure is listed within a specific domain below, though many of these measures yield information that spans various domains. Similarly, the specific domains reviewed below are not exhaustive, nor are they included in every neuropsychological evaluation.

Performing complex tasks—whether in school, in life, in relationships, or at work—requires a person to utilize many different skills at the same time. Imagine entering a biology class for a pop quiz. Here are some of the skills needed to earn a passing grade:

- Notice (see, hear) the social environment of quiet and independent work
- Attend to the directions (spoken and written)
- Move to the right location, put away backpack/books (gross motor skills)
- Use accurate and paced fine motor skills to provide answers in the time allotted
- Read the questions and look at the diagrams in the questions
- Relate the written questions to diagrams, pictures, and other visuals provided
- Recall previously learned information and apply this information to the (new) scenario of the question
- Maintain pace, move from one question to the next, and follow the expected sequence

All of this is expected to happen in smooth coordination! And when one of these skills is weak, like a weak link in the chain, the rest of the chinks depending on it can't function as well. Understanding the strengths and weaknesses of an individual's processing, in order to clarify their current function and determine how to best support success, becomes the ultimate objective of neuropsychological testing.

The goal of neuropsychological assessment is therefore to create a cognitive profile comprised of many areas of functioning, including, but not limited to:

- General intelligence
- Attention
- Executive functions
- Learning and memory
- Fine motor skills
- Language skills
- Visual-perceptual and complex motor abilities
- Academic achievement

Intellectual Functioning

Overall intellectual functioning is assessed by the administration of several subtests that are thought to measure core cognitive abilities (e.g., verbal comprehension, visual spatial, and fluid reasoning skills) as well as areas of cognitive proficiency (e.g., processing speed and working memory). Together, these subtests yield an overall intellectual functioning score, commonly referred to as a child's "IQ." This composite score often gives at least some insight into a child's capabilities and may serve as a comparison when examining other areas of functioning (e.g., adaptive and academic functioning). Table 6.1 lists several measures commonly used to assess intelligence in teenagers.

The descriptions below provide in-depth and sometimes technical information. It is geared for clinicians, who may not have already had focused training on child and adolescent assessment. Parents and teachers may prefer to focus on boxed tips, search this section to understand how *specific domains* are assessed, or *find a specific test* to better understand its function.

For Clinicians

Attention

Attention is a complex construct with no universal operationalization. Neuropsychological assessment can examine many aspects of attention, such as immediate/brief attention, sustained attention or vigilance, selective or focused attention, and divided attention, with tasks that involve auditory and/or visual stimuli.

- *Immediate/brief attention* is often measured using span tests, which expose an individual to increasing amounts of auditory or visual information; after each exposure, the test taker repeats the information auditorily or motorically. Such information may come in the form of strings of digits (e.g., WISC-V and WAIS-IV *Digit Span: Forward*) or visual sequences (WISC-V *Integrated Spatial Span: Forward* [12]; *Wide Range Assessment of Memory and Learning, Second Edition [WRAML2] Finger Windows* [13]).

Table 6.1 Common measures to assess intelligence in teenagers

Common measures to assess intelligence in teenagers
Differential Ability Scales, Second Edition (DAS-II [7])
Wechsler Intelligence Scale for Children, Fifth Edition (WISC-V [8])
Wechsler Adult Intelligence Scale, Fourth Edition (WAIS-IV [9])
Stanford-Binet Intelligence Scales, Fifth Edition (SB-5 [10])
Woodcock-Johnson Tests of Cognitive Abilities, Fourth Edition (WJ IV COG [11])

- *Sustained attention or vigilance* is essentially the ability to remain on task for a prolonged duration while demonstrating readiness to respond (e.g., remaining focused on a teacher's voice while listening for the next instruction). *Selective attention* is associated with distractibility and requires someone to focus on relevant stimuli (i.e., targets) and filter out or ignore distractors. Vigilance tasks also require selective attention given that a target stimulus occurs infrequently. One common method of standardized assessment of these constructs in youth is through a continuous performance test, such as the *Conners Continuous Performance Test, Third Edition (Conners CPT-3* [14]*), the Conners Continuous Auditory Test of Attention (Conners CATA* [15]*)*, and the *Test of Variables of Attention* (T.O.V.A. [16]). Such tasks provide a continuous string of briefly presented (auditory or visual) stimuli, and the test taker is instructed to respond only to a target stimulus (e.g., low tone, the letter "Y"). Additional tests of sustained auditory attention include the *Auditory Attention* task from *A Developmental Neuropsychological Assessment, Second Edition (NEPSY-II* [17]), in which an individual responds every time "blue" is spoken during a string of words, and *Score! on the Test of Everyday Attention for Children (TEA-Ch* [18]), which requires silent counting of "scoring sounds" over several trials. *Cancellation tasks* (e.g., *Cancellation on the WISC-V and WAIS-IV, Map Mission and Sky Search on the TEA-Ch*) can tap visual sustained and selective attention in that a test taker is required to search for and cross out a target that is embedded among distractor stimuli.
- *Divided attention* refers to the ability to attend to two concurrent stimuli or activities simultaneously and allows us to multitask (e.g., listen to a class lecture while taking notes). The *TEA-Ch* includes tests that assess divided and sustained attention: *Score DT and Sky Search DT*; each test requires the simultaneous completion of two different tasks (e.g., count sounds while searching for and circling a visual target).

Executive Functions

Executive functions are a set of mental processes that are required for goal-directed behavior and task completion. These skills include planning and organization, focusing and directing our attention, controlling impulses and emotional responses, and successfully managing multiple tasks. The operationalization of executive functioning is continuing to evolve, and multiple models exist to define and outline specific domains. Common areas of functioning assessed by neuropsychological tests will be reviewed, including working memory, response inhibition, set-shifting/cognitive flexibility, planning/organization, and novel problem-solving.

Working memory is thought of as the capability to hold and manipulate information over a short time period or hold information while focusing on other information. Span tests can be used to assess this domain, but unlike the repetition mentioned when describing brief attention, an examinee is required to manipulate the information by providing the auditory (e.g., *WISC-V Digit Span: Backward and Sequencing*) and visual (e.g., *WISC-V Integrated Spatial Span: Backward*) information in a different order than initially presented by the examiner (e.g., backward,

> There are many types of "attention." Different tests used by neuropsychologists test different types of attention. For example:
>
> - *Immediate attention* is required for a student to listen to teacher directions.
> - *Sustained attention* contributes to a student's ability to stay focused on the teacher's voice and listen for the next instruction.
> - *Divided attention* is required to concurrently take a quiz and attend to teacher's reminders.

ascending order). The *WAIS-IV* includes a working memory test requiring the examinee to complete arithmetic problems without pencil and paper (i.e., mental math) and within a time limit (arithmetic), thus tapping the individual's ability to hold and manipulate information efficiently.

Response inhibition is the ability to control impulses or stop and think before acting. Impulsivity can be measured as commission errors, or response to a nontarget, in the *continuous performance tasks* described above or in the second test condition of the T.O.V.A. In the latter, the individual expects to respond to the majority of targets—as in the first condition—but will need to inhibit the tendency to respond much more often, as the target to nontarget ratio switches. A common measure of inhibition in youth is the third condition of the *Color-Word Interference Test from the Delis-Kaplan Executive Function System (D-KEFS* [19]), a traditional *Stroop task*. A Stroop task presents a participant with color words (e.g., red, blue) that are printed in a different colored ink (e.g., the word "red" printed in green ink). The individual is asked to say the ink color as quickly as possible, thus requiring them to inhibit the brain's natural response to read the word. Difficulties with inhibition can be reflected in response speed and/or error rate. *The inhibition task* on the *NEPSY-II* is also a timed subtest assessing ability to inhibit automatic in favor of novel responses; this task utilizes shapes and arrow direction rather than colors.

Cognitive/mental flexibility refers to the ability to change or revise problem-solving approaches or plans when conditions change. In standardized testing, it refers to the ability to alternate one's attention between two tasks or sets of rules. These set-shifting tasks also require directing attention and maintaining a sequence in working memory. The *Number-Letter Sequencing* condition on the *D-KEFS Trail Making Test* is a pen-and-paper task that involves alternately connecting a sequencing of numbers and letters (e.g., 1-A-2-B). Verbal switching is assessed through the *Category Switching* condition of the *D-KEFS Verbal Fluency Test*, where an individual alternates between (orally) generating a word from two different categories. The *TEA-Ch* also includes *set-shifting tasks*, such as *Creature Counting*, which involves counting "creatures"; when a child reaches an arrow, it cues them to switch the direction in which they were counting.

Novel problem-solving represents a higher-order skill that requires the simultaneous use of multiple basic executive functions. *Tower of London (TOL* [20]*)* and the *D-KEFS Tower Test* require a test taker to plan ahead in order to move rings, balls, or discs to a predetermined position while adhering to rules (e.g., one piece moved at a time, larger piece cannot go on top of smaller piece). In addition to planning, this requires self-monitoring, inhibiting immediate responses or the urge to break rules, directing and sustaining attention, and keeping prior series of completed moves in mind while completing the task. Another popular novel problem-solving measure is the *Wisconsin Card Sorting Test (WCST* [21]*)*. Examinees are provided with one stimulus card at a time, and they must match the card to one of four possible cards that remain displayed throughout the task. There are multiple ways to classify or match each card, and the only feedback provided to the participant is whether the match is correct or incorrect (thus assessing how well the individual can shift a cognitive strategy in response to feedback). In addition to assessing *problem-solving* and *set-shifting*, the WCST requires *working memory* and aspects of *regulating attention*.

There is no standardized measure that attempts to isolate the skills of *planning and organization*, but there are several neuropsychological tests that allow for quantitative and qualitative assessment of these areas of executive functioning. Learning and memory measures provide an opportunity to assess organization by observing how an individual encodes and recalls information. For example, organized approaches are seen when an individual clusters words into categories when recalling word lists (as opposed to in serial order), recalls stories in sequential order (as opposed to seemingly random ordering of details), and identifies the underlying shapes when copying a geometric form (e.g., as opposed to a part-oriented/piece-meal approach). Organization can also be evaluated during cancellation tasks (e.g., top to bottom vs. random search strategy).

Processing Speed

Processing speed is assessed using measures of response speed, which require the test taker to complete tasks quickly and accurately. Several constructs may be examined through these tasks, including how quickly an individual can visually scan,

---

Executive functions contribute to task completion. For example:

- *Working memory* is required for algebra II: a student must recall and apply math facts in order to solve equations.
- *Response inhibition* is called for during group projects, when a student has to stop themselves from jumping in and instead wait for others to reply.
- *Planning/organization* is required when completing long-term projects by the deadline; a student must determine what materials are required, what steps need to be completed in what order, and how long each step will take.

sequence, copy, transcribe, name, or discriminate information (*Symbol Search and Coding from the WISC-V and WAIS-IV; D-KEFS Trail Making Test: Visual Scanning, Number Sequencing, Letter Sequencing, and Motor Speed; D-KEFS Color-Word Interference Test: Color Naming and Word Reading*). As it is challenging to assess processing speed and efficiency in isolation, without tapping into other areas of functioning, it is important for a neuropsychologist to remain cognizant of other factors involved in measures of processing speed when interpreting testing results. For example, youth with fine motor weaknesses may struggle on tasks with such requirements (e.g., *Coding*). Similarly, deficits in rapid naming have been associated with reading and word retrieval difficulties.

Language

While not nearly as in-depth as the information yielded from a comprehensive speech and language evaluation, neuropsychological assessment often includes the measurement of various aspects of language. Such assessment may be split into expressive (i.e., the ability to communicate using spoken language) and receptive (i.e., the ability to understand spoken language) language domains; each of these areas is measured at multiple levels (Table 6.2).

Table 6.2 Neuropsychological measures assessing language

Skill area assessed	Assessment measure(s)
Expressive language	
Confrontation naming ability	*Boston Naming Test [BNT]* [22]
Single-word naming	*Expressive Vocabulary Test, Third Edition [EVT-3]* [23] *Expressive One-Word Picture Vocabulary Test, Fourth Edition [EOWPVT-4]* [24]
Ability to orally define words	*WISC-V and WAIS-IV Vocabulary*
Repetition of orally presented information	*WRAML2 Sentence Repetition*
Verbal fluency	*D-KEFS Verbal Fluency; NEPSY-II Word Generation*
Receptive language	
Single-word receptive vocabulary	*Peabody Picture Vocabulary Test, Fifth Edition [PPVT-5]* [25]; *Receptive One-Word Picture Vocabulary Test, Fourth Edition [ROWPVT-4]* [26]
Ability to comprehend orally presented instructions/stories	*NEPSY-II Comprehension of Instructions; Wechsler Individual Achievement Test, Third Edition [WIAT-III]* [27] *Oral Discourse Comprehension*

Learning and Memory

Memory is not a single process, but a multistage faculty (e.g., encoding, storage, retrieval) that is associated with other cognitive skills such as attention and working memory; this section will focus on tests requiring *new learning and long-term retrieval*. Neuropsychological assessment of a teenager's ability to encode and retrieve novel information generally includes measures involving verbal and visual stimuli. Learning and memory measures also vary depending on the nature of the information that is presented; for example, stimuli may be rote, contextual, or abstract. On some tests, the learning phase includes several exposures to stimuli, which can provide information as to whether the adolescent's encoding of novel information benefits from repetition; other measures involve exposure to new information during a single trial. After an adolescent is exposed to auditory and/or visual information, immediate recall is assessed. Some measures include an interference trial prior to immediate recall or a single exposure to similar information (e.g., a different list of words), which allows for the assessment of proactive interference (i.e., when previously learned information hinders the learning of new information). Following a time period of approximately 20–30 min, the participant is asked to produce the information freely (i.e., delayed recall) and/or in the context of cues or multiple-choice or yes/no format (i.e., recognition).

There are several assessment measures that include multiple measures of *verbal and nonverbal memory*, as well as stand-alone assessments (Table 6.3).

Table 6.3 Neuropsychological measures of verbal and nonverbal memory

Skill area assessed	Assessment measure(s)
Learning and memory of simple verbal information (generally presented in word lists)	*California Verbal Learning Test, Children's Version (CVLT-C* [30]*); California Verbal Learning Test, Third Edition (CVLT-3* [19]*); WRAML2 Verbal Learning and Child and Adolescent Memory Profile (ChAMP* [29]*) Lists*
Learning and memory of contextual verbal information (often provided in the form of stories)	*WRAML2 Story Memory Children's Memory Scale (CMS* [28] *Stories*
Visual learning and memory involving	
Spatial location	*CMS Dots*
Visual content and spatial location	*NEPSY-II Memory for Designs*
Geometric images	*Rey Complex Figure Test and Recognition Trial* [31]*, WRAML2 Design Memory*
Faces	*CMS Faces, NEPSY-II Memory for Faces*
Information presented with context, such as scenes	*CMS: Family Pictures, WRAML2: Picture Memory, ChAMP: Places*

You may see neuropsychological testing assess for processing speed, language, learning, and memory.

- Processing speed is hard to assess, because one's response rate is impacted by a variety of factors, such as fine motor skills.
- Language measures are often included in neuropsychological testing but may be less comprehensive than findings of a full speech and language evaluation.
- Memory requires us to put information into our brains, leave it there, and pull it out when we need it (encoding, storage, retrieval). To assess memory, neuropsychological testing can include content that is taught—either verbally or visually—and then requested 20–30 min later.

Visual, Fine Motor, and Visual-Motor Integration

Neuropsychological assessment of visually based skills may include measures involving visual closure and matching, perception of spatial orientation, figure-ground discrimination, mental rotation, pattern recognition and completion, and visual-motor construction. Some of these constructs are assessed through subtests included in the evaluation of core cognitive abilities (e.g., *Block Design, Visual Puzzles*) and others through stand-alone measures. For example, the *Judgment of Line Orientation Test (JLOT* [32]*)* requires an individual to match the angle and orientation of lines by choosing two matched lines from an array, thus assessing visual-spatial perceptual ability. Utilizing arrows instead of lines, the *NEPSY-II Arrows* task also assesses this area of functioning.

The *Berry-Buktenica Test of Visual-Motor Integration, Sixth Edition (VMI-6* [33]*)* is a screening measure for visual-perceptual and motor abilities, as well as the integration of the two. Each component of the VMI-6 is in paper-pencil form. The *Visual Perception portion of the VMI-6* requires the teen to identify a target from a series of shapes that differ slightly by size or orientation or that have a small component missing. The *VMI-6 Motor Coordination* task attempts to isolate the individual's fine motor control, requiring them to carefully trace the interior of increasingly complex and narrow shapes while remaining within boundary lines. Symbol substitution tests (e.g., *Coding*) act as a measure of graphomotor speed, as the individual is required to quickly transcribe symbols. Fine motor speed and coordination can be assessed through pegboard tasks, in which an individual must place pegs into a board as quickly as possible (e.g., *Grooved Pegboard, Purdue Pegboard*). The integration of motor ability with visual and perceptual skills is often assessed through measures that involve copying shapes (e.g., *VMI-6 Visual-Motor Integration, RCFT Copy trial*).

Academic Achievement

While a neuropsychological assessment often does not include a comprehensive examination of academic skills, administering a screening (at minimum) of core academic abilities is often included. For younger or lower functioning youth, this may involve assessing academics at the skill level (e.g., single-word reading, math calculation, spelling), and for adolescents, it is important to understand their ability to apply these skills (e.g., reading comprehension, math problem-solving, written expression). Fortunately, numerous assessment tools are available that measure achievement across domains, including the *Woodcock-Johnson Tests of Achievement, Fourth Edition (WJ-ACH-IV* [34]); *Wechsler Individual Achievement Test, Third Edition (WIAT-III* [27]); and *Kaufman Test of Educational Achievement, Third Edition (KTEA-3* [35]). Others are designed to specifically focus on one academic skill or domain, such as the *Gray Oral Reading Tests, Fifth Edition (GORT-5* [36]); *Nelson-Denny Reading Test (NDRT* [37]); and *KeyMath Diagnostic Assessment, Third Edition (KeyMath-3 DA* [38]). Across most academic testing measures, the test taker's performance can usually be calculated using age- or grade-based norms, the latter of which may be utilized if an individual has been retained, for example.

Effort

Neuropsychological assessment often includes embedded or stand-alone measures of effort (i.e., *performance validity tests*) to ensure that the test taker's performance is valid [39]. "Effort" does not only mean "*How hard did you try?*" Instead, "effort" refers to the test taker's approach to the tasks offered: how persistent were they? How did they respond to failure? How compliant were they? Measures of effort (aka performance validity tests) determine whether the test taker's approach, such as reduced effort or engagement, impacts how valid the results are. Individuals with ADHD can present as inconsistently motivated or engaged and are sometimes viewed as "lazy" or "unmotivated." Performance validity tests provide objective information about how one's approach to a test impacts the results. This can be very helpful considering that, at times, we see feigned poor performance on testing or overreported symptoms on rating scales. These actions are often motivated by individuals seeking an ADHD diagnosis, in order to access stimulant medication or academic accommodations (e.g., extended time for SATs).

How does neuropsychological testing help figure out who "really has" ADHD from those "faking it?" Look for a validity statement in the report, indicating the evaluator's indication of whether the findings are a valid estimation of the tester's profile.

Comments About Performance-Based Measures and the Adolescent with ADHD

Neuropsychological deficits may vary as a function of chronological and developmental/mental age, and there is no exact cognitive profile for adolescents with ADHD, though literature provides evidence for various areas of weakness. For example, differences in performance (in the expected direction) between youth with and without ADHD have been shown for sustained attention and vigilance, selective attention, and divided attention [40–43]. Similarly, between-group differences have been demonstrated across areas of executive functioning, including working memory, cognitive flexibility, response inhibition, planning, processing speed, and novel problem-solving [44–48]. Importantly, despite studies indicating weaknesses on measures of attention and executive functioning for youth with ADHD, these findings and tests do not offer the sensitivity or specificity to adequately/consistently classify individuals with and without ADHD [48].

> PARENTS: In other words, no single test or combination of tests definitively indicates that a person has—or doesn't have—ADHD. Testing is not *required* to diagnose ADHD, nor are all individuals with ADHD going to perform poorly on tests of attention or executive function.

Scores on neuropsychological measures don't differentiate ADHD subtypes from one another. Classification of an individual subtype/presentation seems fairly straightforward when utilizing standardized report questionnaires, with many funneling individual item responses into composite scores or symptom counts, capturing inattention and hyperactivity/impulsivity as well as specific areas of executive dysfunction. In contrast, these presentations—and ADHD criteria in general—do not neatly emerge from the cognitive profiles yielded by neuropsychological testing. This is in part due to the neuropsychological heterogeneity of ADHD [49, 50]. For instance, some literature outlines group differences in processing speed deficits in the inattentive (but not combined) presentation [46], and there is research suggesting that individuals with ADHD, predominantly inattentive presentation, may have more diffuse cognitive deficits relative to individuals with combined or hyperactive/impulsive presentations [51]. Additionally, executive dysfunction is a prominent feature of ADHD, but not all children and youth who meet ADHD diagnostic criteria demonstrate these deficits [48, 50, 52]. Only about 30% of youth with an ADHD diagnosis have significant executive function impairment on neuropsychological testing [53]. Meaning, we are not surprised to find diffuse cognitive deficits in a child with ADHD, predominantly inattentive presentation, or executive dysfunction in any teen with ADHD, but there are those with ADHD who have no cognitive or executive function deficits on formal testing.

Many children appear relatively unimpaired in the context of standardized testing in a structured one-to-one setting with few distractions.

Parents often ask if the findings on neuropsychological testing correlate to classroom function; just because a student "can do it" in the 1:1 testing environment without any distractions, "doing it" in class may be another story. Ecological validity is a measure of how test performance predicts behavior in real-world settings. A long-standing theme in the neuropsychological testing of ADHD is the ecological validity (or lack thereof) of assessment measures, chiefly seen on performance-based measures of attention and executive functioning. Many norm-referenced neuropsychological measures have only moderate ecological validity [54], including tests assessing domains perhaps most relevant to a diagnosis of ADHD [55]. Additionally, each measure is relatively short in duration as compared to tasks in daily life requiring sustained focus and executive functioning.

As such, clinic-based test performance can provide a useful albeit incomplete assessment of executive functions [56–58]. Standardized questionnaires are a valuable compliment to performance-based measures by providing informant and self-report of day-to-day functioning.

Self-, Parent-, and Teacher-Report Questionnaires

Standardized questionnaires are norm-referenced and compare ratings to other individuals of the same age and, sometimes, gender. These checklists and rating scales are usually designed for multiple raters, including caregivers, teachers, and the adolescent being assessed (Table 6.4). The individual completing the questionnaire reads each item and rates the statement using a Likert scale based on how often or how true the statement is (e.g., 0, not true; 1, sometimes or somewhat true; and 2, very true or often true). A specific time period is generally suggested by each questionnaire when completing the ratings (e.g., within the past 6 months). Standardized score ranges are classified based on severity (e.g., clinically significant, at-risk, average). Raw scores do not typically translate into clinically significant standardized scores, but a response pattern can be informative. For example, while an entire scale may not be clinically elevated, the examination of the items that were endorsed at a high frequency within that scale may provide some insight into the teen's experience or presentation.

There are broad-based questionnaires aimed to assess multiple areas of social, emotional, and behavioral functioning, as well as scales designed to measure specific sets of symptoms or diagnostic presentations (Table 6.4).

Table 6.4 Commonly used self-, parent-, and teacher questionnaires

Domain assessed	Standardized questionnaires
Multiple areas of social, emotional, and behavioral functioning	Behavior Assessment System for Children, Third Edition (BASC-3 [59]) Achenbach System of Empirically Based Assessment (ASEBA [60]) Conners, Third Edition (Conners3 [68]) Disruptive Behavior Disorder (DBD) Rating Scale [66]
Anxiety/depression	Revised Children's Anxiety and Depression Scale (RCADS [61]) Multidimensional Anxiety Scale for Children, Second Edition (MASC-2 [62]) Beck Depression Inventory, Second Edition (BDI-II [63])
ADHD (including symptom count)	Vanderbilt ADHD Rating Scales (VARS [64, 65]) ADHD Rating Scale-5 for Children and Adolescents [67] Conners, Third Edition (Conners3 [68]) Disruptive Behavior Disorder (DBD) Rating Scale [66]
Executive functioning	Behavior Rating Inventory Function, Second Edition (BRIEF2 [69])
Adaptive functioning (independence in daily living skills)	Adaptive Behavior Assessment System, Third Edition (ABAS-3 [70]) Vineland Adaptive Behavior Scales, Third Edition (Vincland-3 [71])

Self-, Parent-, and Teacher-Report: ADHD-Specific Questionnaires

Reviewed in previous chapters, many of the same questionnaires used to gather data for diagnosis in the outpatient clinician setting are used in neuropsychological assessment.

A neuropsychological assessment office is clearly not an environment representative of an adolescent's daily life at home or at school. Similarly, the performance-based measures used to assess attention and executive functions are a poor reflection of how those skills are expressed in everyday tasks. For example, working memory may be gauged by comparing the ability to repeat strings of digits in backward order during standardized testing, while day-to-day indications of working memory dysfunction could be seen in difficulty completing multistep directions or forgetting task directions. Further, the risk-taking activities that illustrate impulsivity in adolescents certainly do not equate to inhibiting the urge to read a word and, instead, name the ink color. As such, while the quantitative and qualitative data gathered during an evaluation are beneficial in diagnostic conceptualization and treatment planning, questionnaires provide an efficient and developmentally referenced assessment of social, emotional, and behavioral functioning outside of the testing environment. This is useful not only in collecting evidence for diagnostic criteria specific to ADHD but also in determining factors that may be accounting for apparent ADHD symptoms (e.g., anxiety) and assessing functional impairment. Further, in addition to their utility in the initial diagnostic process, rating scales can be used as measures of treatment response.

> ADHD-specific questionnaires can be helpful in capturing symptoms in daily life for initial diagnosis as well as evaluating response to treatment (e.g., fewer symptoms following a few months of therapy).

Most questionnaires have versions for parents/caregivers, teachers, and the adolescent themself, which is in line with general recommendations to maximize diagnostic information by gathering data from multiple sources [72, 73]. It is important to get each perspective on an individual's functioning, especially as an ADHD diagnosis requires the presence of several symptoms across settings as well as evidence of impairment. While there is evidence that standardized ratings scales are sensitive to the presence of ADHD in adolescence [74–76], they are not without limitations.

How can subjective ratings by teachers and parents be accurate? Sometimes, they are not. Ratings scales are subject to reporting bias and levels of agreement between raters and across settings are often low [77, 78]. A classroom environment is logically an ideal setting to look for ADHD symptoms, given requirements to inhibit responses (e.g., not speak in class) and sustain auditory (e.g., lectures) and visual (e.g., reading) attention, but it is not always realistic to ask a teacher to rate such symptoms due to large class sizes, varying experience and tolerance, and given that instructors may spend under an hour with a student. As such, it is not surprising that agreement among high school teachers is variable and often poor [79, 80] and parent-teacher discrepancies on ratings scales are high [81, 82]. Unfortunately, adolescents tend to demonstrate poor insight into the presence and severity of their symptom presentation on self-report rating scales [83, 84], and the accuracy of both parents and adolescents is questionable when providing retrospective accounts of behavior [85]. In addition to variable agreement across raters, the DSM-5 symptoms of ADHD are arguably more prominent in younger children; as such, some behavior checklists may not be sensitive to the clinical presentation of ADHD in adolescence. In fact, some argue that the symptom threshold should be less strict when diagnosing ADHD for the first time during adolescence [86].

Clinical Interview and Record Review

As you know from previous chapters, neuropsychological testing is one method for diagnosing ADHD. A comprehensive interview and record review accompany the testing. Knowledge of the components examined through neuropsychological testing should inform any diagnostic interview of an adolescent with a question of

ADHD. In reviewing school history, ask about grade retention, special education services, and presence or history of learning difficulties. Listen for problems that point to specific areas of executive dysfunction. Reviewing previous records (e.g., report cards, developmental evaluations, pediatrician notes) along with conducting a clinical interview with the adolescent can provide evidence of slow processing speed, impaired working memory, inhibition, cognitive rigidity, problems with sustaining or dividing attention, language deficits, and poor fine motor skills. Gathering a developmental history in adolescents with undiagnosed ADHD often reveals long-standing patterns of emotional-behavioral concerns, failed friendships, and variable or poor academic performance [87–89]. Again, ask for the details. Ask about functional impairment as well; for adolescents this typically means school performance that may have declined following the transition to high school, often due to the impact of the executive dysfunction commonly seen in ADHD (e.g., working memory ability is highly related to academic achievement [90]). Further, including an interview with the teenager being assessed is especially important when considering impairment; while adolescents may not be valid reporters of their ADHD symptoms, they are often the best source of information relating to negative social behavior [91]. Interviewing the teen also provides information about their level of insight, which will be relevant to intervention.

Many disorders of childhood and adolescence present with apparent symptoms of ADHD. Moreover, ADHD co-occurs with many medical and psychiatric conditions. As such, gathering background information around the adolescent's history of academic achievement and emotional-behavioral functioning helps to consider coexisting diagnoses and differentiate ADHD from other causes of functional impairment. If an adolescent presents with the report of clinically significant symptoms of inattention, and/or hyperactivity/impulsivity, it must be determined if these features manifested earlier in childhood. For example, the late onset of ADHD symptoms may correspond with a psychosocial stressor or traumatic event or a learning disorder emerging in the context of increased academic demands. Alternatively, characteristics associated with ADHD may reflect other psychopathology or be better accounted for by a different neurodevelopmental disorder.

Emotional-behavioral dysregulation is a common component of the clinical presentation of ADHD [92]; however, it is also observed in separate conditions, as reflected in the high co-occurrence rates of ADHD and oppositional defiant disorder and conduct disorder [93]. Internalizing disorders involving symptoms of anxiety or depression are also highly comorbid with ADHD [89, 94] but can also be the underlying cause of apparent ADHD symptoms (e.g., restlessness due to anxiety, depression resulting in poor focus and motivation). Several of the broad-based screening tools above identify risk for these comorbidities.

ADHD commonly co-occurs in other neurodevelopmental disorders, such as autism spectrum disorder, intellectual disability, and specific learning disorders. ADHD is present in 30–80% of ASD cases [95, 96].

While most individuals with ASD have attentional difficulties, a neuropsychological evaluation helps to determine if symptoms are independently causing significant functional impairment, warranting separate consideration of a co-occurring ADHD along with treatment. ADHD symptoms must be maladaptive, but they also must be inconsistent with the child's developmental level.

Intellectual disability is often accompanied by ADHD [97, 98], but symptoms must be excessive for mental/developmental age. For example, if a 14-year-old has an intellectual age equivalent of a 7-year-old, the attention and behavioral self-control deficits must be immature for a 7-year-old. The measures of intelligence and adaptive functioning that are completed in neuropsychological evaluations allow for standardized assessment of developmental level or mental age. Academic problems are frequently described in youth with ADHD and sometimes accounted for by a separate specific learning disorder [99].

It is also important to rule out a medical cause of ADHD symptomatology, such as traumatic brain injury, substance use, seizures, hypothyroidism, or sleep disturbance, further highlighting the importance of gathering a comprehensive developmental and medical history (see Chap. 2). For example, a recent change in attention and executive functioning could be observed in an adolescent who recently sustained a concussion [100], but they may not otherwise have a significant history of ADHD symptoms. Drug use, which becomes increasingly relevant as youth age, can also result in cognitive and behavioral issues that mimic an underlying neurodevelopmental disorder [101]. ADHD symptomatology and diagnosis also are common in many types of epilepsy [102], and youth with epilepsy are particularly at risk for symptoms associated with ADHD, predominantly inattentive presentation [103]. Another area that is particularly important to assess is sleep. Chronic sleep issues can be difficult to distinguish from ADHD as both are associated with poor focus, mood swings, and hyperactivity. If a teen has experienced chronic sleep issues and has not received proper treatment, it may not be appropriate to diagnose ADHD, even if the symptoms criteria appear to be met. For example, shorter sleep duration is associated with increased teacher-report ratings of ADHD symptoms in healthy and typically developing children [104]. Additionally, several studies indicate inattention, planning issues, and restlessness in patients with obstructive sleep apnea (OSA) [105], and OSA treatment is associated with a reduction—and, sometimes, a disappearance—in ADHD symptoms [106].

Behavioral Observations

Another critical component of a neuropsychological evaluation includes the behavioral observations, which offer qualitative observations of the individual being assessed. Qualitative observations are arguably just as (if not more) valuable as standardized scores. Any clinician diagnosing ADHD should include behavioral observations as essential pieces of information. While ADHD symptoms are not necessarily as overt in the structured clinical setting as they may be in larger settings or with peers, especially in adolescent populations, many test takers show signs of hyperactivity/impulsivity (e.g., interrupting, fidgeting, attempting to start tasks before completion of directions, reaching for object from examiner's hand, quickly responding followed by self-correction) and inattention (e.g., missing prompts, easily distracted by hallway noise and own thoughts, inconsistent pattern of correct and incorrect responses on items of similar difficulty, looking away from visual stimuli, careless errors). These behavioral observations can provide useful information when considering day-to-day functioning. For instance, if a test taker is having trouble attending to directions in a one-on-one structured setting, it is likely that it is even more difficult for that individual to attend to longer durations of spoken language in more distracting environments, such as a classroom.

Testing anxiety can present similarly to ADHD symptoms. One possible distinction between the two causes comes from changes in inattention and hyperactivity/ impulsivity over relatively short periods of time. Given that neuropsychological testing tends to last several hours, individuals with ADHD often show increasing symptoms over the course of the evaluation. In contrast, if an examinee is initially anxious, behavior that looks like ADHD can decline as the test taker becomes more comfortable.

Attention, activity level, and impulse control are just some of the behavior observations noted during a neuropsychological evaluation. Additional areas observed include mood/affect, general appearance (e.g., grooming, dress), and functional hearing and vision. Gross motor functioning is assessed informally based on the examinee's ability to ambulate independently and gait quality (e.g., balance, posture). Handedness is noted as well as lateral dominance on tasks; informal assessment of fine motor functioning may also look for a tremor, pencil grasp, and general control when manipulating small objects and completing pencil-and-paper tasks.

Speech is assessed for qualities such as rate, volume, and intonation. It is noted if expressive language is largely comprised of single words, multiword phrases, or full, complex sentences and if spoken language is logical, coherent, and organized. Comprehension of spoken language is gauged in the context of informal exchanges and an examinee's ability to understand task directions (e.g., required repetition or simplification of task directions, inconsistently provided contingent responses to questions during conversation). It is noted if any modifications are required to understand test demands, such as repetition of directions, use of visual aids, and additional sample/demonstration items, when standardization procedures allow. Pragmatic language and social interaction skills are assessed by observations of the adolescent's ability to modulate eye contact, participate in back-and-forth conversation, coordinate verbal and nonverbal communication, and appropriately respond to the examiner (e.g., returns social smiles).

Recommendations

Regardless of diagnostic outcome, a neuropsychological evaluation yields recommendations specific to the individual. Such recommendations are based on information obtained throughout the evaluation, including the teen's cognitive and academic profile, social/emotional/behavioral functioning, developmental history, medical history, and diagnostic presentation. Often, recommendations are made for school and home environments and include suggested accommodations and/or interventions. In addition, recommendations are provided that highlight the individual's strengths and the ways in which these strengths can be used to support areas of struggle. While a neuropsychological evaluation produces recommendations spanning psychiatric, neurodevelopmental, and medical disorders, the examples provided below will focus on areas most relevant to youth with ADHD.

A common school-based recommendation is the provision of classroom support and/or special education services through a Section 504 Plan or Individualized Education Program (IEP) (Table 6.5). These documents provide a blueprint for services, modifications to the learning environment, and/or special education and related services. The level of support and whether the teenager requires individualized services depends on the degree of impairment caused by their ADHD symptoms. The utility of these recommendations varies based on several factors, such as level of cognitive functioning, the presence of co-occurring disorders, and the ADHD symptom profile (i.e., inattentive, hyperactive/impulsive, or combined presentation).

Depending on the teenager's level of difficulty with task initiation, specific interventions can target areas of weakness (Table 6.6). Those with trouble in working

Table 6.5 Examples of common recommendations for classroom-based supports

Examples of common recommendations for classroom-based supports
Preferential seating
Testing in a distraction-free environment
Regular breaks
Teacher checks for understanding

Table 6.6 Examples of recommendations for those with difficulty with task initiation

Examples of recommendations for those with difficulty with task initiation
External prompting
Working in small groups
Providing assistance with the initial step of a task or assignment

memory and attending classroom lectures may require access to notes or note outlines, particularly as note taking demands increase as the teenager moves through school. Without this type of accommodation, teenagers with ADHD and accompanying difficulties with working memory and organization often find themselves with incomplete or inaccurate notes, interfering with the ability to study for tests or complete assignments. In college, students with ADHD sometimes seek permission to record class lectures, so that they are able to review information on their own time.

Having the teenager attend a structured study hall, where they have access to academic and organizational support, is sometimes beneficial, particularly as individuals with ADHD often fail to use unstructured time effectively. Such executive function "coaching" could include teaching approaches for breaking down tasks into smaller units, improving study habits, building note taking strategies, and effectively using a (daily/weekly/monthly) planner. Teenagers with ADHD also may require check-ins with teachers/counselors to ensure the accurate recording of academic assignments and that they have the materials required to complete these assignments. Of course, the goal should always be to promote independence, but habits and systems that set the student up for success must first be established, which initially requires assistance (i.e., scaffolding). Again, information obtained through a neuropsychological evaluation can help inform intervention targets and level of need.

The implementation of a behavioral intervention within the classroom that targets specific areas of impairment (e.g., work completion, accuracy, and organization) may also be recommended. While the neuropsychologist does not typically assist in the creation and implementation of a behavioral intervention, recommendations provided by the neuropsychologist can help to identify intervention targets. For example, if a neuropsychologist learned that a teenager completes and returns their work in math class but that they lose points for mistakes, accuracy may be an appropriate target of intervention.

Behavioral intervention in the home also is often recommended to families of teens with ADHD. Like at school, specific intervention targets are identified based on areas of impairment or problems reported by the parent or teen (e.g., chore and homework completion, complying with household rules). As other chapters in this book will illustrate, there are specific behavioral concerns that are associated with ADHD during adolescence as opposed to early developmental periods, such as delinquency [107], risky sexual behavior [108], and school dropout [109]. As such, it is often imperative that parents closely monitor their teen(s) with ADHD, particularly during evenings and weekends, when adolescents are relatively less likely to be engaged in structured activities. To combat the potential dangers of unstructured time for teens with ADHD, a neuropsychologist may recommend their involvement in structured activities that they would enjoy (e.g., cooking class, joining the basketball team).

While most neuropsychologists do not have prescribing privileges and thus medication management is outside of their areas of expertise, recommendations yielded from a neuropsychological evaluation may include consultation with a prescribing physician. More specifically, it may be recommended that the teen and parents meet with their primary care provider or specialist to learn about medication options, if pharmacological interventions have not yet been initiated to treat the adolescent's ADHD symptoms. Consultation with a PCP or psychiatrist also may be recommended when there is evidence that a teenager's ADHD symptoms are not optimally controlled on their current medication regimen. Adequate medication management is particularly important given the positive effect on classroom behavior, delinquency, and the parent-teen relationship [110, 111]. A recent study evaluated the added value of neuropsychological assessment to routine care in the identification and treatment of ADHD and found that youth who underwent neuropsychological evaluations were more likely to receive behavioral and pharmaceutical treatment [112].

Recommendations related to health, sleep, and social functioning are frequently included in the neuropsychological evaluation report of a teenager with ADHD (e.g., increase exercise, improve sleep hygiene, attend social skills group), as such youth can demonstrate suboptimal functioning in these areas. Further, it is often important to monitor the emotional functioning of individuals with ADHD given the toll on self-esteem to put forth effort and be eager to perform well yet experience variable performance and underachievement. When information yielded from evaluation suggests the presence of comorbid mood or anxiety symptoms, treatment recommendations (e.g., cognitive behavioral therapy [CBT]) for these areas also will be included. In addition to individual treatment, family therapy, a family-oriented approach to work on problem-solving skills, basic communication, and parenting issues for adolescents, may be suggested.

Finally, the recommendations section of a neuropsychological evaluation can be used to provide psychoeducation to parents and teachers of youth with ADHD, as well as to the teenager themselves. Such information may review evidence-based treatments, managing appropriate expectations, and what we know about impairment often experienced by youth with ADHD. Book or website recommendations are often provided, as are community and treatment resources.

Case Revisited

You tailor your questions to better understand why his grades are dropping and find that he cannot keep up with the volume of reading expected in 9th grade. He is overwhelmed with the number of assignments (nightly homework, lengthy papers, and individual and group projects). You suspect that his history of ADHD and dyslexia are becoming more interfering given the increased demands for independent organization, task management, sustained attention, and reading comprehension with the transition to high school. You explain to the family that neuropsychological testing will help clarify his reading, executive functioning, and attention abilities, along with ruling out other factors contributing to his difficulties, such as anxiety or sleep disturbance. Recommendations may point toward a change in IEP services and whether it might be time to revisit the use of stimulant medication.

Conclusions

ADHD is a chronic and highly prevalent childhood disorder, warranting adequate assessment and treatment. However, complete and accurate assessment of a behavioral diagnosis such as ADHD can be a challenge, particularly in adolescents. The stipulations that symptoms must be inappropriate for one's developmental level and that functional impairment must be present are not clearly defined. Further muddying the diagnostic process is the extremely high rate of comorbid conditions.

Given the inattentive, hyperactive/impulsive, and combined presentations, adolescents with ADHD don't all look the same. A behaviorally defined disorder is subject to controversy, both in classification and diagnosis, and experts don't agree on how the ADHD population looks on neuropsychological testing. Standardized scores can be useful for individualized recommendations and treatment planning, but standardized performance-based measures (such as an IQ test result or reading test level) and rating scales are only one piece of a neuropsychologist's diagnostic conceptualization puzzle.

Despite the limitations of standardized tests assessing attention and executive functioning, neuropsychological evaluations can be useful for identification of adolescents with ADHD. A neuropsychologist does not solely collect data from scores on tests but taps a variety of sources to examine multiple dimensions of everyday life over extended periods of time. This is completed through obtaining a detailed developmental history; administering standardized questionnaires; gathering information on current functioning through interview with the parent, teacher, and/or teenager; and directly observing the individual during the evaluation. A comprehensive evaluation determines relative strengths and weaknesses, how the latter contribute to functional impairment, and results in recommendations for individualized treatment across settings.

> **Tips**
> - When you review neuropsychological testing for adolescents, look for the following areas:
>   Performance-based measures
>
>   - Intellectual function
>   - Attention
>   - Executive function
>   - Processing speed
>   - Language
>   - Learning and memory
>   - Visual, fine motor, visual-motor integration
>   - Academic achievement
>   - Effort
>
>   Standardized questionnaires
>   Clinical interview
>   Record review
>   Behavioral observations
>   Summary and diagnostic conceptualization
>   Recommendations
> - Look for a validity statement in the report, indicating the evaluator's indication of whether the findings are a valid estimation of the tester's profile

References

1. Bishop D, Rutter M. Neurodevelopmental disorders: conceptual issues. In: Rutter M, Bishop DV, Pine DS, Scott S, Stevenson J, Taylor E, Thapar A, editors. Rutter's child and adolescent psychiatry. Oxford: Blackwell; 2008. p. 32–41.
2. Rowland AS, Lesesne CA, Abramowitz AJ. The epidemiology of attention-deficit/hyperactivity disorder (ADHD): a public health view. Ment Retard DevDisabil Res Rev. 2002;8(3):162–70.
3. American Academy of Pediatrics. ADHD: clinical practice guideline for the diagnosis, evaluation, and treatment of attention-deficit/hyperactivity disorder in children and adolescents. Pediatrics. 2011;128(5):1007–22.
4. Visser SN, Zablotsky B, Holbrook JR, Danielson ML, Bitsko RH. Diagnostic experiences of children with attention-deficit/hyperactivity disorder. NatlHealth Stat Rep. 2015;81:1–7.
5. American Psychiatric Association. Diagnostic and statistical manual of mental disorders: DSM-5. 5thed. ed. Arlington: American Psychiatric Publishing; 2013.
6. Pritchard AE, Nigro CA, Jacobson LA, Mahone EM. The role of neuropsychological assessment in the functional outcomes of children with ADHD. Neuropsychol Rev. 2012;22(1):54–68.

7. Elliott CD. Differential ability scales, second edition (DAS-II). San Antonio: Harcourt Assessment; 2007.
8. Wechsler D. Wechsler intelligence scale for children. 5thed ed. Bloomington: Pearson; 2014.
9. Wechsler D. Wechsler adult intelligence scale, fourth edition, administration and scoring manual. San Antonio: Psychological Corporation; 2008.
10. Roid GH. Standford-Binet intelligence scales, fifth edition, examiner's manual. Itasca: Riverside; 2003.
11. Mather N, Wendling BJ. Woodcock-Johnson IV tests of cognitive abilities. Rolling Meadows: Riverside; 2014.
12. Wechsler D, Kaplan E. Wechsler intelligence scale for children, fifth edition, integrated. Bloomington: Pearson; 2015.
13. Sheslow D, Adams W. Wide range assessment of memory and learning. 2nded ed. Wilmington: Wide Range, Inc.; 2003.
14. Conners CK. Conners continuous performance test, third edition, manual. Toronto: Multi-Health Systems Inc; 2014.
15. Conners CK. Conners continuous auditory test of attention, manual. Toronto: Multi-Health Systems Inc; 2014.
16. Greenberg LM. Test of variables of attention. Los Alamitos: The Tova Company; 1991.
17. Korkman M, Kirk U, Kemp S. NEPSY-II: a developmental neuropsychological assessment. San Antonio: The Psychological Corporation; 2007.
18. Manly TI, Robertson IH, Anderson V, Nimmo-Smith I. The test of everyday attention for children, manual. Bury St. Edmunds: Thames Valley Test Company Limited; 1999.
19. Delis DC, Kramer JH, Kaplan E, Ober BA. California verbal learning test. 3rd ed. Bloomington: Pearson; 2017.
20. Shallice T. Specific impairments of planning. Proc R SocLond B Biol Sci. 1982;298(1089):199–209.
21. Heaton RK, Chelune GJ, Talley JL, et al. Wisconsin card sorting test manual. Odessa: Psychological Assessment Resources, Inc; 1993.
22. Kaplan E, Goodglass H, Weintraub S. Boston naming test. Philadelphia: Lea &Febiger; 1983.
23. Williams KT. Expressive vocabulary test. 3rd ed. Bloomington: Pearson; 2019.
24. Martin NA, Brownell R. Expressive one-word picture vocabulary test. 4thed. ed. Novato: Academic Therapy; 2011.
25. Dunn DM. Peabody picture vocabulary test. 5thed ed. Bloomington: NCS Pearson; 2019.
26. Martin NA, Brownell R. Receptive one-word picture vocabulary test. 4thed ed. Novarto: Academic Therapy; 2011.
27. Wechsler D. Wechsler individual achievement test. 3rd ed. San Antonio: Psychological Corporation; 2009.
28. Cohen MJ. Children's memory scale. San Antonio: The Psychological Corporation; 1997.
29. Sherman ES, Brooks BL. Child and adolescent memory profile. Lutz: Psychological Assessment Resources, Inc.; 2015.
30. Delis DC, Kramer JH, Kaplan E, Ober BA. California verbal learning test, children's version. Bloomington: Pearson; 1994.
31. Meyers JE, Meyers KR. Rey complex figure test and recognition trial: professional manual. Odesssa: Psychological Assessment Resources; 1995.
32. Benton AL, Sivan AB, Hamsher K, Varney NR, Spreen O. Contributions to neuropsychological assessment: a clinical manual. 2nd ed. New York: Oxford University Press; 1994.
33. Beery KE, Buktenica NA, Beery NA. The beery–buktenica developmental test of visual–motor integration: administration, scoring, and teaching manual. 6th ed. Minneapolis: Pearson; 2010.
34. Mather N, Wendling BJ. Examiner's manual: Woodcock-Johnson IV tests of achievement. Rolling Meadows: Riverside; 2014.
35. Kaufman AS, Kaufman NL. Kaufman test of educational achievement. 3rded ed. Bloomington: Pearson; 2014.
36. Wiederholt JL, Bryant BR. Gray oral reading tests. 5th ed. Austin: Pro-Ed; 2012.

37. Brown JI, Fishco VV, Hanna GS. Nelson-Denny reading test: technical report, forms G &H. Chicago: Riverside Publishing Company; 1993.
38. Connolly AJ. KeyMath 3: diagnostic assessment. San Antonio: Pearson; 2007.
39. Brooks BL, Ploetz DM, Kirkwood M. A survey of neuropsychologists' use of validity tests with children and adolescents. Child Neuropsychol. 2016;22(8):1001–20.
40. Drechsler R, Brandeis D, Földényi M, Imhof K, Steinhausen HC. The course of neuropsychological functions in children with attention deficit hyperactivity disorder from late childhood to early adolescence. J Child Psychol Psychiatry. 2005;46(8):824–36.
41. Manly T, Anderson V, Nimmo-Smith I, Turner A, Watson P, Robertson IH. The differential assessment of children's attention: the test of everyday attention for children (TEA-Ch), normative sample and ADHD performance. J Child Psychol Psychiatry. 2001;42(8):1065–81.
42. Tucha O, Walitza S, Mecklinger L, Sontag TA, Kuebber S, Linder M, Lange KW. Attentional functioning in children with ADHD-predominantly hyperactive-impulsive type and children with ADHD-combined type. J Neural Transm. 2006;113(12):1943–53.
43. Tucha L, Tucha O, Walitza S, Sontag TA, Laufkötter R, Linder M, Lange KW. Vigilance and sustained attention in children and adults with ADHD. J AttenDisord. 2009;12(5):410–21.
44. Klingberg T, Fernell E, Olesen PJ, Johnson M, Gustafsson P, Dahlström K, Gillberg CG, Forssberg H, Westerberg H. Computerized training of working memory in children with ADHD: a randomized, controlled trial. J Am Acad Child Adolesc Psychiatry. 2005;44(2):177–86.
45. Martel M, Nikolas M, Nigg JT. Executive function in adolescents with ADHD. J Am Acad Child Adolesc Psychiatry. 2007;46(11):1437–44.
46. Mayes SD, Calhoun SL, Chase GA, Mink DM, Stagg RE. ADHD subtypes and co-occurring anxiety, depression, and oppositional-defiant disorder: differences in Gordon diagnostic system and Wechsler working memory and processing speed index scores. J AttenDisord. 2009;12(6):540–50.
47. Tucha O, Tucha L, Kaumann G, König S, Lange KM, Stasik D, Streather Z, Engelschalk T, Lange KW. Training of attention functions in children with attention deficit hyperactivity disorder. Atten DeficitHyperactDisord. 2011;3(3):271–83.
48. Willcutt EG, Doyle AE, Nigg JT, Faraone SV, Pennington BF. Validity of the executive function theory of attention-deficit/hyperactivity disorder: a meta-analytic review. Biol Psychiatry. 2005;57(11):1336–46.
49. Castellanos FX, Sonuga-Barke EJ, Milham MP, Tannock R. Characterizing cognition in ADHD: beyond executive dysfunction. Trends Cogn Sci. 2006;10(3):117–23.
50. Nigg JT, Willcutt EG, Doyle AE, Sonuga-Barke EJ. Causal heterogeneity in attention-deficit/hyperactivity disorder: do we need neuropsychologically impaired subtypes? Biol Psychiatry. 2005;57(11):1224–30.
51. Greimel E, Wanderer S, Rothenberger A, Herpertz-Dahlmann B, Konrad K, Roessner V. Attentional performance in children and adolescents with tic disorder and co-occurring attention-deficit/hyperactivity disorder: new insights from a 2× 2 factorial design study. J Abnorm Child Psychol. 2011;39(6):819–28.
52. Coghill D, Nigg J, Rothenberger A, Sonuga-Barke E, Tannock R. Whither causal models in the neuroscience of ADHD? Dev Sci. 2005;2:105–14.
53. Hervey AS, Epstein JN, Curry JF. Neuropsychology of adults with attention-deficit/hyperactivity disorder: a meta-analytic review. Neuropsychology. 2004;18(3):485–503.
54. Lange KW, Reichl S, Lange KM, Tucha L, Tucha O. The history of attention deficit hyperactivity disorder. Atten DeficitHyperactDisord. 2010;2(4):241–55.
55. Lange KW, Hauser J, Lange KM, Makulska-Gertruda E, Takano T, Takeuchi Y, Tucha L, Tucha O. Utility of cognitive neuropsychological assessment in attention-deficit/hyperactivity disorder. Atten DeficitHyperactDisord. 2014;6(4):241–8.
56. Gioia GA, Isquith PK. Ecological assessment of executive function in traumatic brain injury. DevNeuropsychol. 2004;25(1–2):135–58.
57. Isquith PK, Roth RM, Gioia G. Contribution of rating scales to the assessment of executive functions. ApplNeuropsychol Child. 2013;2(2):125–32.

58. Toplak ME, West RF, Stanovich KE. Practitioner review: do performance-based measures and ratings of executive function assess the same construct? J Child Psychol Psychiatry. 2013;54(2):131–43.
59. Reynolds CR, Kamphaus RW. Behavior assessment for children manual. Bloomington: Pearson; 2015.
60. Achenbach TM. The Achenbach system of empirically based assessment (ASEBA): development, findings, theory, and applications. Burlington: University of Vermont Research Center for Children, Youth, & Families; 2009.
61. Chorpita BF, Yim L, Moffitt C, Umemoto LA, Francis SE. Assessment of symptoms of DSM-IV anxiety and depression in children: a revised child anxiety and depression scale. Behav Res Ther. 2000;38(8):835–55.
62. March JS. Multidimensional anxiety scale for children, second edition: Technical manual. Toronto: Multi-Health Systems; 2013.
63. Beck AT, Steer RA, Brown GK. Beck depression inventory. 2nd ed. San Antonio: The Psychological Cooperation; 1996.
64. Wolraich ML, Lambert W, Doffing MA, Bickman L, Simmons T, Worley K. Psychometric properties of the Vanderbilt ADHD diagnostic parent rating scale in a referred population. J Pediatr Psychol. 2003;28(8):559–68.
65. Wolraich ML, Hannah JN, Baumgaertel A, Feurer ID. Examination of DSM-IV criteria for attention deficit hyperactivity disorder in a county-wide sample. J DevBehav Pediatr. 1998;19(3):162–8.
66. Pelham WE Jr, Gnagy EM, Greenslade KE, Milich R. Teacher ratings of DSM-III-R symptoms for the disruptive behavior disorders. J Am Acad Child Adolesc Psychiatry. 1992;31(2):210–8.
67. DuPaul GJ, Power TJ, Anastopoulos AD, Reid R. ADHD rating scale-5 for children and adolescents: checklists, norms, and clinical interpretation. New York: Guilford Publications; 2016.
68. Conners CK. Conners. 3rd ed. Los Angeles: Western Psychological Services; 2008.
69. Gioia GA, Isquith PK, Guy SC, Kenworthy L. BRIEF-2: behavior rating inventory of executive function. 2nded ed. Lutz: Psychological Assessment Resources; 2015.
70. Harrison PL, Oakland T. Adaptive behavior assessment system. 3rd ed. Torrance: Western Psychological Services; 2015.
71. Sparrow SS, Cicchetti DV, Saulnier CA. Vineland adaptive behavior scales. 3rd ed. San Antonio: Pearson; 2016.
72. De Los Reyes A, Kazdin AE. Informant discrepancies in the assessment of childhood psychopathology: a critical review, theoretical framework, and recommendations for further study. Psychol Bull. 2005;131(4):483–509.
73. Rubio-Stipec M, Fitzmaurice G, Murphy J, Walker A. The use of multiple informants in identifying the risk factors of depressive and disruptive disorders. Soc Psychiatry PsychiatrEpidemiol. 2003;38(2):51–8.
74. Mahone EM, Hagelthorn KM, Cutting LE, Schuerholz LJ, Pelletier SF, Rawlins C, Singer HS, Denckla MB. Effects of IQ on executive function measures in children with ADHD. Child Neuropsychol. 2002;8(1):52–65.
75. Sullivan JR, Riccio CA. Diagnostic group differences in parent and teacher ratings on the BRIEF and Conners' Scales. J AttenDisord. 2007;11(3):398–406.
76. Toplak ME, Bucciarelli SM, Jain U, Tannock R. Executive functions: performance-based measures and the behavior rating inventory of executive function (BRIEF) in adolescents with attention deficit/hyperactivity disorder (ADHD). Child Neuropsychol. 2008;15(1):53–72.
77. Gomez R, Burns GL, Walsh JA, De Moura MA. Multitrait-multisource confirmatory factor analytic approach to the construct validity of ADHD rating scales. Psychol Assess. 2003;15(1):3–16.
78. Mares D, McLuckie A, Schwartz M, Saini M. Executive function impairments in children with attention-deficit hyperactivity disorder: do they differ between school and home environments? Can J Psychiatry. 2007;52(8):527–34.

79. Evans SW, Allen J, Moore S, Strauss V. Measuring symptoms and functioning of youth with ADHD in middle schools. J Abnorm Child Psychol. 2005;33(6):695–706.
80. Molina BS, Smith BH, Pelham WE. Factor structure and criterion validity of secondary school teacher ratings of ADHD and ODD. J Abnorm Child Psychol. 2001;29(1):71–82.
81. Achenbach TM, McConaughy SH, Howell CT. Child/adolescent behavioral and emotional problems: implications of cross-informant correlations for situational specificity. Psychol Bull. 1987;101(2):213.
82. Offord DR, Boyle MH, Racine Y, Szatmari P, Fleming JE, Sanford M, et al. Integrating assessment data from multiple informants. J Am Acad Child Adolesc Psychiatry. 1996;35(8):1078–85.
83. Owens J, Goldfine M, Evangelista N, Hoza B, Kaiser N. A critical review of self-perceptions and the positive illusory bias in children with ADHD. Clin Child FamPsychol Rev. 2007;10(4):335–51.
84. Sibley MH, Pelham WE, Molina BSG, Waschbusch DA, Gnagy E, Babinski DE, et al. Inconsistent self-report of delinquency by adolescents and young adults with ADHD. J Abnorm Child Psychol. 2010;38(5):645–56.
85. Miller C, Newcorn J, Halperin J. Fading memories: retrospective recall inaccuracies in ADHD. J AttenDisord. 2010;14(10):7–14.
86. Sibley MH, Pelham WE Jr, Molina BS, Gnagy EM, Waschbusch DA, Garefino AC, et al. Diagnosing ADHD in adolescence. J Consult ClinPsychol. 2012;80(1):139–50.
87. Efron D, Hazell P, Anderson V. Update on attention deficit hyperactivity disorder. J Paediatr Child Health. 2011;47(10):682–9.
88. Marshall SA, Evans SW, Eiraldi RB, Becker SP, Power TJ. Social and academic impairment in youth with ADHD, predominately inattentive type and sluggish cognitive tempo. J Abnorm Child Psychol. 2014;42(1):77–90.
89. Taylor E, Sonuga-Barke E. Disorders of attention and activity. In: Rutter M, Bishop DV, Pine DS, Scott S, Stevenson J, Taylor E, Thapar A, editors. Rutter's child and adolescent psychiatry. 5th ed. Oxford: Blackwell; 2008. p. 521–42.
90. Thorell LB, Veleiro A, Siu AF, Mohammadi H. Examining the relation between ratings of executive functioning and academic achievement: findings from a cross-cultural study. Child Neuropsychol. 2013;19(6):630–8.
91. Smith BH, Pelham WE Jr, Gnagy E, Molina B, Evans S. The reliability, validity, and unique contributions of self-report by adolescents receiving treatment for attention-deficit/hyperactivity disorder. J Consult ClinPsychol. 2000;68(3):489–99.
92. Barkley RA. Emotional dysregulation is a core component of ADHD. In: Barkley RA, editor. Attention-deficit hyperactivity disorder: a handbook for diagnosis and treatment. 4thed. ed. New York: Guilford Press; 2015. p. 81–115.
93. Wilens TE, Biederman J, Brown S, Tanguay S, Monuteaux MC, Blake C, Spencer TJ. Psychiatric comorbidity and functioning in clinically referred preschool children and school-age youths with ADHD. J Am Acad Child Adolesc Psychiatry. 2002;41(3):262–8.
94. Greene RW, Beszterczey SK, Katzenstein T, Park K, Goring J. Are students with ADHD more stressful to teach? Patterns of teacher stress in an elementary school sample. J EmotBehavDisord. 2002;10(2):79–89.
95. Rommelse NN, Franke B, Geurts HM, Hartman CA, Buitelaar JK. Shared heritability of attention-deficit/hyperactivity disorder and autism spectrum disorder. Eur Child Adolesc Psychiatry. 2010;19(3):281–95.
96. van der Meer JM, Oerlemans AM, van Steijn DJ, Lappenschaar MG, de Sonneville LM, Buitelaar JK, Rommelse NN. Are autism spectrum disorder and attention-deficit/hyperactivity disorder different manifestations of one overarching disorder? Cognitive and symptom evidence from a clinical and population-based sample. J Am Acad Child Adolesc Psychiatry. 2012;51(11):1160–72.
97. Simonoff E, Pickles A, Wood N, Gringras P, Chadwick O. ADHD symptoms in children with mild intellectual disability. J Am Acad Child Adolesc Psychiatry. 2007;46(5):591–600.

98. Lindblad I, Gillberg C, Fernell E. ADHD and other associated developmental problems in childrenwith mild mental retardation: the use of the "Five-To-Fifteen" questionnaire in a population-based sample. Res DevDisabil. 2011;32(6):2805–9.
99. DuPaul GJ, Gormley MJ, Laracy SD. Comorbidity of LD and ADHD: implications of DSM-5 for assessment and treatment. J Learn Disabil. 2013;46(1):43–51.
100. Howell D, Osternig L, Van Donkelaar P, Mayr U, Chou LS. Effects of concussion on attention and executive function in adolescents. Med Sci Sports Exerc. 2013;45(6):1030–7.
101. Dougherty DM, Mathias CW, Dawes MA, Furr RM, Charles NE, Liguori A, et al. Impulsivity, attention, memory, and decision-making among adolescent marijuana users. Psychopharmacology. 2013;226(2):307–19.
102. Parisi P, Moavero R, Verrotti A, Curatolo P. Attention deficit hyperactivity disorder in children with epilepsy. Brain and Development. 2010;32(1):10–6.
103. Reilly C, Ballantine R. Epilepsy in school-aged children: more than just seizures? Support Learn. 2011;26(4):144–51.
104. Gruber R, Michaelsen S, Bergmame L, Frenette S, Bruni O, Fontil L, Carrier J. Short sleep duration is associated with teacher-reported inattention and cognitive problems in healthy school-aged children. Nat Sci Sleep. 2012;4:33–40.
105. Hansen DE, Vandenberg B. Neuropsychological features and differential diagnosis of sleep apnea syndrome in children. J Clin Child Psychol. 1997;26(3):304–10.
106. Youssef NA, Ege M, Angly SS, Strauss JL, Marx CE. Is obstructive sleep apnea associated with ADHD. Ann ClinPsychiatry. 2011;23(3):213–24.
107. Sibley MH, Pelham WE, Molina BS, Gnagy EM, Waschbusch DA, Biswas A, MacLean MG, Babinski DE, Karch KM. The delinquency outcomes of boys with ADHD with and without comorbidity. J Abnorm Child Psychol. 2011;39(1):21–32.
108. Flory K, Molina BS, Pelham WE Jr, Gnagy E, Smith B. Childhood ADHD predicts risky sexual behavior in young adulthood. J Clin Child AdolescPsychol. 2006;35(4):571–7.
109. Kent KM, Pelham WE, Molina BS, Sibley MH, Waschbusch DA, Yu J, Gnagy EM, Biswas A, Babinski DE, Karch KM. The academic experience of male high school students with ADHD. J Clin Child AdolescPsychol. 2011;39(3):451–62.
110. Lichtenstein P, Halldner L, Zetterqvist J, Sjölander A, Serlachius E, Fazel S, et al. Medication for attention deficit–hyperactivity disorder and criminality. N Engl J Med. 2012;367(21):2006–14.
111. Schachar RJ, Tannock R, Cunningham C, Corkum PV. Behavioral, situational, and temporal effects of treatment of ADHD with methylphenidate. J Am Acad Child Adolesc Psychiatry. 1997;36(6):754–63.
112. Pritchard AE, Koriakin T, Jacobson LA, Mahone EM. Incremental validity of neuropsychological assessment in the identification and treatment of youth with ADHD. ClinNeuropsychol. 2014;28(1):26–48.

Part II
ADHD Mimickers and Co-morbidities

Chapter 7
When Learning Disabilities Mask ADHD

Katherine Driscoll

Case Example

Michaela is a 13-year-old girl who showed increased social and academic challenges as she transitioned to middle school. She was not meeting academic expectations in first grade and repeated the year. She was diagnosed with dyslexia in third grade. Michaela receives pull-out reading intervention via her Individualized Education Plan (IEP). She exhibited some social and behavioral challenges in early elementary school but was considered to be a hard worker who always tried her best. School testing in third grade illustrated Michaela's reading challenges relative to her appropriate cognitive skills. She responded fairly well to reading support in elementary school, but her self-esteem and work habits waned as academic demands increased.

Background

Like ADHD, specific learning disorders are a form of neurodevelopmental disorder, but disorders are challenges in one of the three academic areas—reading, writing, and math—that are foundational to students' ability to learn. The DSM-5 defines three forms of specific learning disorders, including impairment in reading, impairment in mathematics, and impairment in written expression. Specific learning disorders are also sometimes referred to as dyslexia (reading disorder), dyscalculia (math disorder), and dysgraphia (writing disorder).

Adolescents with ADHD often experience challenges with academic performance and achievement. In his review of learning disorders in children with ADHD,

K. Driscoll (✉)
Division of Developmental Medicine, Boston Children's Hospital, Boston, MA, USA
e-mail: katherine.driscoll@childrens.harvard.edu

© Springer Nature Switzerland AG 2020
A. Schonwald (ed.), *ADHD in Adolescents*,
https://doi.org/10.1007/978-3-030-62393-7_7

Barkley cited comorbidity rates of 8–60% depending on the definition of learning disorders as well as the achievement areas measured [1]. A large research study found that learning disorders occurred in 71% of children with ADHD, ranging from 26% in math, to 33% in reading, to 63% in written expression [2]. The majority of children and adolescents with ADHD will experience challenges with learning, attention, working memory, processing speed, and graphomotor skills [3]. Students who experience learning challenges may appear to struggle to sustain attention. However, not all students with ADHD have comorbid learning disorders, just as not all adolescents with learning disorders meet full diagnostic criteria for ADHD. Learning disorders can mask ADHD symptoms. The purpose of this chapter is to provide information on the association between learning disorders and ADHD for families, teachers, and clinicians.

Practical Steps to Figuring It Out

1. *Is it ADHD and/or a specific learning disorder?*

It is important to consider the development of your child's challenges with attention and/or learning. Has your child always been more active than their peers? Were they unable to sit at the dinner table as a younger child? Were you unable to ask your child to get two things and meet you by the front door to go to soccer practice? Did your child seem forgetful? Did they struggle to regulate their emotions and behavior when they were upset or frustrated? If the answers to these questions are yes, ADHD might have been emerging from those early years. Did they need more time to pick up new skills in the early grades of school? Were learning and academic achievement always challenging? Has your child experienced any upsetting or difficult times that seemed to coincide with increased challenges with learning and/or attention? If the answers to these questions are yes, then learning disabilities might have been emerging from those early years. The answers to these questions explain the sequence of the trajectory of your child's challenges, helping to clarify what came first.

To gather additional information, talk with your child's teachers about attention and learning. Schedule a meeting (or several) to check in with each teacher about your child's attention and academic performance. Are there trends related to types of academic work or subject areas? For example, do your daughter's teachers tell you that she has excellent ideas but struggles to put her thoughts on paper when writing? Your child may already have an Individualized Education Plan (IEP) or 504 Plan. If so, it may be time to boost accommodations and/or services. If not, it may be time to explore the possibility of putting some additional supports in place for your child.

Even seasoned teachers may have difficulty distinguishing ADHD from a learning disorder. Don't expect it to be the final answer. Instead, concrete examples of where the student shines and where the student struggles are most helpful.

2. *Request further evaluation and support*

The Individuals with Disabilities Education Act (IDEA) supports students who qualify for special education. Parents can request the public school where they live to complete an Individualized Education Program (IEP) evaluation. This testing can quantify a student's level of academic achievement and cognitive potential, indicating whether or not the student qualifies as having a learning disability. When a student is identified with a disability classified under one of the qualifying conditions, the student is eligible to receive special education services under IDEA. According to the Department of Education, every child receiving special education support must have an IEP. An IEP is an individualized document that outlines special educations services and goals. If academic skills are delayed and lower than expected for the child's capacity to learn, then academic interventions (for reading, writing, and/ or math) should be offered. Interventions can also be offered to address communication, social skills, executive function, motor skills, and self-regulation.

> Whether or not your child attends your district public school system for school, the evaluation must be offered there.

Some students do not meet the criteria for IDEA but qualify for support under Section 504 of the Rehabilitation Act of 1973, a civil rights law. This is often referred to as "Section 504" or a "504 Plan." IEPs and 504 Plans share the goal of ensuring that students with disabilities have access to a free and appropriate public education that is comparable to the education available to nondisabled peers. Children with ADHD and no specific learning disability often qualify for a 504 Plan when their ADHD "substantially limits" their ability to learn. While an IEP includes direct support and intervention, a 504 Plan for a student with ADHD generally provides classroom accommodations, such as provision of additional time to complete classroom assignments.

Look at each of the following examples, and think about how distractibility and impulsivity can contribute to the scenarios suggesting learning problems. Each one is an appropriate candidate for referral for special education evaluation.

A. The first student who does not appear to comprehend written material when asked to respond to questions at the end of a chapter. This student should be evaluated for learning and language needs.
B. Another student seems to have mastered a skill during a review session but then fails the test the very next day. This student should be evaluated to better understand their learning profile, including comprehension, working memory, and retrieval.
C. A third student may brain-storm essay ideas easily with a peer. Their ideas are thoughtful and well-articulated, yet the result is a poorly crafted essay submitted the following week. Issues might lie in organization of output, working memory, writing, and/or other executive functions.

3. *The school-home collaboration*

Communication between teachers and families is an important piece of the support provided for students with ADHD and/or learning disorders. This can be a difficult terrain to navigate with adolescents. It is common for teachers or families to feel concerned that providing closer monitoring, such as checking to see that an assignment has been recorded correctly or reminding a student to review responses before submitting an exam, will reduce independence and will be met with resistance. However, many students require this additional support to fully access the curriculum. Therefore, it is important to clearly delineate accommodations and/or goals, and support may be tapered over time as students are able to achieve a goal independently. Student buy-in is equally important. The learner should participate in identifying goals and agreeing to interventions. For example, a student may shift from receiving a printed list of homework for the week to copying down assignments independently with a teacher checking the list for accuracy, as appropriate.

Providing appropriate special education support and/or accommodations is also paramount to student achievement. Students with specific learning disorders will require individual or small-group academic support as a provision of their IEP. For example, a student with dyslexia might work with a reading specialist for 30 min/day using an evidence-based reading intervention. Support and accommodations for students with ADHD vary and should be determined based on the unique needs of each student.

Important for the student with both ADHD and learning disabilities is the ongoing appreciation of how each exacerbates the other and the changes that can evolve with time:

- A second grader who successfully navigates the rote skills of spelling tests and math equations might struggle when reading comprehension expectations increase in third grade.
- Another student with ADHD and dyslexia may succeed relatively well with only reading intervention in early elementary school.

By high school, the demand for sustained attention is far greater, and so untreated ADHD symptoms may interfere with all learning, including reading, more than in the past. Furthermore, puberty and/or increased social demands can also affect an older child's presentation. Parents and teachers should rethink a student's needs as the educational and social environment matures.

> High school classes have a quicker pace and less repetition, magnifying the impact of a student's distractibility.

The Data

It is important for clinicians to consider comorbidity when determining assessment plans and treatment for adolescents. DuPaul and Stoner reviewed 17 studies that reported the percentage of students with ADHD who were also diagnosed with a specific learning disorder [4]. Prevalence of learning disorders varied from 7% to 92%, and the variability was largely due to different methods of identifying learning disorders. The median rate of learning disorder prevalence across the 17 ADHD samples was 31.1%. In contrast, rates of learning disorders among students in the control groups of the 17 studies ranged from 0% to 22% with a median prevalence of 8.9%. Thus, students with ADHD appear to be three times more likely to have a learning disorder as are their classmates who do not have ADHD.

> In other words, one out of every three students with ADHD will also have a specific learning disorder.

Despite comorbidity, most students with ADHD will not have a specific learning disorder, and most students with a learning disorder will not have ADHD [5]. However, clinicians must consider the significant minority of students with comorbid ADHD and learning disorders when planning and conducting assessments and interventions. Educational testing should be conducted across academic subject areas of reading, math, and writing.

> Assessments for ADHD should always include academic testing, and evaluations for learning concerns should always include measures of attention and executive functioning.

It is also important to consider whether interventions for ADHD improve academic performance [4]. Although stimulant medications often reduce ADHD symptoms, medication will not reverse academic skills deficits in students with comorbid ADHD and learning disorders. Stimulant medication is associated with small effects on academic achievement [6]. Students with comorbid learning disorders require intensive, direct instruction beyond medication and behavioral strategies [4].

Executive Functioning

Executive functioning is a critical piece of the relationship between attention difficulties and learning challenges. Executive functioning is an umbrella term that refers to our ability to manage ourselves and our resources to achieve a goal. It involves neurologically based skills related to cognitive control and self-regulation. Executive functioning and self-regulation skills are the mental processes that help us plan, focus our attention, remember, and juggle multiple tasks. In short, executive functioning helps us get things done.

Case Revisited

Remember Michaela who has dyslexia and whose work habits deteriorated in middle school? Information about comorbidity sheds some light on Michaela's increased challenges. Her initial school evaluation highlighted her reading challenges, but no note is made of her attention and executive functioning at that point. Fortunately, Michaela's middle school history teacher referred her for additional school testing. Testing included assessment of attention and executive functioning via parent and teacher report measures, as well as direct assessment with Michaela. Results of this testing illustrated her steady progress in reading, in addition to challenges with working memory, distractibility, organization, shifting attention, and impulsivity that had likely exacerbated her learning challenges throughout her schooling. These difficulties, combined with Michaela's strong desire to do well, had affected her self-esteem and social functioning. This new information will enable her parents, school team, and pediatrician to develop a more comprehensive plan to address her comorbid dyslexia and ADHD.

Conclusions

ADHD and learning disabilities are closely linked, so can be easy to confuse. Both affect how we learn and how we show what we know. Academics are typically affected when a teen has ADHD, unless intentional preparation started early and ongoing support persists. A reasoned approach to gathering data will usually be required to disentangle the two disorders, starting with attention scales but likely building to an assessment of learning and executive function profile as well.

Tips
- Students often experience greater impact of both learning disabilities and ADHD in high school, when greater demands for learning and attention are harder to meet.
- All evaluations for learning disabilities should consider the student's attention profile.
- All evaluations for attention deficits should consider the student's learning profile.

References

1. Barkley RA. Associated cognitive, developmental, and health problems. In: Attention-deficit hyperactivity disorder: a handbook for diagnosis and treatment. 4th ed. New York: Guilford; 2018. p. 122–83.
2. Mayes SD, Calhoun SL. Frequency of reading, math, and writing disabilities in children with clinical disorders. Learn Individ Differ. 2006;16(2):145–57. https://doi.org/10.1016/j.lindif.2005.07.004.
3. Mayes SD, Calhoun SL. Learning, attention, writing, and processing speed in typical children and children with ADHD, autism, anxiety, depression, and oppositional-defiant disorder. Child Neuropsychol. 2007;13(6):469–93. https://doi.org/10.1080/09297040601112773.
4. DuPaul GJ, Stoner G. ADHD in the schools: assessment and intervention strategies. New York: Guilford; 2003.
5. DuPaul GJ, Gormley MJ, Laracy SD. Comorbidity of LD and ADHD: implications of DSM-5 for assessment and treatment. J Learn Disabil. 2013;46(1):43–51. https://doi.org/10.1177/0022219412464351.
6. Van der Oord S, Prins PJ, Oosterlaan J, Emmelkamp PM. Efficacy of methylphenidate, psycho-social treatments and their combination in school-aged children with ADHD: a meta-analysis. ClinPsychol Rev. 2008;28(5):783–800. https://doi.org/10.1016/j.cpr.2007.10.007.

Chapter 8
ADHD and Anxiety Disorders

Devon Carroll

Case Example

Chloe, an 11th grader, who complains that it is hard to focus because she has constant worries running through her head about her upcoming calculus midterm (e.g., Will I fail the exam? And, what if I fail the class? If I don't pass the class, I'm never going to get into college). Chloe's math teacher already knows that she has a 504 Plan for attention-deficit/hyperactivity disorder (ADHD), so she may think that Chloe is "zoning out" when in fact it is her anxiety that is making it difficult for Chloe to pay attention.

Background

All teens experience some amount of anxiety at times. Feeling anxious is as much a part of adolescence as final exams, first dates, and puberty. In a 2013 survey conducted by the American Psychological Association (APA), teens reported their stress level was 5.8 on a 10-point scale compared with 5.1 for adults [1]. Approximately 31% of teens reported feeling overwhelmed, and 30% reported feeling depressed or sad as a result of their stress. More than one-third of teens complained of fatigue or feeling tired, and nearly one-fourth of teens reported skipping a meal due to stress [1].

Anxiety is a normal reaction to the stresses of our everyday lives. In fact, stress can help teens deal with overwhelming or threatening situations. Stressful situations trigger a cascade of stress hormones. As a fight-or-flight response, the body

D. Carroll (✉)
Department of Psychiatry and Behavioral Sciences, Boston Children's Hospital,
Boston, MA, USA
e-mail: devon.carroll@childrens.harvard.edu

© Springer Nature Switzerland AG 2020
A. Schonwald (ed.), *ADHD in Adolescents*,
https://doi.org/10.1007/978-3-030-62393-7_8

mobilizes and prepares to take action—you begin breathing faster, your heart pounds, and your entire body becomes tense. You can see why it can be easy to overlook anxiety because we all experience it in some way, shape, or form.

An anxiety disorder, by contrast, can be debilitating. Highly anxious teens have an overactive fight-or-flight response that perceives threats when often there are none. For these teenagers, anxiety is not protecting them but rather preventing them from fully engaging in typical activities of daily life including school, friendships, and academics. Their anxiety may be terrifying—and, at times, incapacitating—or it may be relatively mild but pervasive for seemingly no reason. According to the National Institute of Mental Health, approximately 32% of adolescents develop an anxiety disorder between the ages of 13 and 18 [2].

> It is normal for teens to feel anxious or to worry. Adolescents with anxiety disorders stand out from their peers whose anxiety is more typical: symptoms are more frequent and interfere with their everyday lives.

Epidemiology of ADHD with Anxiety Disorders

Like ADHD, there is no single cause of anxiety. Anxiety most likely results from a complex interplay of genetic vulnerabilities, biological factors, temperamental qualities, early negative stressors, and sociocultural factors. We know that anxiety runs in families at an unusually high rate. We also know that ADHD tends to run in families. Thus, it is not surprising that ADHD and comorbid anxiety disorders have been shown to occur together in first-degree relatives like children, parents, and grandparents [3]. Family genetic studies show that first-degree relatives of children with comorbid ADHD and anxiety have a similar risk for ADHD but a much higher risk for anxiety than relatives of children with ADHD only [4]. We also think that maternal anxiety or stress during pregnancy may increase the risk for comorbid ADHD and anxiety. Findings have been inconsistent with regard to the gestational age at which these effects are most pronounced, but we think that the first 8–24 weeks of pregnancy are critical [4].

> Any subtype of ADHD may co-occur with any anxiety disorder.

It is important to know that any anxiety disorder, like social anxiety disorder or generalized anxiety disorder, may occur with ADHD. We once thought that the inattentive subtype of ADHD had a higher association with anxiety disorders than the combined and hyperactive/impulsive subtypes, but that no longer appears true.

Recent research shows the rates of comorbid anxiety disorders are similar across subtypes of ADHD [4]. That means that the youngster given detention for goofing off in class with their friends may be just as likely to have an anxiety disorder as the teen who sits anxiously in class hoping not to be called on—aware that they didn't prepare for class or fearful of having the wrong answer.

While we know that anxiety disorders affect significantly more females on average, we think that males and females with ADHD are affected by anxiety disorders at similar rates. The research is conflicting, with some evidence indicating that females with ADHD report higher levels of anxiety than males [5, 6] and other research suggesting just the opposite—that males with ADHD have a higher risk for anxiety than females [7]. The take-home message is that the risk for developing an anxiety disorder appears to be about the same for both females and males with ADHD.

Clinical Course of ADHD with Anxiety

Anxiety symptoms typically wax and wane from childhood into adolescence and even adulthood. They are dynamic and can evolve into other anxiety disorders and conditions like depression. For instance, shyness or behavioral inhibition in very young children may continue into adolescence and progress into an anxiety disorder. In many cases, anxiety disorders persist from teenage years into early adulthood. Interestingly, a large majority of adults with anxiety disorders report that their disorder started in adolescence [8].

Despite the fluctuating nature of anxiety, there is a typical age of onset for the various types of anxiety disorders. For instance, separation anxiety disorder and certain specific phobias, like a fear of dogs or becoming ill, usually start before the age of 12 [8]. These disorders typically begin to decrease in adolescence and continue to do so in adulthood. Social anxiety disorder develops in late childhood or adolescence and very rarely after the age of 25. Agoraphobia, panic disorder, and generalized anxiety disorder usually emerge in adolescence or early adulthood and persist into adulthood [8].

Little is known about the long-term course of comorbid ADHD and anxiety disorders. However, there is literature to support the chronic nature of ADHD and anxiety disorders alone. We can speculate that when these disorders co-occur, they may be likely to persist into adulthood. Studies of anxiety disorders, like panic disorder and generalized anxiety disorder, suggest that the course of the disorder may be influenced by factors like stressful life events, sensitivity, and other comorbid disorders [8]. We also know that teens with anxiety disorders are at a higher risk of developing problems with depression and substance abuse in adulthood [8]. With this in mind, the earlier we can identify these problems and intervene, the better.

Anxiety: Signs and Symptoms

There are many different types of anxiety disorders, including generalized anxiety, social anxiety, separation anxiety, obsessive-compulsive, phobias, and panic. All of these disorders are known to cause significant distress and impair functioning within the home, school, and social settings.

Adolescents with ADHD and anxiety tend to be "worriers"—they worry about school, social situations, their athletic performance, and their behavior. Some teens may not be willing to try new activities and are afraid of taking risks. Other teens may be more likely to engage in risky behaviors like substance abuse or risky sexual behavior to help ease their constant worries. They may seek excessive reassurance from parents or friends and ask "What if?" questions over and over again. Worried teens tend to do less well in school, and this can affect their self-esteem, placing them at risk for depressive disorders. Adolescents often feel that their symptoms are beyond their control, making things feel even more unmanageable.

Some common signs of anxiety in a teenager include:

- Excessive fears and worries
- Feeling nervous or "on edge"
- Feelings of inner restlessness
- Tendency to be wary and vigilant

Many teens also experience physical symptoms of anxiety like muscle tension, stomachaches, headaches, diarrhea, pain, and fatigue. They may visit the nurse's office regularly or ask to see their primary care provider for relatively minor medical complaints. Also common in this age group are sleep disturbances: problems falling asleep, midnight awakening, and nightmares.

> For some adolescents, physical symptoms coincide with anxiety-provoking situations like tests, oral presentations, and athletic competitions, resulting in teenagers missing school or other events on important days.

It's not surprising that anxiety can greatly impact a teenager's social world. Anxious teens uneasy in social situations may experience difficulty participating in school activities (e.g., working in groups, answering questions in front of the class) or avoid social situations (e.g., joining school clubs or sports teams). This can result in teens becoming increasingly isolated and withdrawn, placing them at risk for depressive symptoms.

Again, there are several different types of anxiety disorders that occur in adolescence, including some of the most common anxiety disorders.

Generalized Anxiety Disorder (GAD)

The hallmark of generalized anxiety disorder (GAD) is excessive anxiety or worry about things related to personal health, school, social interactions, and everyday routine life circumstances. A teenager that complains frequently about physical symptoms, like stomachaches, diarrhea, headaches, and muscle tension, may have GAD. The fear and anxiety associated with GAD causes significant problems in areas of the teen's life, such as social interactions, academic performance, and extracurricular activities.

Panic Disorder

Panic disorder is characterized by discrete episodes of excessive fear for no particular reason. Episodes occur seemingly "out of the blue," and teens describe feeling like they are losing control even when there is no actual danger. Adolescents may complain about their heart racing, not being able to catch their breath, and an inability to stop shaking. Adolescents might be fearful of traveling on bridges or roads. It is important to keep in mind that not every teen that has panic attacks will develop panic disorder. Some adolescents develop something called "agoraphobia," a fear and avoidance of places or situations that they worry may cause them to panic.

Social Anxiety Disorder

Adolescents with social anxiety disorder (also called social phobia) have a marked fear of humiliation in social situations. Symptoms may include a fear of meeting and talking to new peers or adults, avoidance of social situations, and having few friends outside of the family. Teens may avoid class presentations or talking to their friends for fear of saying something embarrassing.

When to Seek Help
If any of the following symptoms are reported by a teen, seek immediate assistance from a mental health professional:
   Self-harm or thoughts about death and dying
   Threats of harm to others
   Substance abuse
   Severe aggression
   Hallucinations (e.g., hearing or seeing things) or paranoid thinking

The Interplay Between Anxiety and ADHD

Thinking back to our case example, Chloe, it can be difficult to detect an anxiety disorder in a teenager with ADHD because of overlapping symptoms. Inattention, a core symptom of ADHD, is also a common symptom of adolescent anxiety. For teens with ADHD and anxiety, inattention is often a major concern and can be mistakenly attributed to ADHD only. Fidgety behavior seen in ADHD may be similar to physical restlessness associated with anxiety. Some parents may attribute this solely to ADHD when it may be a telltale sign of anxiety. This is why it is important to have an open conversation with the teen about their symptoms instead of making assumptions based on what we already know.

There is some research to suggest that the presence of an anxiety disorder may actually "protect" against certain symptoms associated with ADHD. For instance, research has shown that children with ADHD and anxiety reliably do better on tasks of inhibitory control [9]. For certain teens, anxiety enhances their performance on tasks that require response inhibition. Some researchers have also found that children with ADHD and anxiety do better on tasks of sustained attention [9]. Unfortunately, these findings have not been widely replicated outside of the laboratory. For many teens with ADHD and anxiety, attentional issues may be even more pronounced than in teens with ADHD alone [10].

We also think that the combination of ADHD and comorbid anxiety may make some things harder for teens. Teenagers with ADHD and comorbid anxiety perform worse on tasks with high demands for remembering and learning information that requires effort and attention. Within the school setting, children with anxiety and ADHD show more impairment in certain areas of functioning. For instance, children with comorbid anxiety have double the frequency of placement in special classes and higher rates of extra help [11]. Low self-esteem has also been associated with anxiety and ADHD [12]. Children with concurrent anxiety disorders report higher levels of co-existing stressful life events than children with ADHD only [13]. Adolescents with anxiety and ADHD may also be at an increased risk for substance abuse problems.

Diagnostic Assessment

Just like ADHD, there is no blood test or x-ray to diagnose anxiety at this time. This means that a careful history and assessment is required by a mental health professional or medical provider. A diagnosis of comorbid anxiety may be made by a mental health clinician (e.g., psychologist, social worker, guidance counselor) or medical provider (e.g., psychiatrist, psychiatric nurse practitioner, pediatrician, developmental behavioral pediatrician, pediatric nurse practitioner). This involves a clinical interview with the adolescent and their parent/guardian as well as collateral feedback. A history should be obtained from both the parent and the adolescent, but it is imperative for the clinician to meet with the adolescent individually if possible. Parents may be better informants than adolescents about externalizing behavior associated with ADHD, but adolescents are usually better able to report their own internalizing symptoms. As we mentioned previously, teens can be good at hiding their thoughts and feelings, making an anxiety disorder difficult to identify.

The clinical interview involves a review of family history, birth and developmental history, medical history, and social history. Given the heritability of anxiety disorders, the evaluation should include a review of any mental health concerns in the immediate and extended family, including a history of anxiety disorders and whether family members received any formal treatment. When considering treatment for a teen, it is helpful to know if their family members have ever received any formal treatment for anxiety (e.g., medication or therapy) and how they responded to this treatment. The developmental history may reveal long-standing patterns of avoidance or shy and inhibited temperament in early childhood. A comprehensive medical history and review of symptoms can help rule out any underlying medical problems that could be causing or contributing to a teenager's anxiety. A clinician may ask targeted medical questions: Has your child had a history of a head injury? Have they seen a neurologist in the past? This is good time to inquire about any reported physical symptoms such as headaches or stomachaches. It also is important to disclose any repeat visits to the school nurse, primary care provider, or emergency department for these or other symptoms in the past. A provider may also ask about appetite changes and whether a teen is getting adequate sleep. Not only can sleep disturbances (e.g., nightmares, difficulty falling asleep, or inability to sleep alone) be symptomatic of anxiety, but sleep problems are also known to intensify anxiety symptoms. Certain medical conditions, like hyperthyroidism, and medications, such as corticosteroids or albuterol, can also mimic anxiety symptoms. Substance use, including abuse of cannabis and alcohol, can also induce anxiety symptoms in teens [14].

In addition to a comprehensive history and clinical interview, clinicians often use rating scales to help diagnose anxiety. These are usually pen-and-pencil scales (or Internet-based scales) that ask the teen about anxiety symptoms. For some of these scales, a parent version is also available. Ratings are summed to help determine whether an anxiety disorder may be likely or to estimate the severity of anxiety symptoms. Some adolescents with ADHD and anxiety will not voice their worries spontaneously and are more likely to be open when asked to complete rating scales (Table 8.1).

Table 8.1 Commonly used rating scales for assessment of anxiety in teenagers	Anxiety Rating Scales
	Multidimensional Anxiety Scale for Children, 2nd Edition (MASC2)
	Screen for Child Anxiety and Related Emotional Disorders (SCARED)
	Revised Children's Manifest Anxiety Scale, Second Edition (RCMAS-2)

Collateral feedback with teachers, staff, and other adults close to the adolescent is an important part of a comprehensive assessment. This information can help provide a richer perspective of the teen's school and social life as well as clarify any discrepancy between reports from the teen and their parents. This may include reaching out to an extended family member, coach, or tutor.

Treatment

An effective treatment plan is tailored to the teenager and their family. The first step is to identify the problem or symptom causing the greatest level of impairment. For some teens, this may be inattention or impulsivity secondary to ADHD. For others, it may be the excessive worries or gastrointestinal symptoms of anxiety. How do you know what condition is most impairing? Parents, teachers, and healthcare providers may not be aware to the extent of the adolescent's anxiety. The best place to start is by asking the teenager first. A teen may be able to provide very important insights into the course of treatment. When the primary symptom or set of symptoms are under better control, treatment for the secondary condition should begin.

There are certain instances in which treatment for the primary concern may prove too challenging, in which case it is better to start treatment for the secondary problem. For example, if a teen's anxiety symptoms, such as phobia of swallowing pills, are impairing their ability to engage in a treatment intervention (e.g., swallowing medication for ADHD), it will be important to treat the other condition first (e.g., start exposure therapy to help the teen overcome their pill swallowing phobia). On the other hand, if ADHD symptoms are impairing a child's ability to engage in psychotherapy (e.g., if a teen is unable to attend long enough to participate in therapy sessions), then treat the attentional problem first. We know that the course of the disorders is variable, and each may require short-term, intermittent, or long-term treatment and follow-up.

> *My kid's anxiety is better, but my pediatrician won't start a stimulant for ADHD.*
> This is, unfortunately, a big misunderstanding among many healthcare professionals. Though your pediatrician or primary care provider may think that stimulants make anxiety worse, the research tells us that this is not necessarily the case.

Anxiety disorders in teenagers are generally treatable. Early identification and treatment can prevent future difficulties, such as loss of friendships, failure to reach academic potential, and feelings of low self-esteem. Additionally, early intervention may help reduce the risk of persistent symptoms into adulthood [2]. Both psychotherapy and medication have been shown to be effective for anxiety problems in adolescence. However, we generally recommend a "multi-modal approach" to treatment for anxiety. This may include a combination of the following interventions, including individual therapy, family therapy, behavioral treatments, medications, and consultation to the teen's school.

For anxiety symptoms that are considered "mild or moderate," in that they do not severely limit the teen's ability to function, first-line treatment includes education (*psychoeducation*) about anxiety disorders, psychotherapy, parent guidance, and consultation to the school to help inform treatment planning and coordination of care.

Behavioral Treatment for Anxiety

Cognitive behavioral therapy (CBT) has gained the most attention for treatment of anxiety in teens because it is the most effective form of therapy and it is as effective if not more effective than medication.

> CBT helps teens identify the link between their thoughts and behaviors and learn effective strategies to minimize anxiety.

The treatment can be administered in an individual or group format. CBT involves several different treatment components including psychoeducation about anxiety, identification of difficult emotions, learning relaxation strategies (e.g., progressive muscle relaxation, diaphragmatic breathing), making the connection between thoughts and feelings, cognitive restructuring strategies, problem-solving, challenging negative emotions, and building positive emotions. For all teens, CBT involves regular practice outside of therapy appointments including weekly homework. Parents also play an important role in treatment as they may meet separately with a therapist to learn about anxiety and develop skills to manage anxiety at home.

There is some research to show that CBT for youth with ADHD and anxiety may require some modification to take into account challenges associated with ADHD. The Child-Adolescent Anxiety Multimodal Study (CAMS), a study funded by the National Institutes of Health, showed that anxious youth with ADHD fared worse than youth with anxiety alone when treated with CBT alone [15]. These findings suggest that CBT for this population may need to be adapted or prolonged to accommodate difficulties associated with comorbid ADHD. This has led some to develop CBT interventions specifically designed for youth with ADHD and comorbid anxiety. A research team in Australia developed a CBT intervention to help reduce levels of anxiety in teens with ADHD and found a significant decrease in anxiety symptoms with this 8-week program [16].

Medication Treatment for Anxiety

For moderate to severe symptoms of anxiety, a combination of therapy and medications is considered the gold standard. The CAMS study shows that youth who received combined medication and CBT treatments had a greater reduction in anxiety symptoms than youth who received medication or CBT alone [17].

> Medication should almost never be used alone and always combined with therapy.

Selective serotonin reuptake inhibitor (SSRI) medications are considered to be first-line medication treatment for anxiety in teens (Table 8.2). There is no strong evidence to suggest one particular SSRI over another. Instead, an SSRI is selected based on a combination of side effect profile, duration of onset, drug-to-drug interactions, and family response. An adequate trial of SSRI involves 4–6 weeks at a therapeutic dose. If a teen does not respond to the first SSRI trial, a second trial of an SSRI is often recommended. After two failed SSRI trials, consideration should be given to a non-SSRI medication, usually a serotonin and norepinephrine reuptake inhibitor (SNRI), along with continued utilization of therapy interventions. SNRIs include Effexor (venlafaxine) and Cymbalta (duloxetine). Cymbalta has been approved for treatment of GAD in children and has been increasingly used for treatment of anxiety in teens [18].

Once effective treatment has been established, medication should be continued for at least 6–12 months to avoid symptoms from returning [14]. We usually recommend that the medication be gradually tapered after this time frame. If any symptoms of anxiety re-emerge, we know that we need to consider restarting the medication at the lowest effective dose or boosting the dose back up to the level that seemed most helpful. Because some anxiety disorders may wax and wane, continuous assessment is needed. In some cases, children might need higher doses around the beginning (August–November) or end (April–June) of the school year [19].

All SSRIs and many other medications used for anxiety have a black box warning on their packaging label. This warning indicates that there is a risk of increased suicidal thoughts and behavior when beginning treatment with the medication. It

Table 8.2 Selective serotonin reuptake inhibitors

Brand name	Generic name
Prozac®	Fluoxetine
Zoloft®	Sertraline
Lexapro®	Escitalopram
Celexa®	Citalopram
Luvox®	Fluvoxamine
Paxil®	Paroxetine

will be important to monitor for worsening sadness, withdrawal, restlessness, elated mood, hostility, agitation, and suicidal ideation. Risk of suicidality may be especially high for patients with a family history of bipolar disorder or attempted suicide. It is important to develop a plan of action in advance should suicidality or aggression develop. Although the risk is small, it is important for parents and providers to take this into account and weigh the risks with the implications of untreated anxiety in the teen.

Atomoxetine, a selective norepinephrine reuptake inhibitor, is often considered for co-occurring anxiety with ADHD. This medication is the first non-stimulant approved for treatment of ADHD in children, adolescents, and adults. The role of atomoxetine in treatment of anxiety disorders has not been studied, but research shows reduction in anxiety and ADHD symptoms with atomoxetine [20]. Because atomoxetine cannot be abused, it may be a good medication for adolescents who are at risk for or have a history of substance abuse. Atomoxetine usually takes a few weeks to see its full benefit, and it may take up to 6 weeks to get to an effective dose.

> We typically do not recommend long-term treatment of anxiety with benzodiazepines due to high risk for abuse and addiction.

Other anxiety medications that may be helpful include anxiety-breaking agents called benzodiazepines, such as Ativan (lorazepam), Klonopin (clonazepam), and Xanax (alprazolam). Side effects of these medications include disinhibition and sedation as well as a potential for abuse and addiction. In general, we are careful with these medications in teens, because they are already at an increased risk for substance abuse and these medications can be highly addictive. Buspar (buspirone) is another medication that is used for everyday anxiety, whereas medications like propranolol or vistaril (hydroxyzine) are used for acute episodes of anxiety.

> *How do I talk to my child about medication?*
> Adolescents can be difficult because they may be distrustful of medication based on stories they've heard from friends or in the media. It is important to have an honest and open conversation with your teen.

One of the major reasons for medication failure in adolescents is non-adherence. Teens should be involved in their treatment from the early stages of assessment and onward. They should be educated about what to expect from the treatment and to recognize common side effects. By educating and empowering your teen, they are more likely to participate in their treatment.

Some tips to improve medication adherence include:

- Simplify the regimen (e.g., switch from twice-per-day dosing to single-day dosing)
- Set an alarm on your cell phone or use a medication reminder app
- Request school nurses to administer medication at school

> **Common problems that interfere with compliance in a teen:**
> They may think that they don't have a problem.
> They may think that their problem doesn't necessitate medication.
> They may be worried that the medication will change their personality.

Treatment of Anxiety: The Role of the School

Anxious teens may benefit from special accommodations at school to help minimize symptoms. Children spend most of their time in school, approximately 1000 h/year, so the school setting can be an important place for intervention. Every adolescent has different needs, so no one plan will work for every teen. Given the wide range of symptoms experienced by adolescents with anxiety disorders and ADHD, it is important to identify the teen's unique needs and develop a plan accordingly. Accommodations may change over time and regular check-ins with the treatment team are recommended to help assess what is working and what isn't (Table 8.3).

Special Considerations for Treatment of ADHD with Anxiety

We previously thought that teens with ADHD and comorbid anxiety responded differently to treatments for ADHD, but recent research shows that this is not true for most. The MTA study reported that children with ADHD and anxiety responded just as well to a program of medication and CBT for ADHD as children without an anxiety disorder [21, 22]. It was long believed that stimulants were less effective for treatment of ADHD in teens with comorbid anxiety compared with ADHD alone.

Table 8.3 Examples of school accommodations for adolescent anxiety

School accommodations for adolescent anxiety
Regular check-ins with the school guidance counselor or psychologist to help monitor anxiety and provide a "safe space" to discuss difficult feelings
Taking a break from class to get a drink of water or stretch can help reduce building pressure throughout the day and help the teen reenter class feeling calmer
Extended time on tests may help alleviate anxiety, and just knowing that the time is available may be enough for some teens
Having access to a separate and quiet environment for tests can ease stress and reduce distraction

Specifically, it was felt that the response to stimulants was blunted in this population making researchers question whether ADHD and anxiety constituted an entirely different subtype of ADHD [4]. However, data from longer-term studies show that children with and without anxiety have similar rates of improvement in ADHD symptoms with stimulants [4, 23]. One study showed that the presence of an anxiety disorder predicted better response to treatment as measured by teachers [24].

In the case that a teen develops worsening anxiety on stimulants, the first-line medication treatment for ADHD, a trial of atomoxetine or an alpha agonist may be helpful. The short-acting alpha agonists, Tenex (guanfacine) and Catapres (clonidine), may be preferred over the long-acting agonists, Intuniv (guanfacine) and Kapvay (clonidine), or vice versa. In general, non-stimulants are thought to be less effective than the stimulants in treating ADHD symptoms, but they do provide coverage throughout the day with fewer side effects in some cases.

Case Revisited

It can be tricky to disentangle teen inattention from anxiety, but Chloe makes it easier by telling us the content of her thoughts. Chloe's evaluation should include a comprehensive update of her academic, social, and emotional functioning. Current ADHD symptoms should be reviewed, understanding that untreated ADHD symptoms might contribute to her current anxiety. Using a rating scale will help gather her symptoms in a standardized manner. Chloe may benefit from behavioral treatments for anxiety, such as from cognitive restructuring and relaxation techniques. If her anxiety persists, escalates, or interferes with function, Chloe may also benefit from an SSRI.

Tips
- Screen for anxiety occurring with ADHD from a young age. Early intervention may help reduce the risk of persistent symptoms into adulthood.
- Though anxiety disorders affect significantly more females on average, males and females with ADHD are affected by anxiety disorders at similar rates.
- Medication is often not the first intervention for anxiety with ADHD in teens. Consider behavioral or other therapies and school accommodations.

Conclusions

Anxiety disorders are very common in adolescents and occur even more frequently in teens with ADHD than teens without the diagnosis. Early identification and treatment of anxiety may improve functioning in youth with ADHD and reduce the persistence of anxiety disorders into adulthood. The assessment of anxiety disorders and ADHD involves a careful history and assessment including a detailed history of the presenting problems, developmental history, medical history, social history, and family history. It is essential to remember that teens may be better able to report symptoms of anxiety than their parents and should be involved in their treatment from the very beginning. Both disorders should be considered in the treatment plan, and the teen should help identify which problem areas should be addressed first. The course of treatment may vary from teen to teen, and it is important to monitor treatment effects for both disorders.

References

1. American Psychological Association. Stress in America: are teens adopting adults' stress habits? 2014. https://www.apa.org/news/press/releases/stress/2013/stress-report.pdf. Accessed 15 Feb 2019.
2. Merikangas KR, He JP, Burstein M, Swanson SA, Avenevoli S, Cui L, et al. Lifetime prevalence of mental disorders in U.S. adolescents: results from the National Comorbidity Survey Replication--Adolescent Supplement (NCS-A). J Am Acad Child Adolesc Psychiatry. 2010;49(10):980–9.
3. Biederman J, Faraone SV, Keenan K, Knee D, Tsuang MT. Family-genetic and psychosocial risk factors in DSM-III attention deficit disorder. J Am Acad Child Adolesc Psychiatry. 1990;29(4):526–33.
4. Tannock R. ADHD with anxiety disorders. In: Brown TE, editor. ADHD comorbidities: handbook for ADHD complications in children and adults. Arlington, VA, USA: American Psychiatric Publishing, Inc.; 2009. p. 131–55.
5. Biederman J, Faraone SV, Spencer T, Wilens T, Mick E, Lapey KA. Gender differences in a sample of adults with attention deficit hyperactivity disorder. Psychiatry Res. 1994;53(1):13–29.
6. Rucklidge JJ, Tannock R. Psychiatric, psychosocial, and cognitive functioning of female adolescents with ADHD. J Am Acad Child Adolesc Psychiatry. 2001;40:530–40.
7. Tai YM, Gau CS, Gau SS, Chiu HW. Prediction of ADHD to anxiety disorders: an 11-year national insurance data analysis in Taiwan. J AttenDisord. 2013;17(8):660–9.
8. Beesdo K, Knappe S, Pine DS. Anxiety and anxiety disorders in children and adolescents: developmental issues and implications for DSM-V. Psychiatr Clin North Am. 2009;32(3):483–524.
9. Jarrett MA, Wolff JC, Davis TE III, Cowart MJ, Ollendick TH. Characteristics of children with ADHD and comorbid anxiety. J Atten Disord. 2016;20(7):636–44.
10. Maric M, Bexkens A, Bögels SM. Is clinical anxiety a risk or a protective factor for executive functioning in youth with ADHD? A meta-regression analysis. Clin Child Fam Psychol Rev. 2018;21(3):340–53.
11. Angold A, Costello EJ, Erkanli A. Comorbidity. J Child Psychol Psychiatry. 1999;40(1):57–87.
12. Bussing R, Levin GM. Methamphetamine and fluoxetine treatment of a child with attention-deficit hyperactivity disorder and obsessive-compulsive disorder. J Child Adolesc Psychopharmacol. 1993;3(1):53–8.
13. Newcorn JH, Miller SR, Ivanova I, Schulz KP, Kalmar J, Marks DJ. Adolescent outcome of ADHD: impact of childhood conduct and anxiety disorders. CNS Spectr. 2004;9(9):668–78.
14. Connolly SD, Bernstein GA. Practice parameter for the assessment and treatment of children and adolescents with anxiety disorders. J Am Acad Child Adolesc Psychiatry. 2007;46(2):267–83.
15. Halldorsdottir T, Ollendick TH, Ginsburg G, Sherrill J, Kendall PC, Walkup J, et al. Treatment outcomes in anxious youth with and without comorbid ADHD in the CAMS. J Clin Child Adolesc Psychol. 2015;44(6):985–91.

16. Houghton S, Alsalmi N, Tan C, Taylor M, Durkin K. Treating comorbid anxiety in adolescents with ADHD using a cognitive behavior therapy program approach. J Atten Disord. 2017;21(13):1094–104.
17. Walkup JT, Albano AM, Piacentini J, Birmaher B, Compton SN, Sherrill JT, et al. Cognitive behavioral therapy, sertraline, or a combination in childhood anxiety. N Engl J Med. 2008;359(26):2753–66.
18. Strawn JR, Welge JA, Wehry AM, Keeshin B, Rynn MA. Efficacy and tolerability of antidepressants in pediatric anxiety disorders: a systematic review and meta-analysis. *Depress Anxiety*. 2014;32(3):149–57.
19. Pine DS. Treating children and adolescents with selective serotonin reuptake inhibitors: how long is appropriate? J Child AdolescPsychopharmacol. 2002;12(3):189–203.
20. Geller D, Donnelly C, Lopez F, Rubin R, Newcorn J, Sutton V, et al. Atomoxetine treatment for pediatric patients with attention-deficit/hyperactivity disorder with comorbid anxiety disorder. J Am Acad Child Adolesc Psychiatry. 2007;46(9):1119–27.
21. MTA Cooperative Group. A 14-month randomized clinical trial of treatment strategies for attention-deficit/hyperactivity disorder. Multimodal treatment study of children with ADHD. Arch Gen Psychiatry. 1999;56:1073–86.
22. Jensen PS, Hinshaw SP, Kraemer HC, Lenora N, Newcorn JH, Abikoff HB, et al. ADHD comorbidity findings from the MTA study: comparing comorbid subgroups. J Am Acad Child Adolesc Psychiatry. 2001;40:147–58.
23. Abikoff HB, Jensen PS, Arnold LL, Hoza B, Hechtman L, Pollack S, et al. Observed classroom behavior of children with ADHD: relationship to gender and comorbidity. J Abnorm Child Psychol. 2002;30(4):349–59.
24. van der Oord S, Prins PJ, Oosterlaan J, Emmelkamp PM. Treatment of attention deficit hyperactivity disorder in children.Predictors of treatment outcome. Eur Child Adolesc Psychiatry. 2008;17(2):73–81.

Chapter 9
ADHD and Depression

Olivia Carrick and Rachel Tunick

Case Example

Courtney, an active and vivacious 14-year-old ninth grader, had been diagnosed with ADHD (with a predominantly inattentive presentation) during the early elementary school years. After some deliberation, her family had made the decision to pursue psychopharmacological treatment when increasing academic demands, in combination with Courtney's attentional difficulties, began to take a toll on her academic performance, when she was in the fourth grade. Over recent years, her parents were very pleased with their daughter's continued educational progress. Courtney had also chosen to pursue several extracurricular interests, joining a dance class and a community swim team, and she had a close group of friends.

However, since Courtney's transition to high school earlier in the year, her parents began to notice concerning changes in their daughter. She seemed increasingly reluctant to participate in her swim and dance practice, frequently complaining about being too tired or preferring to stay alone in her room at home instead. At home she was often irritable and cranky; she frequently picked fights with her younger brother or argued over petty matters during family dinners. On her second-semester report card, several of Courtney's teachers indicated concern about her attention during classroom instruction, and she was missing homework assignments in several of her classes.

O. Carrick (✉) · R. Tunick
Department of Psychiatry, Boston Children's Hospital, Harvard Medical School,
Boston, MA, USA
e-mail: olivia.carrick@childrens.harvard.edu; rachel.tunick@childrens.harvard.edu

© Springer Nature Switzerland AG 2020
A. Schonwald (ed.), *ADHD in Adolescents*,
https://doi.org/10.1007/978-3-030-62393-7_9

Background

All teenagers can be moody, and adolescence is a period of time which is fairly notorious for emotional turmoil and drama. For many youngsters, intermittent sadness, mood swings, and emotional turbulence are not all that unusual and may in fact be developmentally normative. However, if accompanied by other changes, such as sudden or marked social withdrawal, decline in academic performance or motivation, and/or changes in sleep or appetite, these mood changes may be signs of clinical depression. While all teens are vulnerable toward experiencing such difficulties, teenage girls are especially susceptible; beginning in adolescence, depression is about twice as common in females, relative to males.

Depression can strike at any age across the lifespan, but the incidence of this disorder increases profoundly during adolescence and young adulthood.

There are two main types of clinical depression: major depressive disorder (MDD; Table 9.1) in which defining symptoms are present for at least 2 weeks and persistent depressive disorder (or dysthymia; Table 9.2) where symptoms are more

Table 9.1 DSM-5 criteria for major depressive disorder

Major depressive disorder	
Five or more of nine symptoms for at least 2 continuous weeks (one symptom must be either depressed/irritable mood or diminished interest and pleasure):	
	1. Depressed mood most of the day, nearly every day. In children and adolescents, can substitute "irritable" mood
	2. Diminished interest and pleasure
	3. Significant decrease in weight (5%). In children, failure to make expected weight gains
	4. Sleep disturbances (difficulty falling or staying asleep, early waking, sleeping more than usual)
	5. Psychomotor agitation or retardation
	6. Fatigue or loss of energy
	7. Feelings of worthlessness or excessive guilt
	8. Diminished ability to think or concentrate or indecisiveness
	9. Thoughts of death or suicidal ideation
Symptoms cause meaningful impairment	
Symptoms are not caused by substance use or another medical condition	

Adapted from American Psychiatric Association [37]

Table 9.2 DSM-V diagnostic criteria for persistent depressive disorder (dysthymia)

Persistent depressive disorder (dysthymia)	
A. Depressed mood (or irritability for children and adolescents) for most of the day, for more days than not for at least 1 year for children and adolescents (2 years in adults)	
B. Presence while depressed of two or more of the following:	1. Poor appetite/overeating
	2. Insomnia or hypersomnia
	3. Low energy or fatigue
	4. Low self-esteem
	5. Poor concentration or difficulty making decisions
	6. Feelings of hopelessness
During the 1 year period of the disturbance, the person has never been without symptoms in Criteria A or B for >2 months at a time	
There has never been a manic or hypomanic episode	
The symptoms do not occur exclusively in the context of a chronic psychotic disorder, and symptoms are not due to the effects of a substance or a general medical condition	

Adapted from American Psychiatric Association [37]

intermittent or less severe but can persist for a year or longer. Both of these types of depression can lead to significant impairment with regard to an individual's emotional, social, and academic functioning and (particularly if unaddressed) may lead to far-reaching and at times devastating consequences at this developmental stage. Even when symptoms of depression are below threshold to meet diagnostic criteria for either of these disorders, they can create significant disruption and disarray in one's overall health and well-being.

Prevalence

Adolescents with attention-deficit/hyperactivity disorder (ADHD) are at higher risk for developing depression, compared to their peers who do not have ADHD. While ADHD is a neurodevelopmental disorder that begins in childhood, with symptoms that typically persist across the lifespan into adulthood, the incidence of major depressive disorder (MDD) peaks during the adolescent and young adult years. Moreover, though a single lifetime episode of MDD is certainly possible, most commonly MDD relapses following its initial occurrence. In those with ADHD and MDD, MDD usually presents several years after the onset of symptoms of ADHD [1, 2].

MDD alone has been found to occur in approximately 2% of children and 8% of adolescents [3]. The rate of MDD in youths with ADHD is over five times higher, compared to youths without ADHD [4]. A prospective longitudinal study of children diagnosed with ADHD in early childhood found that youth with ADHD were at significantly greater risk for single and multiple episodes of adolescent depression and suicidal behavior prior to age 18 than comparison children [5]. Furthermore, youth with both ADHD and depression have been found to have more severe symptoms, as well as higher rates of long-term impairment, compared to youth with either disorder alone. Importantly, early treatment of ADHD has been associated with lower risk of the development of subsequent symptoms of MDD [6]. This finding underscores the benefits of early identification and intervention to prevent or mitigate the onset of depressive symptoms and associated consequences.

Prevalence rates regarding the co-occurrence of ADHD and MDD have been found to be quite variable across studies. Estimates regarding the prevalence of depression in youngsters with a diagnosis of ADHD have been found to range from 12% to 50% [1, 4]. These numbers also vary markedly across sex and age [7]. For example, Beiderman et al. found that 11% of girls with ADHD had comorbid MDD, but by adulthood, 72% of women with ADHD also met diagnostic criteria for MDD [3]. The same authors found that in males, the rate of comorbid ADHD and depression was more stable across development, with 21% of boys with ADHD, and 35% of adult men with ADHD, also meeting diagnostic criteria for comorbid MDD. There is also evidence to suggest that prevalence rates of the two disorders diverge over the course of development. For example, in a longitudinal community study, the prevalence of ADHD symptoms was found to diminish with age, while in contrast, symptoms of depression were found to increase over the course of development [8].

Etiology

Given the potential for significant lifetime consequences related to having both disorders, it is important to consider the various factors that may be involved in the development of depression in the context of ADHD. Recognition and understanding regarding the various environmental, familial, and other risk factors for the development of comorbid depression in youth with ADHD may help to inform and guide prevention and intervention strategies for adolescents at risk for the development of both disorders. Why certain adolescents with ADHD are more vulnerable toward developing depression is not fully understood, and the reasons for the overlap between these two disorders are likely multifactorial and complex. However, a number of risk factors have been identified.

1. *Academic performance deficits* (which often may be either caused or exacerbated by symptoms of ADHD or related problems) may increase risk for the development of symptoms of depression. When children enter school, they are met with various demands regarding compliance, concentration, and participation in cooperative peer activities, all of which may present particular difficulties for youngsters with ADHD. The associated increased risk of academic failure, conflict with teachers, and general school dissatisfaction may in turn predispose youths with ADHD to the subsequent development of depressive symptoms.

2. Children and adolescents with ADHD are known to have various *difficulties across the social functioning domain*, and such impairments have also been implicated as risk factors for the development of depressive symptoms, for a range of reasons. For example, hallmark characteristics of ADHD, such as hyperactivity and impulse control problems, may contribute to peer rejection, particularly in later childhood and adolescence. Additionally, symptoms of inattention may make it more difficult for kids to adequately notice and attend to subtle social cues which are important in the context of the development and maturation of interpersonal skills, and as a result, social interactions may suffer. In such circumstances, it has been posited that peer rejection and social isolation may lead to the development of depressive symptoms.

3. Beyond the academic and social vulnerabilities that have been associated with ADHD, core ADHD symptoms in a child or adolescent may impact upon parenting practices and ultimately *parent-child relationships*, which may in turn increase risk for a child with ADHD to develop symptoms of depression. For example, symptoms associated with ADHD including impulsivity, hyperactivity, and inattention may inadvertently provoke more negative and inconsistent parenting practices [9]. Such parenting interactions have been found to be associated with negative cognitions that tend to be characteristic in children and adolescents with depression [10].

4. *Internal factors such as irritability and emotion regulation* have been studied as a link between ADHD and depression [11]. Emotion dysregulation is common in ADHD and contributes to the severity of impairment [12]. A study of adolescents with ADHD found emotion regulation to be a mediator in the relationship between ADHD and depression in youth [13].

5. The development of depression in youth with ADHD may also be influenced by factors pertaining to other *psychiatric comorbidities*. Both anxiety and disruptive behavior disorders have been found to increase one's risk of developing depressive disorder [14]. Roy and colleagues collected data from Tracking Adolescents' Individual Lives Survey (TRAILS) and examined the effects of ADHD, anxiety, and disruptive behaviors on the development of depression. They found that in adolescents who met diagnostic criteria for ADHD, as well as those with subthreshold ADHD symptoms, there was increased risk for the development of symptoms of depression. These researchers concluded that the pathway from ADHD to depression is at least partially mediated by symptoms of anxiety and the presence of disruptive behavior problems.

6. Another variable that has the potential to impact development of depressive symptoms in youth with ADHD relates to the pharmacological treatment of this disorder. While there have been reports of mood changes with medications for ADHD, there is at least one study that found that *delayed pharmacotherapy for ADHD* increased the likelihood of later developing depression [14], and the authors suggest that treating ADHD in childhood may be protective against developing depression later in life. With regard to this topic, more research is needed to determine how other factors, such as female sex, may influence the treatment course and development of depression in youth with ADHD.

Morbidity

ADHD is a developmental disorder that begins in childhood. The symptoms of ADHD change throughout the life cycle. Most typically, symptoms of impulsivity and hyperactivity associated with ADHD are at their worst during the school-age years, but inattention persists and can worsen as cognitive demands increase, and as such these symptoms often persist into adulthood. Depression typically first manifests itself years after the onset of ADHD.

While it can occur as a single episode, depression is a chronic disorder for many patients, with a significant likelihood for relapse after first episode of major depression. While having either of these disorders individually may be associated with significant effects across various domains of development, when the two disorders co-occur, the symptom severity and accompanying impairment may be far worse. In addition, the rate of self-injurious behavior and suicide is higher in adolescents with ADHD and MDD relative to those with MDD alone [15]. Beiderman and colleagues followed adolescent and young adult females over a 5-year period and found that patients with both depression and ADHD tend to have earlier onset of depression, longer durations of depressive episodes, and higher rates of suicidality and psychiatric hospitalizations compared to those with depression alone [3].

Additional psychiatric comorbidity is common with both ADHD and depression. Oppositional defiant disorder (ODD) and conduct disorder (CD) are commonly diagnosed with ADHD, and anxiety disorders are frequently diagnosed with depression. When ADHD and depression occur together, they are often associated with one or more of these added other disorders, further complicating the presentation and treatment course.

> Depressive episodes in youth with ADHD can be more prolonged and harder to treat, compared to such episodes in others who do not have ADHD.

Impairment often persists across the lifespan. Level of impairment later in life may be associated with the severity of the condition at onset, other comorbidities, or other environmental factors. Adults who have both ADHD and depression have been found to experience higher overall healthcare costs compared to those with depression alone [16]. Given the severity of symptoms and impairment when depression and ADHD occur together, it is important to understand effective assessment and intervention strategies in adolescents in order to optimize outcomes across a range of domains.

Assessment

If you suspect that your teenager is struggling with symptoms of depression, it is important to take some thoughtful next steps in order to better understand the nature of these difficulties:

- As a first step, parents are encouraged to initiate dialogue with their child in a gentle and nonjudgmental manner, noting symptoms that they've observed and soliciting input from their child regarding their sense about what might be going on. These conversations can certainly be challenging and fraught and may be optimized by parent efforts to focus on listening to their child and acknowledging and validating their perspectives.
- Reaching out for professional help may be warranted particularly if your child's current difficulties appear to be getting in the way of their daily functioning (e.g., interfering with social and/or family relationships, negatively affecting academic performance), represent a notable shift from their typical presentation, and/or are accompanied by thoughts about self-harm.
- Meeting with your child's pediatrician is a recommended next step in the evaluation process. The pediatrician may conduct preliminary assessment, including administering standardized parent- and self-report screening measures and talking with you and your child about your concerns. A thoughtful review about these matters may help to rule out any potentially contributing medical factors, and begin to shed some light on whether current difficulties may reflect an exacerbation of the child's ADHD (as the presentation of this developmental disorder can vary over time), or may be suggestive of concerns beyond the ADHD domain. Depending on the level and nature of concern, the pediatrician may recommend further, more in-depth assessment by a behavioral health professional. Some pediatric practices are staffed by behavioral health providers who can complete such assessment on-site, and others will refer your child to a child psychologist, psychiatrist, or similar professional in your community.
- A comprehensive and evidence-based evaluation is crucial in order to clarify the specific nature of teens' difficulties [17, 18]. Optimally, a thorough assessment is closely tied to subsequent treatment, and will be used to help inform and guide decisions about when and how to treat, as well as regarding specific targets of intervention [17]. Assessments typically consist of various components:
  - Interview (with both parents and adolescent) regarding current concerns and pertinent history (e.g., family, developmental, medical, school, social).
  - Completion of additional self- and parent-report symptom rating scales and questionnaires. These measures will typically include questions about both broadband and narrowly focused domains of functioning as symptoms of depression (particularly in overlap with ADHD) may mimic other concerns such as effects of substance use or other disorders of emotion or behavior regulation such as anxiety or disruptive behavior disorders [1]. Multi-informant perspectives (including input from teachers or other individuals working closely with your child) are often included in a comprehensive evaluation as well. Across parents, teachers, and the adolescents, there may not always be agreement about current concerns [19], and as such the integration and consolidation across information from multiple perspectives will help the clinician to derive a thorough and comprehensive understanding about your

child and to generate a nuanced conceptualization about the nature of their current difficulties.
- Formal assessment typically concludes with a feedback session, together with the adolescent and their parents, at which point the clinician will share their conceptualization and initiate discussions about treatment recommendations.

Ideally, over the course of treatment, more informal ongoing assessment will continue in order to monitor for the development of any new or changing symptoms, gauge progress, and modify treatment recommendations as needed.

Treatment

The recommended treatment for co-occurring depression in teens with ADHD will vary depending upon the specific circumstances, symptoms, and history of each individual. Ideally, your child's treatment course will be informed and guided, in a customized manner, by a thorough and comprehensive evaluation, in order to optimize its effectiveness. The behavioral health professional working with your child will generally conclude their assessment by meeting together with you and your child, in order to review assessment findings and to discuss treatment planning and goal-setting. In general, treatment for comorbid depression and ADHD will typically involve psychotherapy, pharmacological management, or a combination of these two approaches [20].

> Thoughts about suicide and/or self-harm may at times accompany other symptoms of depression. Should you be concerned about such symptoms, a more acute assessment such as in a hospital emergency department or via a psychiatric emergency response program may be warranted.

Psychotherapy

Cognitive behavioral therapy (CBT) is a therapeutic approach with a strong evidence base for the treatment of symptoms of depression across a wide age range, and as such this is most often the psychotherapeutic approach of choice for teens with depression. This is a short-term treatment modality with roots in both cognitive and behavioral approaches. Beck's classic cognitive vulnerability model [21] identifies maladaptive thinking patterns (e.g., tendency to selectively attend to negative rather than positive attribute of situations) as major causal and maintaining factors in the context of depression, while behavioral theories [22] emphasize the role of maladaptive actions. CBT combines elements from both approaches and focuses on the interrelations and connections among one's thoughts, feelings, and behavior, particularly in the context of the onset and maintenance of behavioral health problems such as depression. This therapeutic approach aims to promote self-awareness and self-understanding, particularly around one's tendency to get "stuck" in negative cycles, and entails structured sessions with active, collaborative goal-setting and skill-building, homework assignments for additional practice and skill-building outside of sessions, and continual efforts around treatment monitoring. CBT for depression in teenagers typically involves various specific components including behavioral activation (e.g., encouraging social connections, encouraging participation in pleasurable activities); bolstering of problem-solving skills; identifying and challenging of negative, maladaptive thoughts; and supporting the development of new, more adaptive coping strategies [23, 24].

Across many studies, including the large-scale Treatment for Adolescents with Depression Study (TADS), CBT has been found to have a moderate effect size for the treatment of depression in adolescents, to have a positive effect on suicidal ideation, and to facilitate the maintenance of therapeutic gains. Adolescents with moderate to severe depression who are treated with both medication and CBT have been found to show more rapid improvements in the early stages of treatment and to have a diminished risk of emerging suicidality [20, 25]. CBT has been found to be a well-established intervention for the treatment of adolescent depression in both individual and group formats [23].

To our knowledge, no CBT treatments have been specifically developed or tested for adolescents with comorbid ADHD and depression. There have been some studies in teens with both diagnoses, in which CBT alone or in combination with medication management was associated with more positive outcomes, compared to those who underwent placebo treatment [26]. More recently, a study examining the effects of various treatments for depressed adolescents found that improvement in depressive symptoms (either in the context of medication management alone or in combination with CBT) also led to improvement in terms of comorbid ADHD symptoms, even though those symptoms were not specifically targeted in treatment [27]. These findings underscore the importance of treatment of comorbid depressive symptoms in adolescents with ADHD and suggest that such approaches may in fact lead to amelioration of both disorders.

While there is very limited evidence to support the effectiveness of CBT for those with ADHD alone, a relatively recent study [28] found that adolescents with ADHD and comorbid depression showed greater improvement (compared to those with ADHD alone) following a CBT-based intervention specifically targeting ADHD symptoms. Specific components of this intervention are listed in Table 9.3.

These findings suggest that treatment for teens with both ADHD and depression may be optimized through the thoughtful targeting of prominent symptoms of each disorder. More broadly, there has been some recent attention across the field of child and adolescent psychology around the targeting of general principles of therapeutic change in psychotherapeutic protocols, as opposed to the delivery of focal treatments for specific diagnostic presentations [29]. Such "transdiagnostic" approaches (which include CBT-based interventions targeting diagnostically cross-cutting

Table 9.3 Common components of CBT for ADHD

Common components of CBT for ADHD
Psychoeducation about ADHD
Training in organization and planning skills
Skills aimed at reducing procrastination, bolstering communication skills, and improving anger/frustration management

domains such as emotion regulation, problem-solving, and motivation) hold promise for the treatment of comorbid ADHD and depression, but will require further
investigation and study in youths with symptoms of both disorders.

As noted above, adolescents with comorbid depression and ADHD are at elevated risk for problems across various academic and interpersonal domains, and in
fact social difficulties (including parent-child and peer relationship problems) in
youths with ADHD have been associated with the subsequent development of
symptoms of depression [30]. These areas of functioning may thus be important
treatment targets as well, beyond treatment aimed at alleviating specific symptoms.
Such aims may be included within the broader framework of CBT. As an alternative, interpersonal psychotherapy (IPT) is another approach that is viewed as a well-
established intervention for the treatment of adolescent depression, and which may
be of particular benefit in circumstances where interpersonal conflict and problematic peer relationships are central characteristics of an adolescent's presentation
[31]. In this approach (which has its roots in interpersonal theory of depression), the
fluctuating nature of interpersonal relationships during adolescence (such as changing relationships with parents and peers and increasing autonomy) is conceptualized
as contributing to the development of depressive symptoms. For those with ADHD,
this may be particularly pertinent, given susceptibility toward social functioning
problems of various natures [30]. Treatment within the IPT modality aims to
decrease depressive symptoms by targeting the interpersonal context in which it
unfolds through psychoeducation, interpersonal skill-building, and a supportive
therapeutic relationship [31].

With regard to elevated risk for problems in the domain of academic functioning,
families are encouraged to be in communication with staff at their children's school
in order to discuss potential eligibility for a 504 Plan or Individualized Educational
Plan (IEP) through the Individuals with Disabilities Act, in order to support the
development of customized school-based supports and accommodations [1, 6].
These may include adjustments or modifications in assignments or tasks (such as
allotment of extra time for assignment completion or extra help around breaking
down complex assignments and setting up schedules or study habits), consultation
with a school-based behavioral health professional (school psychologist, counselor,
or social worker) as needed, and engaging with the student in a collaborative relationship, in order that they may play an active role in their own support planning.

Given the high risk for the development of symptoms of depression in adolescents with ADHD, routine screening for depressive and related symptoms in those
with ADHD is strongly encouraged [32]. Furthermore, it has been suggested that in

some cases, the adaptation and incorporation of more formalized depression prevention programs within existing ADHD treatment programs for adolescents may
be warranted, even in the absence of the emergence of depressive symptoms [33].
Such prevention programs may be particularly beneficial for those known to be at
elevated risk for depression, such as through a strong family history of depression
or other known risk factors. Application of the cognitive behavioral model in a pre-
ventative manner is an area that is undergoing active research and one which holds
great promise for a meaningful clinical and public health impact [24].

Medication Management

There are few studies to inform medication treatment recommendations for youth
with ADHD and comorbid depression. For ADHD alone, psychostimulants
(methylphenidate-based, dextroamphetamine-based medications) are the first-line
treatments of choice in most cases with second-line choices being atomoxetine and
long-acting alpha-agonists (long-acting formulations of clonidine and guanfacine).
In the case of depression, there is evidence supporting the use of selective serotonin
reuptake inhibitors (SSRIs) as first-line medication treatments in adolescents. There
are two SSRIs that have FDA approval for depression in the pediatric population:
fluoxetine (ages 8+) and escitalopram (ages 13+).

A consensus conference was held in 1998 in Texas, and from this algorithms
were developed informing the treatment of MDD and comorbid conditions. The
Texas Children's Medication Algorithm Project revised their recommendations in
2006 [34] and provided updated recommendations for treatment of ADHD and
comorbid depression. The group recommended that in the context of both disorders,
but where depressive symptoms are milder, there should be a trial of a psychostimulant for 2 weeks at a sufficient dose. If both depressive and ADHD symptoms
improve, the stimulant alone should be continued. If after the stimulant is started,
though, the ADHD or depressive symptoms worsen, the stimulant should be discontinued. In the case that ADHD symptoms improve but depressive symptoms do not
improve, the addition of an SSRI medication should be considered while continuing
the stimulant. If in a patient with ADHD and MDD/dysthymia, the depressive
symptoms are the most prominent or more severe (i.e., marked loss of appetite,
weight loss, severe sleep disturbance, suicidal intent or plan), starting with antidepressant medication is recommended.

While there are a few reports that stimulants can cause depressive symptoms or
that potential side effects of stimulant medication could mimic symptoms of depression [1], there is evidence that treatment for ADHD may reduce likelihood of depression. Stimulant medication used in treatment of ADHD may reduce symptoms of
depression in ADHD [35]. It is also possible that depressive symptoms present as a
consequence of untreated ADHD. If depression symptoms resolve after stimulant
treatment alone, the validity of the depression diagnosis should be reconsidered. In
addition, at least one study indicated that in those with ADHD and comorbid

depression, there is an increased risk of treatment resistance to antidepressants (treatment failure in ≥ 2 different antidepressants) and that in those that had regular ADHD treatment there was a lower likelihood of antidepressant resistance [36].

> While two medications may be indicated to treat both disorders, it is best not to start with both treatments at the same time; new medications should always be added one at a time.

Increased suicidality (suicidal behavior, suicidal ideation, and suicide attempts) has been reported in children, adolescents, and young adults who are prescribed antidepressants. In the studies documenting this rare risk, the average risk of increased suicidality was 4% (risk of increased suicidality with placebo medication was 2%). In the studies that were pooled that resulted in this data, suicidal ideation was the most common event, and there were no completed suicides among the youth included in the trials (Food and Drug Administration 2004). When antidepressant medication is indicated, it should be used, and there should be close follow-up after these medications are started. The FDA recommends following up weekly during a medication titration due to this rare but potential increase in suicidality linked with starting or titrating doses of antidepressants. It is important to educate parents to look for mood worsening, increased agitation, or suicidal behaviors/thoughts when antidepressants are being initiated or titrated.

Case Revisited

Courtney is displaying symptoms of depression (decreased interest in participating, fatigue, irritability), but some of her symptoms (inattention during classroom instruction, missing homework assignments in several of her classes) are explained by untreated ADHD as well. The first step is for her parents to initiate a dialogue about their observations, seeking Courtney's input and perspective. She may next visit with her primary care provider, where a comprehensive clinical interview helps clarify her current needs. Standardized parent and self-report measures will help gather detailed information, and depending on the level and nature of concern, the pediatrician may recommend further, more in-depth assessment by a behavioral health professional.

Conclusion

The presence of depressive disorders in the context of ADHD in adolescents is common, and often these youth present with more severe symptoms and greater functional impairment. Thorough assessment, including information from multiple sources, is important to yield accurate diagnosis and prompt treatment initiation. While evidence-based recommendations are available based on preliminary studies, more research is needed to help guide treatment of youth with ADHD and comorbid depression.

> **Tips**
> - Adolescents with ADHD should be screened systematically for depression, since the rate of major depressive disorder in youths with ADHD is over five times higher compared to youths without ADHD.
> - Try to find quality therapy for adolescents with ADHD and depression. Cognitive behavioral therapy has been found to have a moderate effect size for the treatment of depression in adolescents, to have a positive effect on suicidal ideation, and to facilitate the maintenance of therapeutic gains.

References

1. Daviss WB. A review of comorbid depression in pediatric ADHD: etiologies, phenomenology, and treatment. J Child Adolesc Psychopharmacol. 2008;18(6):565–71.
2. Jerrell JM, McIntyre RS, Mark Park YM. Risk factors for major depressive disorder in children and adolescents with attention-deficit/hyperactivity disorder. Eur Child Adolesc Psychiatry. 2015;24:65–73.
3. Beiderman J, Ball SW, Monuteaux MC, Mick E, Spencer TJ, McCreary M, Cote M, Faraone SV. New insights into the comorbidity between ADHD and major depression in adolescent and young adult females. J Am Acad Child Adolesc Psychiatry. 2008;47(4):426–34.
4. Angold A, Costello EJ, Erkanli A. Comorbidity. J Child Psychol Psychiatry. 1999;40(1):57–87.
5. Chronis-Tuscano A, Molina BG, Pelham WE, Applegate B, Dahlke A, Overmyer M, Lahey BB. Very early predictors of adolescent depression and suicide attempts in children with attention-deficit/hyperactivity disorder. Arch Gen Psychiatry. 2010;67(10):1044–51.
6. Daviss WB, Bond JB. Comorbid ADHD and depression: assessment and treatment strategies. Psychiatr Times. 2016;33(9). http://www.psychiatrictimes.com/special-reports/comorbid-adhd-and-depression-assessment-and-treatment-strategies/
7. Carlson GA, Meyer S. ADHD with mood disorders. In: Brown T, editor. ADHD comorbidities handbook for ADHD complications in children and adults. Arlington: American Psychiatric Publishing; 2009. p. 97–109.
8. Costello EJ, Mustillo S, Erkanli A, Keeler G, Angold A. Prevalence and development of psychiatric disorders in childhood and adolescence. Arch Gen Psychiatry. 2003;60:837–44.
9. Ostrander R, Herman KC. Potential cognitive, parenting, and developmental mediators of the relationship between ADHD and depression. J Consult Clin Psychol. 2006;74(1):89–98.
10. Rudolph KD, Kurlakowsky KD, Conley CS. Developmental and social-contextual origins of depressive control-related beliefs and behavior. Cogn Ther Res. 2001;25:447–75.
11. Eyre O, Langley K, Stringaris A, Leibenluft E, Collishaw S, Thapar A. Irritability in ADHD: associations with depression liability. J Affect Disord. 2017;215:281–7.
12. Shaw P, Stringaris A, Leibenluft E. Emotional dysregulation and attention-deficit/hyperactivity disorder. Am J Psychiatr. 2014;171(3):276–93.
13. Seymour KE, Chronis-Tuscano A, Halldorsdottir T, Stupica B, Owens K, Sacks T. Emotion regulation mediates the relationship between ADHD and depressive symptoms in youth. J Abnorm Child Psychol. 2012;40:595–606.

14. Roy A, Oldehinkel AJ, Verhulst FC, Ormel J, Hartman CA. Anxiety and disruptive behavior mediate pathways from attention-deficit/hyperactivity disorder to depression. J Clin Psychiatry. 2014;75(2):e108–13.
15. Turgay A, Ansari R. Major depression with ADHD in children and adolescents. Psychiatry (Edgmont). 2006;3(4):20–32.
16. Fishman PA, Stang PE, Hogue SL. Impact of co-morbid attention deficit disorder on the direct medical costs of treating adults with depression in managed care. J Clin Psychiatry. 2007;68:248–53.
17. Youngstrom EA, Van Meter A. Empirically supported assessment of children and adolescents. Clin Psychol Sci Pract. 2016;23(4):327–47.
18. Youngstrom EA, Van Meter A, Frazier TW, Hunsley J, Prinstein MJ. Evidence-based assessment as an integrative model for applying psychological science to guide the voyage of treatment. Clin Psychol Sci Pract. 2017;24(4):331–63.
19. Hawley KM, Weisz JR. Child, parent and therapist (dis)agreement on target problems in outpatient therapy: the therapist's dilemma and its implications. J Consult Clin Psychol. 2003;71:62–70.
20. Reinecke MA, Curry JF, March JS. Findings from the Treatment for Adolescents with Depression Study (TADS): what have we learned? What do we need to know? J Clin Child Adolesc Psychol. 2009;38(6):761–7.
21. Beck AT. Depression: clinical, experimental, and theoretical aspects. New York: Harper & Row; 1967.
22. Lewinsohn PM. A behavioral approach to depression. In: Friedman RJ, Katz MM, editors. The psychology of depression: contemporary theory and research. New York: Wiley; 1974. p. 157–78.
23. Weersing VR, Jeffreys M, Do MCT, Schwartz KTG, Bolano C. Evidence base update of psychosocial treatments for child and adolescent depression. J Clin Child Adolesc Psychol. 2017;46(1):11–43.
24. Rohde P. Cognitive-behavioral treatment for adolescent depression. In: Weisz JR, Kazdin AE, editors. Evidence-based psychotherapies for children and adolescents. 3rd ed. New York: Guilford Press; 2017. p. 49–65.
25. Emslie G, Kratochvil C, Vitiello B, Silva S, Mayes T, McNulty S, et al. Treatment for Adolescents with Depression Study (TADS): safety results. J Am Acad Child Adolesc Psychiatry. 2006;45(12):1440–55.
26. Kratochvil CJ, May DE, Silva SG, Madaan V, Puumala SE, Curry JF, et al. Treatment response in depressed adolescents with and without co-morbid attention-deficit/hyperactivity disorder in the Treatment for Adolescents with Depression Study. J Child Adolesc Psychopharmacol. 2009;19(9):519–27.
27. Hilton RC, Rengasamy M, Mansoor B, He J, Mayes T, Emslie GJ, et al. Impact of treatments for depression on comorbid anxiety, attentional, and behavioral symptoms in adolescents with selective serotonin reuptake inhibitor-resistant depression. J Am Acad Child Adolesc Psychiatry. 2013;52(5):482–92.
28. Antshel KM, Faraone SV, Gordon M. Cognitive behavioral treatment outcomes in adolescent ADHD. J Atten Disord. 2014;18(6):483–95.
29. Weisz J, Bearman SK, Santucci LC, Jensen-Doss A. Initial test of a principle-guided approach to transdiagnostic psychotherapy with children and adolescents. J Clin Child Adolesc Psychol. 2017;46(1):44–58.
30. Humphreys KL, Katz SJ, Lee SS, Hammen C, Brennan PA, Najman JM. The association of ADHD and depression: mediation by peer problems and parent-child difficulties in two complementary samples. J Abnorm Psychol. 2013;122(3):854–67.
31. Jacobson CM, Mufson LH, Young JF. Treating adolescent depression using interpersonal psychotherapy. In: Weisz JR, Kazdin AE, editors. Evidence-based psychotherapies for children and adolescents. 3rd ed. New York: Guilford Press; 2017. p. 66–82.

32. Yoshimasu K, Barbaresi WJ, Colligan RC, Voigt RG, Killian JM, Weaver AL, Katusic SK. Childhood ADHD is strongly associated with a broad range of psychiatric disorders during adolescence: a population-based birth cohort study. J Child Psychol Psychiatry. 2012;53(10):1036–43.
33. Meinzer MC, Pettit JW, Viswesvaran C. The co-occurrence of attention-deficit/hyperactivity disorder and unipolar depression in children and adolescents: a meta-analytic review. Clin Psychol Rev. 2014;34:595–607.
34. Pliska SR, Crismon ML, Hughes CW, Conners CK, Emslie GJ, Jensen PS, McCracken JT, Swanson JM, Lopez M. The Texas consensus conference panel on pharmacotherapy of childhood attention-deficit/hyperactivity disorder. The Texas Children's Medication Algorithm Project: revision of the algorithm for pharmacotherapy of attention-deficit/hyperactivity disorder. J Am Acad Child Adolesc Psychiatry. 2006;45(6):642–57.
35. Gürkan K, Bilgiç A, Türkoglu S, Kiliç BG, Aysev A, Uslu R. Depression, anxiety and obsessive-compulsive symptoms and quality of life in children with attention-deficit hyperactivity disorder (ADHD) during three-month methylphenidate treatment. J Psychopharmacol. 2010;24(12):1810–8.
36. Chen M, Pan T, Hsu T, Huang K, Su T, Cheng-Ta L, Lin W, Tsai S, Change W, Chen T, Bai Y. Attention deficit hyperactivity disorder comorbidity and antidepressant resistance among patients with major depression: a nationwide longitudinal study. Eur Neuropsychopharmacol. 2016;26:1760–7.
37. American Psychiatric Association. Diagnostic and statistical manual of mental disorders: diagnostic and statistical manual of mental disorders. 5th ed. Arlington: American Psychiatric Association; 2013.

Chapter 10
When Autism Spectrum Disorder Masks ADHD in Adolescents

Laura Weissman

Case Examples

1. AJ is a 13-year-old male with Autism Spectrum Disorder (ASD). He had been doing well in school but over the past year has been experiencing increased difficulty paying attention in class, with homework completion and with school projects. He has a few friends but struggles to read social cues. Transitioning into new situations remains hard for him. Explicit teaching has helped him develop strategies for social understanding and emotional regulation, but he still becomes overwhelmed by transitions and new situations. This past year, he has started to argue more frequently with family members, often because of his rigid thinking. He often insists activities occur at a specific time and in a particular way, and that family members behave as expected.

2. Caren is a 14-year-old ninth-grade girl previously diagnosed with ASD. She is not on an Individualized Educational Plan (IEP). She has an above average IQ, always earned good grades, and never had behavioral concerns at home or school. Caren has always kept to herself, satisfied to be alone, and focused on her specific area of interest (which is currently Anime). However, she is more emotional as of late and resists going to school, saying she feels overwhelmed by the noise, work, pace, and expectations for group work. Her grades are dropping, as she is having difficulty completing homework and handing in assignments.

L. Weissman (✉)
Division of Developmental Medicine, Boston Children's Hospital, Boston, MA, USA
e-mail: laura.weissman@childrens.harvard.edu

© Springer Nature Switzerland AG 2020
A. Schonwald (ed.), *ADHD in Adolescents*,
https://doi.org/10.1007/978-3-030-62393-7_10

Background

It is well understood tht Autism Spectrum Disorder (ASD) is a neurobiological disorder characterized by social, communication and behavioral challenges based on the Diagnositic and Statistical Manual of Mental Disorders Fifth Edition (DSM-5). Individuals with ASD often present with executive functioning and attentional issues related to the diagnosis. However, sometimes these attentional issues reach a threshold beyond the diagnosis and warrant an additional diagnosis of Attention-deficit/hyperactivity disorder (ADHD). Current statistics estimate that up to 40% or more individuals with ASD **also** meet DSM 5 diagnostic criteria for Attention-Deficit/Hyperactivity Disorder (ADHD) [1–3].

However, prior to 2013, ADHD was often unrecognized or undiagnosed in individuals with ASD. The *Diagnostic and Statistical Manual of Mental Disorders, Fourth Edition* (DSM-IV), which provides diagnostic criteria for psychiatric and neurodevelopmental disorders and was in use until 2013, specifically stated that ADHD and ASD could not be diagnosed together [4]. In other words, until 2013, an individual diagnosed with one of these disorders could not be diagnosed with the second simultaneously. This resulted in suboptimal treatment of many individuals, and research on the population with both disorders was limited; what research existed was not always clincially relevant.

Published in 2013, the DSM-5 allowed for both ADHD and ASD to be diagnosed in the same individual [5]. However, even as these diagnoses have become recognized as co-occurring, many individuals are not diagnosed appropriately. This is concerning as individuals who present with co-occurring diagnoses have a higher level of need and a higher level of impairment than those with a single diagnosis. Additionally, as these individuals move into adolescence and young adulthood, and face increased executive functioning and social demands, the impairment and level of need increases resulting in poorer outcomes emotionally and cognitively compared to individuals with just one of these diagnoses, further stressing the importance of accurate diagnosis. Moreover, the diagnosis remains a clinical one, as we are yet to fully understand the neural basis of overlaps and differences between these two disorders [6].

Difficulties in Recognizing a Co-occurring ADHD and ASD Diagnoses

1. We lack the range of empiric studies of children and adolescents with co-occurring ADHD and ASD to guide care. This means clinicians, teachers, and providers have less evidence on which to base diagnosis, treatment, and prognosis. There was no uniformity in diagnosing until 2013, making long-term studies simply unavailable.

2. Severity and intensity of symptoms can be a factor. Individuals with severe symptomology of either ASD or ADHD are more likely to be diagnosed early, but those with subtler symptoms or those with other compensatory skills (higher cognition, better regulation) may not. It is easy to miss or misattribute less problematic symptoms.
3. The two diagnoses can share overlapping symptoms, making distinction difficult. Individuals with ASD are often distracted by their own thoughts or stimuli related to perseverative interests so may look distractible. Observation alone may be insufficient to clarify whether such distractibility stems from autism or a separate attention deficit. Alternately, an individual with ADHD may present with social difficulties, the primary deficit in individuals with ASD. However, the impulsivity and inattention of ADHD can interfere with response to social cues and social situations. This makes it particularly challenging to disentangle attentional and social difficulties in individuals with ASD and/or ADHD.
4. Both disorders also present with executive functioning deficits. Executive functioning describes the ability to organize information mentally and to control one's emotions. Isolated neuropsychological measures of executive function do not clarify the cause of the deficit, just its presence or absence. Although comprehensive neuropsychological testing can be used to diagnose ASD and ADHD, it cannot clarify diagnoses based on executive function profiles alone.
5. Risk factors for both of these diagnoses overlap, including being male, a history of prematurity, and other perinatal factors (such as use of medications, exposures, and illnesses). The contribution of these risk factors does not aide in the clarification of ADHD versus ASD.
6. Finally, even if an individual with ASD presents with symptoms of inattention, at what point does this meet the threshold for a secondary diagnosis? The cutoff is subjective, based on observations and report of impact.

ASD and ADHD and Adolescence: A Confusing Complex

Problems with executive functioning may first become apparent in adolescence. Through elementary school, students are learning self-restraint, management of multistep tasks, study skills, and navigation of group work. However, as individuals move into adolescence, school success requires real mastery of these skills and workload intensifies. Additionally, executive functioning demands and expectations simultaneously, students are given more social and academic independence by both parents and teachers.

Beyond academics, social demands escalate for most adolescents. They face increased social pressure, more complex social relationships, and more abstract social information to interpret. Adolescence can be hard for the typically developing teen, harder for the teen with either ASD or ADHD, and particularly taxing for the individual with both ASD and ADHD.

Not surprisingly, individuals with both ASD and ADHD are more likely to present with comorbid mental health disorders such as anxiety or depression. These diagnoses can be either primary or secondary, further complicating the presentation and diagnosis [8, 9].

Diagnosis

How can we differentiate these as individual or co-occurring diagnoses? Although neuropsychological testing can assist in this process, it requires consequent careful interpretation by a skilled clinician along with correlation to the clinical presentation.

Some patterns can be helpful in discriminating ASD from ADHD. As described above, both patients with ASD and ADHD can demonstrate difficulties with executive functioning which includes planning, organizing, fluency, cognitive flexibility, working memory, and inhibition. On direct testing, there can be subtle differences between these populations.

- Whereas individuals with ADHD are more likely to demonstrate executive functioning deficits related to impulsivity, sustained attention, working memory, and the ability to inhibit (to stop doing something when they are supposed to), those with ASD are more likely to demonstrate a wider range of difficulties with lower performance in all areas of executive functioning.
- Both groups can have difficulties shifting set. That is to say, when individuals are completing a task, they can have difficulty moving to the next task or have difficulty transitioning to a different type of task. It appears that the brain is fixed in the pattern of the previous task. Clinicians, parents, and teachers sometimes describe this as "sticky thinking." You can imagine how this could impact functioning at school, where students are required to move quickly from one classroom activity to another and from class to class. We don't currently have a lot of information about what executive functioning testing looks like for individuals with both disorders to help us with diagnostic clarification at an individual level with consistency and accuracy.
- Externally both ADHD and ASD can cause a person to appear distractible, so the next step is to find out where and why the distractibility occurs. Is the distractibility worse in social settings, with high sensory loads, or when higher order language is expected? This can be explained by the social challenges of the teen with ASD. On the other hand, is the distractibility worse when tasks are less interesting or engaging or have no social context or during periods when sustained attention is expected? This can be explained by the common symptoms of ADHD in a teen. Clinicians need to hone in on the details of the symptoms. Teachers, therapists and other providers can be an essential resource in describing when and how the student appears distracted in class, while parents and students themselves can give details about extracurricular time.

- Theory of mind tasks (those which ask an individual to understand the perspective of another individual) are more likely to be difficult for individuals with ASD than ADHD. Sometimes a person with ASD starts talking "in the middle," as if the listener knows the story from beginning without clarifying the context. Sometimes, the person with ASD seems to think that the listener knows about a person or television show or character without asking first. Teaching these skills is often central to educating a person with ASD. In contrast, a person with ADHD may also speak as if the listener knows more, but due to inattention or impulsivity rather than reduced social perception.

> Theory of mind requires a person to understand that what I think is not what you think and that what I know is different from what you know.

Using these concepts, a comprehensive neuropsychological assessment can be helpful in finding diagnostic clarity. Looking at measures of attention, executive functioning, working memory, and social cognition helps understand the nature of an individual's struggle. However, as stated, no single test or result is definitive.

That being said, most individuals don't undergo comprehensive neuropsychological testing to aid in this diagnosis. Testing can be hard to access and harder to afford. When clinicians and families consider both of these diagnoses, a combination of careful history and familiar measures (such as Vanderbilt Attention Scales or Conners' Rating Scales) can be helpful. Information about functioning should be gathered from a multitude of sources including parents, teachers, therapists, and in adolescents or those where developmentally appropriate, the student directly. The results of this investigation might not suggest that the individual has reached a diagnostic threshold, but still can provide evidence to inform a therapeutic treatment plan. In fact, in some cases, clinicians use medication to treat the ADHD symptoms in those with ASD even when the full ADHD criteria are not met. Likewise, social skills training is often recommended for those with ADHD who fail to meet full ASD criteria.

Treatment

For individuals with ASD and suspected or confirmed ADHD, treatment aims to support behavioral, academic, social, and executive functioning skills [10]. If symptoms are sufficiently problematic or persist after introduction of behavioral educational and other therapeutic interventions, a medication trial is often warranted.

Behavioral interventions are paramount to supporting individuals with both ASD and ADHD and may look similar across these disorders. Interventions and accomodations need to be appropriate to the students cogntive and developmental level. The goals of intervention in all settings are promoting attention to task, increasing compliance, improving study skills, addressing social skills and improving emotional regulation. This should include supports at home and school. At home, students likely will benefit from utilizing postive behavioral support plans and accomodations around homework. At school this includes interventions as part of an IEP or 504 plans which addresses the students needs (see table 10.2).

Having the support at home and school of a behavioral specialist with experience in both disorders can be very helpful. Optimally, school teams should include participation of a consultant familiar with ADHD and ASD. That provider should participate in IEP meetings, consult to the school team at scheduled intervals, and be available to consult to the family so that skills are generalized to the home setting Table 10.1.

Academic accommodations should also match the learner's individual profile. Some examples are listed in Table 10.2.

Direct support for executive functioning deficits can include organizational tutors or study skills sessions in school, when a student meets with a teacher to work on organizational and other executive function competencies.

Most students with ASD will need social supports through high school and sometimes beyond. This can be in the form of a structured group where individuals are coached systematically on areas of deficit or as part of individual social coaching.

In addition, as is the need for treatment of ASD alone, parents should be involved in the treatment plan. Parent education around dual diagnoses and successful behavioral strategies along with direct parental support is recommended.

Although medication can be a useful part of comprehensive treatment program, those with both ASD and ADHD may respond less robustly to standard ADHD medication and tend to experience more side effects compared to those with ADHD alone [10]. This underscores the importance of additional therapeutic supports in the home and school along with a good monitoring system. If medication is used, the same treatment algorithm is followed as for those with ADHD alone. Stimulants are used first line, more commonly starting with methylphenidate preparations, and adjustments are made as needed. Individuals with ASD and ADHD need to be monitored closely for side effects and response to medication.

> Given the risk for more medication side effects, start treatment of ADHD in those with ASD with a low dose of medication, and increase slowly until you reach a meaningful therapeutic effect with minimal or tolerable side effects.

Table 10.1 Sample IEP goals for a student with ADHD and ASD	Sample IEP goals for a student with ADHD and ASD
	Prolonged attention to task
	Increased compliance
	Improved emotional regulation
	Use of organizational strategies

Table 10.2 Sample IEP accommodations for students with ADHD and ASD

Sample IEP accommodations for students with ADHD and ASD
Allow extra time on all academic exercises.
Reduce the volume work and focus on quality rather than quantity. For students with ADHD, time and reduced volume can be the most beneficial (and easiest to implement) accommodations to promoting their learning success.
Use preferential seating to help reduce distractibility.
Keep oral directions clear and simple and demonstrate (i.e., model) an instruction or skill whenever possible.
The teacher should check in with the student after giving instructions, to make sure that they have understood.
Tasks should be broken down into smaller, easy-to-complete units, with positive feedback at the completion of each.
Attempt to use multi-sensory presentations of new concepts: combine oral, visual, and tactile activities whenever possible. Also, continue to encourage discovery, demonstration, and practice of new concepts within a meaningful context by using manipulatives (e.g., blocks, tiles, pie charts).
Allow the student "down time" or short breaks on a fairly regular basis to ensure retention and improve their productivity.
The teacher may want to check in frequently as the student does independent work, so that they are getting attention and feedback for being on-task rather than only when they go off-task.
Extra time on tests
Explicit language when teaching and explaining assignments
Immediate feedback to course correct misunderstandings
Limited quantity of classwork and homework
Increased support around academics with high executive functioning demands (such as projects and writing)
Provision of notes, note-taking support for lectures
Minimized environmental sensory stimuli

Use of interval standardized measures (Vanderbilt's, Conners', etc.) and/or other regular data collection (through ABA or other behavioral methodologies) can be helpful in monitoring response to both therapeutic and medication interventions.

Individuals should be closely monitored for other mental health comorbidities, especially anxiety and depression.

Cases Revisited

Plan for AJ: Remember, there can be many reasons that students experience difficulties sustaining attention. His increasing distress in managing expectations at school may be fueling his rigidity at home. Next steps are to gather information that will help distinguish the potential causes of his deteriorating attention and increasing rigidity.

- Parents and teachers should be given attention rating scales for more objective data collection. Clarify whether inattention is only in the school setting or whether there are issues elsewhere.
- Investigate for comorbid mental health diagnoses as well; screening tools for anxiety and depression might be appropriate.
- A meeting with school providers can be helpful, as can Individualized Education Program (IEP) testing (or updated testing) to determine the current needs in school.
- Due to the potential contribution of rigid thinking, he may benefit from individual sessions with a behavioral health clinician, using various strategies to improve his social cognition.
- If in the context of school and home supports, AJ is still struggling, a medication trial could be initiated, targeting the diagnosis identified.

Plan for Caren: Again, remember there can be many reasons that students experience difficulties with mood and school function. As students transition to high school, the expectations are increased. Individuals who were previously compensating for their difficulties may no longer have capacity. This can sometimes manifest behaviorally, emotionally, as well as academically. Next steps are to gather information that will help distinguish the potential causes of their deteriorating attention.

- Although, at first glance, one would consider many other issues besides a comorbid diagnosis of ADHD for Caren, this should be considered in the differential. Collection of attention scales contributes to comprehensive history. ADHD in girls with fewer externalizing symptoms may be missed.
- Specifically evaluate for mood issues and substance use, again with focused history and diagnosis-specific screening tools.
- Puberty onset can align with increase of moodiness. Investigate any temporal relationship with menses that could be clarifying.
- Ask about potential bullying. Involving school personnel and educating parents about interventions might be appropriate.

Interestingly, some characteristics inherent to the diagnosis of ASD may have helped an individual compensate to this point: preference for routines, rigidity, and a preference for following rules could have supported on task behavior. In high school, new skills might be needed to support task completion when the demands become overwhelming.

Conclusions

When pateints with ASD or ADHD present with challenges in the teen years, it may be appropriate to consider an additional diagnosis. Adolescents with dual diagnoses of ASD and ADHD are particularly vulnerable to the challenges of their academic and social worlds. Although difficult, identification and treatment in this population is essential to success. Use screening tools to gather information from teachers, parents, therapist and the student themselves. Involve outside specialists when you need. Generally, a comprehensive intervention includes social skills training, behavioral interventions, classroom accomodations, executive functioning supports and consideration for medication. It is essential that interventions are integrated into both home and school environments for an optimal outcome.

Tips

- Look for possible ASD in adolescents with ADHD who are struggling socially. Strong language and cognitive skills could have masked this diagnosis earlier.
- In adolescents with ASD who are struggling with attention consider evaluation for co-occurring ADHD. Use ADHD monitorning instruments to assisist in assessing for ADHD symptoms in those with ASD.
- Treatment for ADHD and ASD will require a comprehensive treatment plan both medically and behaviorally in the home and school settings.
- ADHD medications may cause more side effects in those with ASD than those without. A good rule of thumb is to start low and go slow.

References

1. https://www.cdc.gov/ncbddd/adhd/data.html. Accessed 18 July 2020.
2. Leitner Y. The co-occurrence of autism and attention deficit hyperactivity disorder in children – what do we know? Front Human Neurosci. 2014;8:268. Published 2014 Apr 29. https://doi.org/10.3389/fnhum.2014.00268.
3. https://www.cdc.gov/ncbddd/autism/data.html.Accessed 18 July 2020.
4. American Psychiatric Association. Diagnostic and statistical manual of mental disorders. 4th ed., Text Revision. Washington, DC: American Psychiatric Association; 2000.
5. American Psychiatric Association. Diagnostic and statistical manual of mental disorders. 5th ed. Washington, DC: American Psychiatric Association; 2013.
6. Lau-Zhu A, Fritz A, McLoughlin G. Overlaps and distinctions between attention deficit/hyperactivity disorder and autism spectrum disorder in young adulthood: systematic review and guiding framework for EEG-imaging research. NeurosciBiobehav Rev. 2019;96:93–115. Epub 2018 Oct 24.
7. Hartman C, Geurts H, Franke B, Buitelaar J, Rommelse N. Changing ASD-ADHD symptom co-occurrence across the lifespan with adolescence as crucial time window: illustrating the need to go beyond childhood. NeurosciBiobehav Rev. 2016;71:529–41.
8. Jang J, Matson JL, Williams LW, Tureck K, Goldin RL, Cervantes PE. Rates of comorbid symptoms in children with ASD, ADHD, and comorbid ASD and ADHD. Res DevDisabil. 2013;34(8):2369–78. https://doi.org/10.1016/j.ridd.2013.04.021.
9. Mansour R, Dovi AT, Lane DM, Loveland KA, Pearson DA. ADHD severity as it relates to comorbid psychiatric symptomatology in children with Autism Spectrum Disorders (ASD). Res DevDisabil. 2017;60:52–64. https://doi.org/10.1016/j.ridd.2016.11.009.
10. Young S, Hollingdale J, Absoud M, et al. Guidance for identification and treatment of individuals with attention deficit/hyperactivity disorder and autism spectrum disorder based upon expert consensus. BMC Med. 2020;18(1):146. Published 2020 May 25.

Chapter 11
ADHD and Tics

Anisha Srinivasan and Samuel Zinner

Case Example

Robert is a 15-year-old with attention-deficit/hyperactivity disorder (ADHD) diagnosed when he was 7 years old. He has been treated with stimulant medication for several years. He has an eye-blinking tic, which worsens when he is tired or anxious. As his tic persists, he now asks to stop his stimulant medication to see if the tic will stop as well.

Background

Fidgeting, squirming, and shifting are behaviors that may come to mind when thinking of an individual with ADHD. However, seemingly restless behaviors in adolescents with ADHD may have other causes as well, including tics. Tics are unwanted, frequent, repetitive, and non-rhythmic movements (motor tics) or noises (phonic tics including voice, or "vocal", tics). In this chapter, we use the term "vocal" to refer to tics that produce noise from the throat, mouth, and/or nose. Up to 20% of all children have a *short-lived* course of tics (i.e., lasting less than 1 year, never to return) before their 10th birthday [1].

In contrast, tic disorders that last more than 1 year are called *chronic* tic disorders (CTDs). These are much less common. CTDs occur in about 4% of all children, and their tics will likely persist into adolescence [2]. CTDs may be limited to either motor *or* vocal tics, but when both types occur, the CTD is called Tourette syndrome

A. Srinivasan (✉) · S. Zinner
Division of Developmental Medicine, University of Washington and Seattle Children's Hospital, Seattle, WA, USA
e-mail: Anisha.Srinivasan@seattlechildrens.org; Samuel.zinner@seattlechildrens.org

© Springer Nature Switzerland AG 2020
A. Schonwald (ed.), *ADHD in Adolescents*,
https://doi.org/10.1007/978-3-030-62393-7_11

(also called Tourette's disorder) [3]. For the purposes of this chapter, the term CTD will be used to refer to all three types of chronic tic disorders: motor, vocal, and motor-plus-vocal.

Most children who develop tics do not have ADHD. However, children with ADHD are much more likely than children without ADHD to have a CTD. In fact, up to 30% of youth with ADHD also have a CTD [4]. While tics may or may not be problematic for the adolescent with a CTD, youth with ADHD+CTD are very likely also to develop additional often problematic symptoms, often rising to the level of further diagnosable coexisting conditions. Frequent coexisting conditions may include anxiety and mood disorders, obsessive-compulsive disorder (OCD), learning disabilities, sleep difficulties, rage or outbursts of anger, problems with fine motor coordination skills, and/or autism spectrum disorder [5]. These conditions can interfere with learning, personal relationships, general health, and well-being.

Tic Severity Varies Widely

Tics may be very mild in some people while very severe or overwhelming in others. When describing how severe a person's tics are, many experts and researchers evaluate the following different dimensions of the tics [6]:

- *Number*: How many different individual tic varieties can be identified in the person. Some people have just one type of tic at a time. Others have too many types to count.
- *Frequency*: How often the person performs tics, ranging from less than once per day to nearly constantly.
- *Intensity*: The strength or force of the tic movement or noise. Some tics are weak and would not be noticed by other people. Very intense tics look exaggerated and can sometimes be so strong that they cause injury.
- *Complexity*: How complicated the tic appears to be. When complexity is low, the tic is usually brief and involves one muscle group, such as the muscles of the eyes or of the eyelids, such as looking to the side or blinking or making a simple noise such as a grunt or a sniff. When complexity is high, tics may involve many parts of the body at once or in a repeating sequence, so the tic often looks purposeful (such as reaching for something or making a sudden leap) or the tic sounds like speech (such as repeating part of a word or uttering an entire sentence, sometimes multiple times). While complex tics may look or sound purposeful, they do not actually serve the apparent purpose.
- *Interference*: How much the tics interrupt what the person is otherwise trying to do or say. Tics with mild interference may not interrupt anything at all, whereas tics with severe interference can make it impossible for the person to do what they intend until the tic or tics are finished.
- *Impairment*: How much the tics seem to result in problems with self-esteem, schoolwork, family life, and friendships.

Examples of Motor Tics:	Examples of Vocal Tics:
Eye blinking	Sniffling
Facial expressions	Throat clearing
Nodding	Coughing
Neck jerking	Huffing
Head turning	Tongue-clicking
Shoulder shrugging	Whistling
Arm jerking	Humming
Finger tapping	Grunting
Abdomen muscles tightening	Shouting
Jumping	Barking
Making socially inappropriate gestures	Repeating another's words or phrases
	Saying socially inappropriate words or phrases

Fig. 11.1 Examples of common motor and vocal tics

There are different kinds of tics, organized by motor and vocal types (Fig. 11.1).

Another feature of tics is that their severity is not constant. Rather they tend to increase and diminish over minutes, days, weeks, months, or even years and often unpredictably. Periods of emotional stress or excitement, as well as complete relaxation, tend to increase tic severity. Some tic expressions may last a lifetime, while others begin and then disappear quickly, never to return.

Sensory Urges Linked to Tics

Importantly, there is more to tic behaviors than meets the eye. Tics are a blend of movement patterns and sensory experiences. A key feature of tics is a peculiar, uncomfortable sensation that emerges and builds in intensity in the face or other body locations, wherever the tic occurs [7]. Performing the tic relieves the discomfort. While these sensations are involuntary, the tic behaviors can be controlled, in the same way that scratching is a somewhat controllable response to an involuntary, intolerable itch. The urge builds and becomes unbearable, essentially forcing the youth to complete the tic in order to feel relief. While a tic behavior may be somewhat controllable, efforts to prevent the tic can be incredibly distracting and exhausting.

Many people with tics say that the sensation is similar to the feeling that builds in the eyelids when trying not to blink.

Adolescents, unlike younger children with tics, are almost always able to notice and describe these sensations [8]. This ability makes adolescents more suitable candidates for behavior treatment to reduce their tics (described later in this chapter), as well as more likely to try to hide their tics from other people, including from their peers. Adolescents may also try to hide their tics from healthcare providers, so providers who treat adolescents with tics may underestimate the severity of the condition, if they are aware of them at all.

Time Courses of Tics and Coexisting Conditions in ADHD Are Different for Each Condition

Although youth with ADHD+CTD usually have additional coexisting conditions, symptoms of each of these conditions generally begin at different stages during childhood and adolescence [5]. Symptoms of one condition may influence symptoms of other conditions, but each condition should be considered separately.

Tic Symptoms in Relation to ADHD Symptoms

Tics typically first emerge later than ADHD symptoms do, but almost always before the start of adolescence. Tics may be overlooked, particularly if mild or short-lived, or if mistaken for some other concern, such as seasonal allergies or the fidgetiness of ADHD. Tics usually first show up in the head and neck (although tics can occur anywhere on the body) and are usually mild in severity. In CTDs, tics often progress to include lower parts of the body such as the chest, arms, abdomen, pelvis, and legs and often increase in severity.

For children who go on to develop a CTD, tic severity usually peaks around the beginning of puberty, between 9 and 12 years of age. By the mid to late teens, tic severity usually reduces, and for some with a CTD, tics may disappear completely [1]. As with ADHD, tic disorders are diagnosed by gathering information from the patient and caregiver and by completing a physical examination. CTDs may exacerbate ADHD symptoms, as tics and efforts to hide them can be distracting.

Coexisting Conditions in Youth with ADHD+CTD

Among adolescents with ADHD, the presence of a CTD, whether mild or severe, should raise a red flag for the possible presence of coexisting conditions, and that possibility should be re-explored periodically. Figure 11.2 shows typical age ranges for onset of tics and for other coexisting conditions [5, 9–11]. Symptoms of such

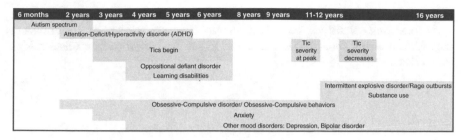

Fig. 11.2 Typical age ranges of symptom onset for coexisting conditions in those with chronic tic disorders [5, 9–11]. Time course of tics is highlighted in blue to illustrate their timeline relative to that of coexisting conditions

conditions may first become apparent or grow in severity during adolescence or even in adulthood. It is important to understand that each adolescent with ADHD+CTD is a unique individual who may have some, all, or none of these other coexisting symptoms.

How to Live Well in Adolescence with ADHD+CTD and Coexisting Conditions

The keys to success are building positive relationships with others while prioritizing the treatment of the most challenging symptoms. Tic severity usually decreases by late adolescence, so quality of life for teens tends to be affected most by symptoms of ADHD and other coexisting conditions rather than by tics themselves [12]. In general, adolescents with ADHD+CTD with or without additional coexisting conditions have poorer self-esteem and social adjustment than their peers with CTDs alone [13]. Below, we explore common challenges and their management approaches to help youth with ADHD+CTD live and function well.

Build Supportive Relationships

The quality of peer and family relationships both affects, and is affected by, severity of coexisting conditions [14]. Supportive environments at home and school and positive relationships with peers, family, and teachers can serve as protective factors even for those with severe symptoms. Teens and their families benefit from building skills in resilience, communication, and self-advocacy. These skills may enhance the benefits of medical and counseling treatments and academic supports. The Tourette Association of America (www.Tourette.org) provides skill-building supports to teens and their families through its many resources including its Youth Ambassador Program. This program is specifically designed for adolescents with

CTDs to strengthen and use these skills to educate others about tic disorders and their coexisting conditions. Teens who communicate confidently, respectfully, and clearly with others about CTDs can reduce stigma and improve their relationships with others.

School

Tics and the efforts to suppress them may worsen ADHD symptoms. For example, performing eye-rolling tics can make it difficult to write or to keep focused and on track while reading. At the same time, holding back the tics can lead to fatigue, discomfort, or poor concentration. Additionally, these interferences may make it more difficult for the adolescent to interact socially, which can damage academic, social, and home life.

While tics pose academic and social challenges to some adolescents with ADHD, it is ADHD and frequent coexisting conditions, rather than tics, that cause most school-based difficulties.

The impacts of learning disabilities or difficulties with executive functions, for example, may intensify in adolescence as academic demands increase. Anxiety and mood disorders including depression are common in adolescents with CTDs and can interfere with sleep, learning, and memory. Obsessive-compulsive behaviors occur in most adolescents with CTDs and may first emerge or intensify in adolescence [15]. Youth with these coexisting conditions may appear socially withdrawn or unfriendly to their peers. Victimization by bullying, also common in youth with CTDs, may compound these problems [16].

Every adolescent with coexisting CTDs will experience a unique combination of these conditions, and their symptoms may vary through adolescence. Other chapters within this book address many of these conditions more fully.

> For adolescents with disruptive tics, accommodations at school may be needed.

Adolescents themselves should take the lead in the discussions and decision-making, and parents and school personnel can work together with the adolescent to determine how to best manage tic behaviors at school. Teachers and other school personnel benefit from learning about tic disorders: hearing the adolescent share their own experiences can be most powerful and effective. Educational accommodations may include allowing the student to take private "tic breaks" when needed, sitting close to the classroom exit door, and taking exams in a separate room to allow the student to express tics without fear of disturbing others [17]. These and other ideas for accommodations, when qualifying, may be incorporated into either an individualized education program (IEP) or Section 504 accommodation plan. The Tourette Association of America (www.tourette.org) provides tools for educators, clinicians, and adolescents with tics and their parents to help support the adolescent with CTDs at school and in the community.

Home

Tics, hyperactivity, and anger outbursts can often be most severe at home. Adolescents may feel at ease when at home to unleash pent-up tension created by holding back their tics in public. Furthermore, CTDs and their related disorders, with or without ADHD, usually run in families. Family members related by birth to youth with CTDs often themselves are challenged with ADHD and CTDs and/or with the range of other coexisting conditions. These factors add layers of burden to families. Tics, oppositional behavior, and other coexisting conditions add significantly to a family's stress levels. Caregivers may respond to their adolescent's tic increases with frustration (which can increase the teen's distress) or with sympathetic attention or pity (which can unintentionally serve as a reward, leading to greater likelihood of future tic behaviors during periods of distress). Battling or giving in to demands may take over more reasonable, respectful, and disciplined measures of communicating with each other.

> The social pressures to conform may compel teens with CTDs to hold back their tics in public, resulting in mounting physical urges to perform tics, sometimes called a "tic debt."

An authoritative (not authoritarian!) parenting style that blends compassion and collaborative problem-solving with consistent and clear expectations promotes the adolescent's ability to make and carry out independent and responsible decisions. Comprehensive Behavioral Intervention for Tics (CBIT) (discussed later in this chapter) is a behavioral treatment strategy for tic reduction that helps parenting caregivers build on authoritative parenting approaches when interacting with their teen.

Treating Coexisting Tics and ADHD Symptoms May Include Non-medication, Medication, or Combined Approaches

> For most adolescents with ADHD+CTD, ADHD and coexisting neuropsychiatric conditions cause more impairment than tics do, so those conditions will be the focus of treatment.

Tics do not require any treatment unless they are bothersome or disruptive. When treating tics, management is designed specifically for each patient, but generally includes educating the adolescent and caregivers about tic disorders, including their natural course during adolescence and beyond, embracing lifestyle practices that reduce anxiety and tics including adequate sleep and physical exercise, and providing a tic-reducing intervention either via a behavioral treatment approach and/or with a prescription medication.

Behavior Therapy to Reduce Tics

Comprehensive Behavioral Intervention for Tics (CBIT) is a non-medication treatment that may be just as effective at reducing tics as many of the medications used for treating tic disorders [18].

CBIT takes advantage of the sensory urge that warns of an approaching tic. Through awareness training, the adolescent practices paying attention to this urge. The adolescent then attempts to consciously hold back the tic until the urge goes away or to perform a "competing response" to the urge. This response is a behavior that is selected in advance that, when performed, "competes" with, or makes it difficult or impossible to, physically perform the tic. For example, an adolescent with a barking tic might respond to the urge to bark by breathing in deeply rather than barking. Because barking can only occur when one is breathing out, this competing response makes it difficult to bark. Over time with sustained practice, the urge to perform the tic decreases. Parents or other caregivers also participate in their adolescent's CBIT. Their role is to encourage and praise their adolescent when practicing CBIT. This manner of authoritative parenting provides incentive to the adolescent by rewarding with approval, rather than by punishing with shame. This approach is more effective in helping to reduce tics than is telling the adolescent to "stop it" or to "calm down."

Medications to Reduce Tics and ADHD Symptoms

For most adolescents with ADHD+CTD, treatment of ADHD takes priority over treatment of tics because ADHD usually has a more serious impact on functioning. This is also generally true for many of the frequent coexisting conditions, when such conditions are present. Therefore, when including medication as part of an overall management approach, the possible presence and impact of each of these conditions must be thoughtfully examined and considered.

Until recently, the stimulant medications methylphenidate and amphetamine preparations that are used as first-line medication to treat ADHD were thought to induce or worsen tics. However, we now know that most adolescents with ADHD+CTD can be treated safely with stimulant medications to treat ADHD without worsening their tics [19]. It's important to realize, however, that tics naturally increase and decrease over time. Therefore, an increase in tic severity that coincides with the starting of an ADHD medication should not be assumed to have been caused by that medication.

There is no precise formula when choosing a medication, although as a general rule of thumb it's usually wise to "start low, go slow." In other words, select just one medication, begin with a low dose, and increase the dose slowly, watching for improvement in target symptoms as well as for side effects. Table 11.1 lists common ADHD medication options and their relative effects on tic and ADHD symptoms.

> When targeting ADHD symptoms, the stimulant medications remain the first-line options (whether or not the youth has a CTD).

A non-stimulant medication is selected when there is a specific reason not to use a stimulant medication, such as a medical contraindication. We often meet patients

Table 11.1 Treatment options for adolescents with tics and ADHD [19, 20]

Treatment Type*	Treatment Example	Medication Class	Effect on ADHD Symptoms**	Effect on Tics**
Behavioral	Comprehensive Behavioral Intervention Training (CBIT)	N/A	None known	++++
Medication	Methylphenidate	Psychostimulant	++++	++
	Dextroamphetamine	Psychostimulant		+/-
	Clonidine	Alpha-2 agonist	++++	++++
	Guanfacine	Alpha-2 agonist	++++	++++
	Atomoxetine	Selective norepinephrine reuptake inhibitor	+++	++
	Methylphenidate + Clonidine	Combination psychostimulant + Alpha-2 agonist	+++++	++++

* The table describes the effect of each treatment example based on current scientific evidence, but the quality of this evidence is low. The effect of any particular treatment will vary and cannot be predicted in a given adolescent. Some commonly used medications for ADHD are not listed because there is currently limited scientific information available for their use in ADHD+CTD. Therefore, the choice of treatment type should be discussed with a medical professional who is experienced in treating adolescents with ADHD+CTD

** Plus (+) signs describe effect of each treatment type. More plus signs indicates greater improvement of symptoms. +/− for dextroamphetamine indicates that there is a possibility of increase in tics for some individuals, but this is only seen at very high doses of the medication and is not well studied

who have experienced a tic severity increase during a past stimulant medication trial and feel leery of using a stimulant. Important non-stimulant medication options targeting ADHD symptoms include clonidine, guanfacine, atomoxetine, and desipramine. No medication is guaranteed to improve symptoms in any particular patient, and all medications may cause side effects. The medication choice is based on a variety of considerations, including symptom severity of ADHD, tics, and other coexisting conditions.

The stimulants are usually very effective at treating ADHD symptoms. While stimulants are very unlikely to influence tics, dextroamphetamine at high doses may exacerbate tics in some adolescents [20]. As a result, methylphenidate is a reasonable first choice when prescribing a stimulant for ADHD in those with a CTD.

If tic symptoms are more problematic than ADHD symptoms, treatment prioritizes tic-reduction management via tic disorders education, CBIT (described earlier in this chapter), and/or a tic-reducing medication (usually an "alpha-2 agonist": clonidine or guanfacine). These alpha-2 agonists have the advantages of generally tolerable side effects and while reducing some symptoms of hyperactivity and impulsive tendencies in those with ADHD. Other medication options targeting tic reduction are outside the scope of this chapter. Atomoxetine may also be moderately effective at treating symptoms of both ADHD and tics. Atomoxetine is used if alpha-2 agonists are not tolerated or effective. Desipramine may also be effective in treating symptoms of both ADHD and tics but is used infrequently because of side effect risks including to the heart rhythm. For adolescents with a high burden of both ADHD and tic symptoms, a combination of a methylphenidate derivative and clonidine may be particularly effective.

Case Revisited

Robert reports being bothered by his ongoing tics. The first step is to provide psychoeducation about factors to worsen and alleviate tics, explaining that ADHD medication discontinuation may not provide the relief he expects, but he may suffer from untreated ADHD-related behaviors. Investigate whether Robert is suffering from an additional disorder, such as anxiety or depression, requiring specific treatment. If Robert's tics cause social distress, work toward school accommodations and access CBIT. As stimulant medication is thought not to worsen tics, a trial of adjunctive alpha-2 agonist such as guanfacine may be warranted.

Conclusions

While there is currently no cure for tics, adolescents living with ADHD+CTDs and its frequent coexisting conditions can thrive and live well. These youth do best when they are supported by positive relationships with others, can speak confidently about their tics and the related challenges if they choose to do so, have appropriate accommodations at school when needed, follow effective management of ADHD and coexisting conditions, and, for some of these adolescents, receive tic-reduction treatments. The Tourette Association of America provides tools to assist healthcare clinicians and counselors, educators, and youth with ADHD+CTD and their families.

Tips
- Chronic tic disorders (CTDs) are very common in adolescents with ADHD.
- Tic severity often subsides or disappears during adolescence or young adulthood, a fact that can be reassuring to youth with CTD and their families.
- Adolescents with CTDs may be very skillful in suppressing or masking tics, although often at a cost of increased physical discomfort and distraction.
- Adolescents with coexisting tics and ADHD should be screened for additional frequent coexisting conditions, including obsessive-compulsive behaviors, learning disabilities, anxiety, depression, intermittent explosive disorder, and sleep difficulties.
- Coexisting conditions usually cause more interference than tics.
- Tics often do not require treatment.
- Tic treatments may reduce tic severity but will not eliminate tics.
- The Tourette Association of America (www.Tourette.org) offers updated information and support to teachers, families, and clinicians about tic disorders and management.

References

1. Scahill L, Specht M, Page C. The prevalence of tic disorders and clinical characteristics in children. J Obsessive CompulsRelatDisord. 2014;3(4):394–400.
2. Ogundele MO, Ayyash HF. Review of the evidence for the management of co-morbid Tic disorders in children and adolescents with attention deficit hyperactivity disorder. World J Clin Pediatr. 2018;7(1):36–42.
3. American Psychiatric Association. Diagnostic and statistical manual of mental disorders. 5th ed. Arlington: American Psychiatric Association; 2013.
4. Spencer TJ, Biederman J, Faraone S, et al. Impact of tic disorders on ADHD outcome across the life cycle: findings from a large group of adults with and without ADHD. Am J Psychiatry. 2001;158(4):611–7. https://doi.org/10.1176/appi.ajp.158.4.611.
5. Hirschtritt ME, Lee PC, Pauls DL, et al. Lifetime prevalence, age of risk, and genetic relationships of comorbid psychiatric disorders in Tourette syndrome. JAMAPsychiat. 2015;72(4):325–33.
6. Leckman JF, Riddle MA, Hardin MT, Ort SI, Swartz KL, Stevenson J, Cohen DJ. The Yale Global Tic Severity Scale: initial testing of a clinician-rated scale of tic severity. J Am Acad Child Adolesc Psychiatry. 1989;28(4):566–73.

7. Woods DW, Piacentini J, Himle MB, Chang S. Premonitory Urge for Tics Scale (PUTS): initial psychometric results and examination of the premonitory urge phenomenon in youths with Tic disorders. J DevBehav Pediatr. 2005;26(6):397–403.
8. Zinner SH, Coffey BJ. Developmental and behavioral disorders grown up: Tourette's disorder. J DevBehav Pediatr. 2009;30(6):560–73.
9. Walkup JT. Newly diagnosed seminar. Lecture presented at the: https://tourette.org/resource/newly-diagnosed-seminar-1-4/. Accessed 22 Nov 2018.
10. Steiner H, Remsing L. Practice parameter for the assessment and treatment of children and adolescents with oppositional defiant disorder. J Am Acad Child Adolesc Psychiatry. 2007;46(1):126–41.
11. Kessler RC, Coccaro EF, Fava M, Jaeger S, Jin R, Walters E. The prevalence and correlates of DSM-IV intermittent explosive disorder in the National Comorbidity Survey Replication. Arch Gen Psychiatry. 2006;63(6):669–78.
12. Pringsheim T, Lang A, Kurlan R, Pearce M, Sandor P. Understanding disability in Tourette syndrome. Dev Med Child Neurol. 2009;51(6):468–72.
13. Silvestri PR, Baglioni V, Cardona F, Cavanna AE. Self-concept and self-esteem in patients with chronic tic disorders: a systematic literature review. Eur J Paediatr Neurol. 2018;22(5):749–56.
14. Cohen E, Sade M, Benarroch F, Pollak Y, Gross-tsur V. Locus of control, perceived parenting style, and symptoms of anxiety and depression in children with Tourette's syndrome. Eur Child Adolesc Psychiatry. 2008;17(5):299–305.
15. Peterson BS, Pine DS, Cohen P, Brook JS. Prospective, longitudinal study of tic, obsessive-compulsive, and attention-deficit/hyperactivity disorders in an epidemiological sample. J Am Acad Child Adolesc Psychiatry. 2001;40(6):685–95.
16. Eapen V, Cavanna AE, Robertson MM. Comorbidities, social impact, and quality of life in Tourette syndrome. Front Psych. 2016;7:97.
17. Conners S. The Tourette syndrome & OCD checklist: a practical reference for parents and teachers. San Francisco: Jossey-Bass; 2011.
18. Piacentini J, Woods DW, Scahill L, et al. Behavior therapy for children with Tourette disorder: a randomized controlled trial. JAMA. 2010;303(19):1929–37.
19. Osland ST, Steeves TD, Pringsheim T. Pharmacological treatment for attention deficit hyperactivity disorder (ADHD) in children with comorbid tic disorders. Cochrane Database Syst Rev. 2018;6:CD007990.
20. Bloch MH, Panza KE, Landeros-Weisenberger A, Leckman JF. Meta-analysis: treatment of attention-deficit/hyperactivity disorder in children with comorbid tic disorders. J Am Acad Child Adolesc Psychiatry. 2009;48(9):884–93.

Chapter 12
When Bipolar Disorder Mimics ADHD

Rebecca Baum and Lauren Lindle

Case Example

Anna is a 12-year-old female with increasingly difficult behavior at home and school. For the last few years, she has had trouble paying attention in class and completing homework, but recently, her behavior has become more disruptive. She corrects her teachers during class and talks excessively to the students around her. She can't seem to complete assignments but reports that she has already mastered the material. Her parents have noticed similar behavior at home. She stays up late and seems to have plenty of energy despite getting only a few hours of sleep. Her teacher suspects that Anna may have ADHD, but Anna's behavior reminds her mother of a close relative who was diagnosed with manic depression. Anna's parents aren't sure how best to proceed.

Background

Anna's case highlights the similarities between attention-deficit/hyperactivity disorder (ADHD) and bipolar disorder (BD), as well as the distinctions. Although the two conditions can have similar presentations, their prognosis and treatment are

R. Baum (✉)
The Olson Huff Center, Mission Children's Hospital, Asheville, NC, USA
e-mail: Rebecca.baum@hcahealthcare.com

L. Lindle
Developmental and Behavioral Pediatrician, Advocate Children's Hospital,
Oak Lawn, IL, USA

Department of Clinical Sciences at Rosalind Franklin University of Medicine and Science,
Oak Lawn, IL, USA
e-mail: lauren.lindle@aah.org

© Springer Nature Switzerland AG 2020   163
A. Schonwald (ed.), *ADHD in Adolescents*,
https://doi.org/10.1007/978-3-030-62393-7_12

markedly different, so determining the correct diagnosis is important. Between the two conditions, ADHD is far more common, affecting around 8% of children [1], and is most often diagnosed in childhood. BD occurs much less frequently, with a prevalence of around 2% [2]. Fewer than a third of BD cases are diagnosed in childhood, around a third in adolescence, and between a third and a half in adulthood [3, 4]. Although most cases of BD are diagnosed in older age groups, there is increasing awareness that symptoms can first appear in childhood, even before a definitive diagnosis can be made [5]. Genetics play a role in the etiology of both ADHD and BD, likely more so for ADHD than for BD, although precise estimates can be challenging to determine [6–9]. Their presentations can also overlap: some children (1%–17%) initially diagnosed with ADHD will eventually receive a BD diagnosis [10–14]; of those children, both disorders will persist in about 50% [15]. Given these complexities, it can be challenging – and important – to identify the correct diagnosis.

An understanding of the varied presentation of BD is helpful in identifying the overlap and differences between ADHD and BD. The American Psychiatric Association defines several distinct conditions as being part of the BD spectrum: bipolar disorder I (BD-I), bipolar disorder II (BD-II), cyclothymic disorder, bipolar disorder related to other factors (substance use, underlying medical conditions), and two less specific presentations that also fall under the classification of "bipolar disorder and related conditions" [16]. In order to be diagnosed with BD-I, individuals must experience at least one period of characteristic symptoms, called mania, that lasts for 1 week or longer during their lifetime. A manic episode is a discrete period when the individual's mood changes significantly; they may appear excessively happy or "up" or irritable with rapid changes in mood. Common symptoms include excessive silliness, distractibility, or feelings of invincibility and overconfidence (also called "grandiosity"), often paired with a marked increase in energy and decreased need for sleep. These behaviors occur despite the risk for harm and their effect on other aspects of the individual's life, like relationships and school functioning. Specific criteria have been developed to define mania in order to help clinicians make an accurate diagnosis (Table 12.1).

> When thinking about BD, the condition that first comes to mind for many people is BD-I, which is sometimes referred to as "manic depression."

Diagnostic Criteria of Mania

Although the varied presentations of BD and the terminology used to describe them can be somewhat confusing, these criteria have been developed to help clinicians distinguish typical mood or behavioral fluctuations from a serious condition. However, in some circumstances, a child's mood may be abnormal but to a lesser degree than the criteria listed in Table 12.1. The term "hypomania" is used to define

Table 12.1 List of symptom criteria for mania with examples relevant for teens, adapted from Diagnostic and statistical manual of mental disorders, 5th ed. and Bipolar disorder in children and teens: NIH Publication No. QF 15–6380 [16, 17]

Symptom criteria	Examples in teens
Inflated self-esteem or grandiosity	"I'm the best basketball player ever. I don't need to graduate from high school because I'll be drafted in the first round to play professionally"
Decreased need for sleep	Sleeping only 2–3 hours per night for several nights yet having boundless energy during the day
More talkative than usual	Speech is changed from baseline such that others have difficulty getting a word in; speech is loud or sounds pressured as if the individual can't stop
Racing thoughts	Thoughts come and go quickly and are difficult to control
Distractibility	Difficulty maintaining a line of thinking without changing topics frequently
Increased either goal-directed or non-goal-directed activity	Working obsessively and through the night for several days on a term paper (goal-directed) or on recopying twelfth century manuscripts despite having other overdue assignments (non-goal-directed)
Excessive involvement in activities that could result in harm (e.g., to relationships, education, finances)	Uncontrolled interest or involvement in sexual activity, dropping out of high school to pursue an unlikely career, donating excessive amounts of money to charities despite having financial difficulties

Note: Three or more symptoms must be present, most of the time, for at least a 1-week period to be classified as a manic episode; four symptoms must be present if the mood is irritable and not elevated

a mood state characterized by manic symptoms that last for a shorter period of time (at least 4 days) or that is not severe enough to cause marked impairment in functioning [16]. Individuals with BD-I may experience episodes of hypomania or major depressive disorder in addition to manic episodes, which contributes to the wide range presentations. In contrast, individuals with BD-II experience at least one episode of hypomania in addition to at least one episode of major depressive disorder; if mania is present, a diagnosis of BD-I would be warranted instead. Individuals with cyclothymic disorder experience symptoms of hypomania and major depressive disorder but do not meet diagnostic criteria for either condition. See Table 12.2 for a summary of the presentations of bipolar disorder and related conditions.

Summary of Presentations for Bipolar Disorder and Related Conditions

A few key points further complicate this picture and bear mentioning:

- First, comorbidity in BD is common [15], and ADHD or other mental health conditions may develop first [11].
- Second, there has been some concern that medications used to treat ADHD may rarely precipitate mania or hypomania [18, 19], and this presents a particular

Table 12.2 Summary of presentations for bipolar disorder and related conditions, modified from Diagnostic and statistical manual of mental disorders, 5th ed. [16]

Bipolar disorder and related conditions	Presentations		
Condition	Mania	Hypomania	Major depressive disorder
Bipolar disorder I	+	+/−	+/−
Bipolar disorder II	−	+	+
Cyclothymia	−	+ But subclinical	+ But subclinical
Substance/medication-induced bipolar and related disorder	+ But due to substance use or medication		
Bipolar and related disorder due to another medical condition	+ But due to underlying medical condition		
Other specified bipolar and related disorder	Subclinical symptoms that do not meet other specific definition(s)		
Unspecified bipolar and related disorder	Symptoms that cause significant difficulties but that do not meet other specific definition(s)		

Note: For cyclothymia, symptoms must be present over half the time for at least 1 year with a minimum of 2 months at a time symptom-free

challenge for children diagnosed with both ADHD and BD. More recent studies suggest that ADHD medication can be used safely with close monitoring once mood has been stabilized, although it may be wise to proceed cautiously in individuals who have a close family relative with BD [20].

- And last, some symptoms seen in ADHD and BD overlap, such as distractibility, increased energy level, and impulsivity. Similarly, irritability can be present in children with ADHD who may experience a low tolerance to frustration, and it is also common in children with BD. One of the important considerations in distinguishing between the two disorders is the episodic nature of the mood changes in BD and the recognition that a change has occurred that is distinctly different from the child's baseline.

Diagnosis and Treatment Are Harder in Adolescence!

Adolescence is a time when children are becoming more independent, often spending more time with friends than parents and navigating social pressures. They may also experience moodiness or the effects of stress related to relationships, school, and other factors [21]. In some cases, typical adolescent behavior can be difficult to distinguish from irritability, grandiose thinking, risk-taking, and other behaviors seen in BD. Factors such as the duration and severity of symptoms can be helpful in this regard. In addition, experimentation with substance use, which is relatively common in teens [22], can occasionally masquerade as mania or hypomania.

However, the behavioral changes that occur as a result of psychoactive substances should clear quickly, as opposed to those seen in BD. Teens with BD may use psychoactive substances in an attempt to reduce distressing symptoms, and substance use disorders are relatively common in teens with BD [15]. Thus, substance use is an important consideration when assessing mood and behavioral changes in teens.

> Often, these mood changes occur in conjunction with sleep disturbance; while sleep problems may occur in children with ADHD, they are typically more persistent than the episodic sleep difficulties seen in BD.

What You Need to Know

BD is a serious condition. Once symptoms develop, the condition typically persists and continues into adulthood [16]. Individuals with BD require specialized counseling and long-term treatment with antipsychotic mediations or mood stabilizers [19, 23]. Suicidal ideation and suicide attempts are relatively common in individuals with BD [24], so close monitoring is warranted. With proper treatment, individuals with BD may experience a return to their baseline functioning between episodes [16]. Because of the potential severity of BD, involvement of mental health professionals, such as child and adolescent psychiatrists, psychologists, and therapists, is recommended.

This fact can be important to remind concerned parents who may have BD themselves or who have experienced it in a close relative. Parents should consult with health professionals if concerns about BD are present so that assessment and treatment can occur promptly.

> It is important to remember that BD is a relatively uncommon condition in children. While highly heritable, the majority of children who have a close family relative with BD will not develop it [19].

Case Revisited

Anna's case highlights many of the complexities faced by parents, teachers, and clinicians when considering the possibility of BD. She has had trouble staying focused for a few years and is disrupting the class by talking excessively. Her symptoms now seem to be worsening. While these symptoms can be seen in ADHD, BD should also be a consideration. Correcting her teacher and talking excessively may represent grandiose thinking. Similarly, she appears to have excessive energy with a decreased need for sleep. A positive family history further increases her risk.

Given the information provided, it would be wise to recommend that Anna be evaluated for the possibility of a mental health condition, including consideration of BD.

Conclusions

The overlapping symptoms of ADHD, BD, substance use, and adolescent risk-taking can challenge parents, teachers, and clinicians faced with struggling teens. Every case will require a careful history with detailed family history, investigation for discreet episodes of manic thinking and behavior notably different from baseline, and assessment for substance use. Fortunately, for those with isolated or comorbid BD, medication and therapy can be highly effective treatment options.

> **Tips**
> - BD is less common than ADHD.
> - Although BD may run in families, most children who have a family member with BD do not develop it.
> - While symptoms of ADHD and BD can appear similar, their time course is different. Symptoms are usually persistent in ADHD but are episodic in BD.
> - Sleep disturbance in BD usually occurs in conjunction with changes in mood.
> - Effective treatments for BD exist. Teens should be evaluated as soon as concerns are identified so that treatment can be started early.

References

1. Subcommittee on Attention-Deficit/Hyperactivity D, Steering Committee on Quality Improvement and Management, Wolraich M, Brown L, Brown RT, et al. ADHD: clinical practice guideline for the diagnosis, evaluation, and treatment of attention-deficit/hyperactivity disorder in children and adolescents. Pediatrics. 2011;128(5):1007–22.
2. Van Meter AR, Moreira AL, Youngstrom EA. Meta-analysis of epidemiologic studies of pediatric bipolar disorder. J Clin Psychiatry. 2011;72(9):1250–6.
3. Leverich GS, Post RM, Keck PE Jr, Altshuler LL, Frye MA, Kupka RW, et al. The poor prognosis of childhood-onset bipolar disorder. J Pediatr. 2007;150(5):485–90.
4. Perlis RH, Dennehy EB, Miklowitz DJ, Delbello MP, Ostacher M, Calabrese JR, et al. Retrospective age at onset of bipolar disorder and outcome during two-year follow-up: results from the STEP-BD study. Bipolar Disord. 2009;11(4):391–400.
5. Lish JD, Dime-Meenan S, Whybrow PC, Price RA, Hirschfeld RM. The National Depressive and Manic-depressive Association (DMDA) survey of bipolar members. J Affect Disord. 1994;31(4):281–94.
6. Sullivan PF, Daly MJ, O'Donovan M. Genetic architectures of psychiatric disorders: the emerging picture and its implications. Nat Rev Genet. 2012;13(8):537–51.
7. Burt SA. Rethinking environmental contributions to child and adolescent psychopathology: a meta-analysis of shared environmental influences. Psychol Bull. 2009;135(4):608–37.

8. Bienvenu OJ, Davydow DS, Kendler KS. Psychiatric 'diseases' versus behavioral disorders and degree of genetic influence. Psychol Med. 2011;41(1):33–40.
9. Song J, Bergen SE, Kuja-Halkola R, Larsson H, Landen M, Lichtenstein P. Bipolar disorder and its relation to major psychiatric disorders: a family-based study in the Swedish population. Bipolar Disord. 2015;17(2):184–93.
10. Wang LJ, Shyu YC, Yuan SS, Yang CJ, Yang KC, Lee TL, et al. Attention-deficit hyperactivity disorder, its pharmacotherapy, and the risk of developing bipolar disorder: a nationwide population-based study in Taiwan. J Psychiatr Res. 2016;72:6–14.
11. Chen MH, Su TP, Chen YS, Hsu JW, Huang KL, Chang WH, et al. Higher risk of developing mood disorders among adolescents with comorbidity of attention deficit hyperactivity disorder and disruptive behavior disorder: a nationwide prospective study. J Psychiatr Res. 2013;47(8):1019–23.
12. Jerrell JM, McIntyre RS, Park YM. Correlates of incident bipolar disorder in children and adolescents diagnosed with attention-deficit/hyperactivity disorder. J Clin Psychiatry. 2014;75(11):e1278–83.
13. McIntyre RS, Kennedy SH, Soczynska JK, Nguyen HT, Bilkey TS, Woldeyohannes HO, et al. Attention-deficit/hyperactivity disorder in adults with bipolar disorder or major depressive disorder: results from the international mood disorders collaborative project. Prim Care Companion J Clin Psychiatry. 2010;12(3):PCC.09m00861.
14. Nierenberg AA, Miyahara S, Spencer T, Wisniewski SR, Otto MW, Simon N, et al. Clinical and diagnostic implications of lifetime attention-deficit/hyperactivity disorder comorbidity in adults with bipolar disorder: data from the first 1000 STEP-BD participants. Biol Psychiatry. 2005;57(11):1467–73.
15. Frias A, Palma C, Farriols N. Comorbidity in pediatric bipolar disorder: prevalence, clinical impact, etiology and treatment. J Affect Disord. 2015;174:378–89.
16. American Psychiatric Association. Diagnostic and statistical manual of mental disorders [Internet]. 5th ed. Washington, DC: American Psychiatric Association; 2013. Bipolar and related disorders; [cited 2019 Feb 3]. Available from https://dsm.psychiatryonline.org/doi/abs/10.1176/appi.books.9780890425596.dsm03.
17. National Institute of Mental Health [Internet]. Bethesda, MD: National Institute of Mental Health; 2015. Bipolar disorder in children and teens: NIH Publication No. QF 15–6380 [cited 2019 Feb 3]. Available from: https://www.nimh.nih.gov/health/publications/bipolar-disorder-in-children-and-teens/index.shtml.
18. Goldsmith M, Singh M, Chang K. Antidepressants and psychostimulants in pediatric populations: is there an association with mania? Paediatr Drugs. 2011;13(4):225–43.
19. Goldstein BI, Birmaher B, Carlson GA, DelBello MP, Findling RL, Fristad M, et al. The international society for bipolar disorders task force report on pediatric bipolar disorder: knowledge to date and directions for future research. Bipolar Disord. 2017;19(7):524–43.
20. Schneck CD, Chang KD, Singh MK, DelBello M, Miklowitz DJ. A pharmacologic algorithm for youth who are at high risk for bipolar disorder. J Child Adolesc Psychopharmacol. 2017;27(9):796–805.
21. Centers for Disease Control and Prevention [Internet]. Atlanta, GA: Centers for Disease Control and Prevention; 2017. Child development: positive parenting tips; 2017 Jan 3 [cited 2019 Feb 3]. Available from: https://www.cdc.gov/ncbddd/childdevelopment/positiveparenting/adolescence.html.
22. Kann L, Kinchen S, Shanklin SL, Flint KH, Hawkins J, Harris WA, et al. Youth risk behavior surveillance – United States, 2013. MMWR Suppl. 2014;63(4):1–168.
23. Peruzzolo TL, Tramontina S, Rohde LA, Zeni CP. Pharmacotherapy of bipolar disorder in children and adolescents: an update. Braz J Psychiatry. 2013;35(4):393–405.
24. Hauser M, Galling B, Correll CU. Suicidal ideation and suicide attempts in children and adolescents with bipolar disorder: a systematic review of prevalence and incidence rates, correlates, and targeted interventions. Bipolar Disord. 2013;15(5):507–23.

Chapter 13
When Trauma Mimics ADHD

Anna Chaves McDonald and Kida Ejesi

Case Example

Ryan is a 13-year-old boy in the seventh grade who exhibits difficulties with behavioral regulation. His teachers report that he sometimes has difficulty focusing, often acts impulsively, and is restless. At home, Ryan's mother also observes that he has difficulty paying attention and is fidgety. Ryan's teachers as well as his mother have discussed having him evaluated for ADHD.

At Ryan's next well-child visit, his mother discussed teacher concerns with his pediatrician. According to Ryan's mother, he was a highly energetic toddler and preschooler. She recalls that he had some difficulty learning early academic concepts as a result, but overall, few concerns were raised by his early teachers. Standard measures of ADHD completed by his mother and current middle school teachers revealed clinically significant concerns for inattention and hyperactivity/impulsivity within the home and school settings.

During the visit, Ryan's pediatrician also inquired about the role of potential psychosocial stressors in his life. Upon inquiry, the pediatrician learned that Ryan's father died suddenly in a car accident when Ryan was 9 years old. Following his death, Ryan's mother was diagnosed with depression. Given financial instability and his mother's mental health, Ryan and his mother moved away from the town he grew up in to be closer to his grandparents. In his new town, Ryan has had a hard time adjusting and making friends.

A. C. McDonald (✉)
ASK Program, Primary Care Center, Boston Children's Hospital, Boston, MA, USA
e-mail: Anna.ChavesMcDonald@childrens.harvard.edu

K. Ejesi
Developmental Medicine Center, Boston Children's Hospital, Boston, MA, USA
e-mail: kida.ejesi@childrens.harvard.edu

© Springer Nature Switzerland AG 2020
A. Schonwald (ed.), *ADHD in Adolescents*,
https://doi.org/10.1007/978-3-030-62393-7_13

Background

Attention-deficit/hyperactivity disorder (ADHD) is the most common neurobehavioral disorder among youth, and the diagnosis of ADHD as well as stimulant medication use in children and adolescents has become increasingly prevalent over time [1]. Diagnoses of ADHD, however, may sometimes be confounded by life experiences, which contribute to inattention and/or behavioral dysregulation in adolescents. Scholars have suggested the importance of evaluating for and taking into consideration potential contributions that may influence ADHD symptom onset and progression [2]. Exposure to trauma is just one important potential contribution. Associations between exposure to traumatic occurrences and ADHD are well documented [3, 4]. It is important, therefore, to consider the potential contribution of trauma when diagnosing ADHD in adolescents, in order to accurately diagnose and provide effective treatment.

Trauma

Although the term *trauma* is most often used to describe adolescents' reactions to catastrophic events (such as in the case of post-traumatic stress disorder), trauma actually casts a much wider net. According to the most recent definition of childhood trauma from the National Child Traumatic Stress Network, trauma can be conceptualized as a frightening, violent, or dangerous event that poses a threat to a child's bodily integrity or, more severely, a child's life. Youth's safety and well-being depend on the perceived safety and well-being of their attachment figures [5].

> Unique to trauma in childhood and adolescence is that *witnessing* a traumatic event that threatens the physical security or life of a parent or caregiver can be as traumatic as experiencing the threat directly.

One can see by this definition that what is described as "trauma" can vary widely from the chronic, to the acute, to the stressful, to life-threatening. For example, an adolescent who has experienced persistent homelessness can be conceptualized as having undergone *trauma*, as can the adolescent who witnessed domestic violence between their parents. An adolescent whose family survived an earthquake may have undergone *trauma*, as well as the adolescent who is coping with chronic food insecurity. To add further complexity to the conceptualization of trauma, adolescents' reactions to the different forms of trauma can vary widely: siblings who are exposed to the same single event or series of events may experience entirely different reactions in the moment and can also have differing long-term effects [6].

Common Symptoms of Trauma

Trauma can cause a multitude of symptoms that vary widely between children and adolescents. Some of the most commonly seen symptoms according to the Diagnostic and Statistical Manual of Mental Disorders (DSM-5) are highlighted in the diagnostic criteria for PTSD and the stressor-related disorders. These diagnostic criteria include anger, persistent feelings of sadness or hopelessness, flashbacks, unpredictable emotions (ranging from emotional withdrawal to rage), physical symptoms such as headaches or stomach aches, sleep disturbances, shame, guilt, and feelings of isolation. Currently, the DSM-5 conceptualizes the most severe reactions to trauma as post-traumatic stress disorder, with less severe forms of PTSD listed as well. Other stressor-related disorders include reactive attachment disorder, acute stress disorder, adjustment disorders, and other specified and unspecified trauma- and stressor-related disorders [7].

Post-traumatic Stress and Trauma- and Stressor-Related Disorders

Although the definition of trauma includes many symptoms that overlap with post-traumatic stress disorder (PTSD), they are not mutually exclusive. While every adolescent who has been diagnosed with PTSD has experienced or witnessed some sort of trauma (in fact, it is one of the diagnostic criteria), not all adolescents who are exposed to trauma will go on to develop PTSD. It is impossible to predict with certainty which adolescents will later develop PTSD and which adolescents will not. Individual factors such as gender, socioeconomic status, ethnicity, and age or ages when the trauma occurred can vary widely in their risk or protective nature.

In a nod to the variability in trauma presentations and to better capture the types of trauma that have not been historically captured by PTSD (e.g., chronic interpersonal trauma, environmental instability, unpredictability), the DSM-5 introduced a new diagnosis of trauma- and stressor-related disorder. These diagnoses (there is an *other specified* and *unspecified* version) allow providers to capture the presentation of adolescents who experience significant trauma-related symptoms (below the level that would be expected for a diagnosis of PTSD) in the context of ongoing "low-scale" danger, maltreatment, and/or inadequate caregiving systems. Per the DSM-5, these symptoms persist beyond what would be expected for an adjustment disorder (6 months) and may not include symptoms of dysfunctional attachment that would classify a disorder of reactive attachment disorder or disinhibited social engagement disorder [7].

Traumatic Childhood Events

According to the National Survey of Children's Health (NSCH), as of 2013, almost half (48%) of all youth in the United States had experienced at least one or more types of childhood trauma [8]. In looking at the scope of what this one national survey included as a "traumatic childhood event," we can see how outcomes may be completely different for any one adolescent depending on the event and number of total events in the adolescent's lifetime, as well as any protective factors that may serve to dampen negative outcomes of trauma. These events included (but were not limited to) socioeconomic hardship, divorce/separation of a parent, death of a parent, parent served time in jail, witness to domestic violence, living with a mentally ill individual or someone with a drug/alcohol abuse problem, and being treated unfairly due to race or ethnicity.

Perhaps even more concerning, especially when considering that frontal lobe brain development continues well into adolescence and early adulthood, the NSCH reported that nearly one-third (23%) of 12–17 year olds had experienced two or more adverse family experiences. Although neuroimaging research is still limited on the ranging effects of psychological trauma to the brain [9], we do know that the frontal lobe is the last to develop completely (in the early twenties). Although it has many roles, most research to date implicates the frontal lobe in executive functioning (memory, planning, organization), impulse control, attention, and anticipation of consequences [10]. The high comorbidity of trauma with other psychiatric diagnoses that include impairments in executive functioning is understandable, considering the later development of the frontal lobe.

Comorbidity

The inclusion of an unspecified category of trauma- and stressor-related disorders helps to capture many of the symptoms that were once considered subthreshold for a PTSD diagnosis. However, researchers and clinicians alike contend that there are still symptoms of complex trauma that are not captured by these diagnostic categories, primarily because the symptoms are already captured by other disorders. Disorders that are likely to co-occur with PTSD include, but are not limited to, anxiety disorders (separation anxiety, obsessive-compulsive disorder, specific phobias, social phobia), conduct disorder, major depressive disorder, bipolar disorder, and schizophrenia [11].

Although many psychiatric disorders overlap with PTSD and other stressor-related disorders, they fail to capture the full extent of the self-regulatory and relational impairments caused by low-scale trauma [12].

The Centers for Disease Control and Prevention coined the term "adverse childhood events (ACEs)" in their wide-scale epidemiological study that matched ACEs against adolescent and adult health risks, health status, and social functioning. The original study (which later inspired many smaller-scale studies across the United States) measured ACEs in 17,000 adults in San Diego. Similar to the NSCH study, the CDC's ACE study characterized types of childhood adversity as physical, sexual, or verbal abuse; physical or emotional neglect; having a parent who is an alcoholic, addicted to other drugs, or diagnosed with a mental illness; witnessing domestic violence; losing a parent to abandonment or divorce; and having a family member in jail. Among many negative outcomes, one of the most important outcomes to the context of this chapter concluded that adolescents who experienced one or more ACE had more difficulty with self-regulation, emotional competence, and behavioral control. These effects persisted well into adulthood and systematically increased the likelihood of other mental health diagnoses [13].

Not only does trauma in childhood (ACEs, PTSD, or other trauma- and stressor-related disorders) substantially increase the risk for comorbid disorders in adolescence, but also childhood trauma increases the risk for other mental health disorders and other adverse outcomes in adulthood. Wu and colleagues reported that greater exposure to ACEs in childhood significantly increased the odds of several adverse health outcomes in adulthood including PTSD, alcohol dependence, tobacco use and drug abuse, medical problems, sex work, and poor quality of life [14]. In a study conducted by Famularo and colleagues, youth who had undergone childhood maltreatment exhibited greater instances of ADHD, oppositional defiant disorder (ODD), and PTSD as compared to typically developing children [15]. Further, McLeer et al. found that the most frequent diagnosis of sexually abused children was not in fact PTSD, but ADHD [16]. A more recent study found that children with ADHD were more than two times more likely to be diagnosed with PTSD than children without ADHD [17].

Common Symptoms of Trauma and ADHD

Exposure to traumatic experiences can have a profound impact on development. Exposure to adverse experiences is associated with difficulties related to self, emotional, and behavioral regulation. Exposure to traumatic experiences can lead to emotional distress causing difficulty with concentration, motor restlessness, and outbursts of explosive behavior. In many cases, therefore, adolescents who have been exposed to trauma may present with symptoms that are classically seen in children with ADHD. Several symptoms are common among trauma-exposed youth and ADHD. The National Child Traumatic Stress Network highlighted some of these common symptoms in the figure below [18] (Fig. 13.1).

Based on the illustration, some common symptoms include difficulty concentrating and learning in school, proneness to distraction, difficulty listening, disorganization, hyperactivity, restlessness, and difficulty sleeping. Exposure to traumatic

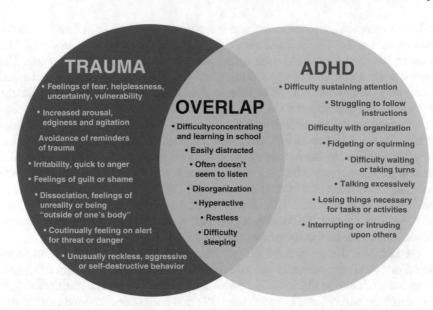

Fig. 13.1 Common symptoms of child traumatic stress and ADHD (Siegfried et al. [18], with permission from the National Center for Child Traumatic Stress)

experiences can lead to the presentation of similar symptoms noted in the inattention and hyperactivity/impulsivity clusters of ADHD as outlined in the DSM-5 [7]. The overlap between trauma exposure and ADHD suggests that it is important to understand the potential role of trauma in an adolescent who presents with inattention and/or hyperactivity and impulsivity.

> Treatment of adolescents with trauma histories and ADHD-like symptoms can be complex, particularly as there are no established guidelines regarding which condition to treat first or whether both conditions should be treated simultaneously [18].

Relationship Between Trauma and ADHD

The coexistence of ADHD and trauma- and stressor-related disorders has been well documented in the literature [19, 20]. Youth who are diagnosed with ADHD are more likely to have been exposed to ACEs compared to youth without an ADHD diagnosis [3]. Exposure to childhood traumatic events may increase symptoms that result in a diagnosis of ADHD [4]. Life stressors such as low socioeconomic status, reduced stimulation and support within the home setting, parental discord, parental psychopathology, and child maltreatment have been found to be associated with an increased risk of ADHD symptoms [21, 22]. Adolescents with a history of childhood physical abuse are more likely to self-report inattentive and hyperactive symptoms, and adolescents with a history of sexual abuse are more likely to self-report symptoms of inattention [23]. While studies have found associations between exposure to various traumatic or stressful occurrences and ADHD, the directionality and causality of these associations are not clearly understood [3, 7].

The nature of the relationship between the exposure to traumatic occurrences in adolescents and ADHD remains a subject of debate. There is disagreement, for instance, as to how to diagnostically understand these youth. Some scholars believe that exposure to childhood trauma can lead to a misdiagnosis of ADHD [24]. Avoidance symptoms of trauma- and stressor-related disorders may mirror inattentive behaviors seen in ADHD such as poor focus, distractibility, and avoidance of activities. Similarly, hyperactive symptoms of trauma- and stressor-related disorders may mirror hyperactive behaviors seen in ADHD such as fidgetiness and restlessness [25]. Additionally, confusion and agitated behavior due to intrusive thoughts may mirror impulsive behaviors seen in ADHD [18]. Trauma-exposed adolescents presenting with symptoms such as hyper-vigilance, disassociation, and hyper-arousal, therefore, may be presenting with the normal effects of traumatic stress suggesting that, for some youth, their symptoms may be entirely secondary to the trauma.

Yet, others suggest that the diagnosis of ADHD can be part of a trauma-exposed adolescent's diagnostic presentation. These adolescents may have an increased risk for ADHD given genetic and familial risk factors and may have exhibited difficulties with regulation prior to the occurrence of their traumatic experience. ADHD symptoms are not necessarily a sequela of PTSD, but can result from the cumulative impact of the two diagnoses and lead to a more complicated course and outcome [17].

In other words, diagnoses of ADHD and trauma- and stressor-related disorders can co-occur and should be diagnosed as such, when appropriate.

Early traumatic stress can lead to changes in neural development and brain functioning consistent with ADHD [26, 27]. For instance, there is evidence that early exposure to traumatic occurrences can lead to changes in brain development contributing to hyperactivity [28]. Additionally, research from the toxic stress literature, defined as the excessive or prolonged activation of stress response systems in the body and brain, found that exposure to ACEs increases the risk of toxic levels of stress in the body, which can change the structure and function of the developing brain. Toxic stress has been associated with higher rates of executive function deficits and an increased risk for ADHD [29].

Further complicating the understanding of the relationship between trauma and ADHD is the debate over ADHD as a risk factor for experiencing trauma or stressful life occurrences and for the development of PTSD in youth [19]. Deficits in behavioral regulation, specifically impulsivity, may contribute to a youth's susceptibility to engage in risk-taking and dangerous behavior. Additionally, youth diagnosed with ADHD may be at risk for experiencing trauma, particularly if their caretakers have been diagnosed with ADHD or have experienced trauma themselves. The stress that vulnerable caregivers may face in parenting a child or adolescent with ADHD increases the likelihood of traumatic experiences such as childhood physical abuse due to poor parental impulse control [30, 31]. Furthermore, having a child with ADHD may also contribute to increased socioeconomic hardship for families, thereby adding additional stress within the home setting [32]. Youth with ADHD may be vulnerable to stressful life events, some of which may be traumatic and lead to a trauma- and stressor-related diagnosis.

Assessment of Trauma and ADHD in Adolescents

Are symptoms such as inattention and hyper-arousal secondary to trauma? Do these symptoms reflect an underlying disorder of ADHD? Should trauma-exposed adolescents presenting with inattention and/or hyperactivity and impulsivity be diagnosed with ADHD, a trauma- and stressor-related disorder, or both? Given the relationship between trauma and ADHD as well as their overlapping symptoms, it is important that a comprehensive assessment is conducted to understand the etiology of an adolescent's presenting concerns. Each adolescent is unique and possesses their own set of genetic and familial risk factors and life experiences. A thorough and well-informed assessment will increase the chances of an accurate diagnosis being made.

Given the overlap in symptomatology between ADHD and trauma exposure, diagnosing trauma-exposed adolescents presenting with inattention and regulation difficulties may be challenging.

> All adolescents presenting with symptoms of ADHD should be screened for exposure to adverse experiences.

This is important so that providers do not misattribute symptoms of trauma exposure exclusively to ADHD [3]. Ultimately, while ADHD and trauma-related disorders can coexist, it is critical for clinicians to ascertain whether or not presenting concerns are best explained by one or both diagnoses [31].

Parents who are concerned about their adolescent's development might first seek consultation from their child's pediatrician. In order to improve the accuracy of diagnosis, when pediatricians are consulted, they are advised to consider the potential contribution of other conditions, such as trauma, which commonly co-occur with ADHD [2]. In addition to obtaining an understanding of an adolescent's history and onset of core symptoms, best practice is to also conduct a complete biopsychosocial assessment when assessing for ADHD, which includes the potential contribution of traumatic event symptoms [33]. In order to assist pediatricians in identifying trauma, the American Academy of Pediatrics has developed a trauma toolbox for use within the primary care setting [34]. Use of the trauma toolbox is particularly important among youth who present with behavioral concerns commonly seen in ADHD, as most ADHD rating scales focus solely on the behavioral presentation of the individual. Typical ADHD rating scales do not assess for ACEs that may have contributed to the onset and progression of ADHD-like symptoms [3].

If an adolescent presenting with inattention and/or behavioral regulation difficulties is suspected to have been exposed to trauma, a referral to an outside health-care professional may be indicated [33]. These professionals, such as psychiatrists, psychologists, and clinical social workers, can help decipher whether or not an adolescent's behavior is indicative of ADHD, a trauma- and stressor-related presentation, or both.

According to the National Child Traumatic Stress Network, a comprehensive assessment of traumatic stress in youth should include the assessment of the following:

- Occurrence of traumatic events
- Presence of a wide range of symptoms (e.g., high-risk behaviors, family environmental factors, functional impairments, trauma reminders and triggers)
- Protective factors (e.g., the youth's strengths, talents, abilities, availability of emotional support, capacity for resilience)

A comprehensive assessment should also utilize multiple methods to gather information including clinical interviews, behavioral observations, and standardized measures; the assessment should also include multiple sources of information including the adolescent, caregivers, teachers, and other providers. Multiple sources can help shed light on an adolescent's functioning to obtain a clearer diagnostic picture [18].

Importantly, when screening for trauma in adolescents who present with ADHD-like symptoms, the assessment must be culturally sensitive. In other words, clinicians must strive to understand how culture (e.g., race, ethnicity, gender) can impact how an adolescent and their family express psychological distress and define trauma, as well as their comfort level in disclosing trauma [35]. A culturally informed assessment will enhance the likelihood of arriving at an accurate understanding and diagnosis of the adolescent.

Implications for Treatment and Service Planning

Having ADHD as well as a trauma history contributes to greater impairment in youth than having ADHD or experiencing trauma alone [19]. Having been exposed to adverse childhood occurrences may increase susceptibility for or exacerbate symptoms of ADHD [20]. Having a clear diagnostic understanding of an adolescent's presenting concerns, therefore, will contribute to the identification and implementation of a treatment and service plan that is sensitive and responsive to the needs of the adolescent. Treatment of adolescents with symptoms of ADHD and trauma histories requires multifaceted interventions. These adolescents will require interventions that target their emotional functioning (i.e., trauma-specific therapies) as well as their behavioral presentation.

Classic adolescent therapies for ADHD utilize interventions that target the symptoms of ADHD; these typically include medication as well as behavioral interventions. Classic ADHD therapies, however, do not address emotional functioning. Therefore, clinicians must exercise caution and consider the impact of trauma when generating and implementing treatment recommendations for ADHD as they may not have the intended benefit for adolescents who experienced traumatic occurrences. Typical treatments for adolescents with ADHD, which include psychopharmacological interventions, may not be appropriate for those with exposure to trauma: these medications may have unintended results. For instance, stimulant medication may contribute to increased sleep difficulties and agitation in adolescents whose symptoms are better accounted for by trauma exposure [31].

Trauma-specific interventions, in contrast, target an adolescent's emotional functioning. Many trauma-focused interventions are available. The National Child Traumatic Stress Network suggests that these interventions share core components with respect to intervention objectives and practice elements. Some of the core components of trauma-focused interventions [36] are listed in Table 13.1. Trauma-focused interventions, therefore, are multifaceted and address the needs of youth at multiple levels.

Depending on the adolescent's symptoms and trauma history, they may benefit from interventions initially targeting their trauma histories rather than their ADHD symptoms. Once symptom stabilization and safety for trauma are achieved, however, the associated ADHD symptoms should be addressed [19]. For some adolescents, symptoms of inattention and hyperactivity may interfere in their ability to participate in trauma-specific interventions, and therefore, it may be necessary to initially target their ADHD symptoms [18]. Overall, clinicians are advised to use information gathered from a comprehensive assessment to guide individualized

Table 13.1 Core components of trauma-focused interventions

Core components of trauma-focused interventions
Motivational interviewing
Risk screening
Psychoeducation about trauma and loss reminders, stress, and grief reactions
Teaching of emotional regulation skills
Parenting skills and behavior management
Construction of a trauma narrative
Teaching of safety skills
Advocacy at school or within the community
Teaching of relapse prevention skills

treatment recommendations. Clinicians are also urged to continually monitor the adolescent's functioning, assess effectiveness of specific interventions, and modify interventions as needed.

In addition to psychopharmacological interventions, behavioral supports, and/or trauma-specific treatment modalities, adolescents with trauma histories and ADHD symptoms should receive school-based interventions that support their behavioral and emotional functioning at school. Depending on the needs of the adolescent, these may include special education services, a 504 Plan, and/or school-based counseling. In some instances, it may be prudent to share the adolescent's trauma history with school personnel in order to prevent exposure to experiences which may be retraumatizing for the individual.

Case Revisited

There are several factors highlighted in this case example that are important to parents, teachers, and clinicians working with youth like Ryan. First and foremost, Ryan's diagnostic presentation is not straightforward. Although he presents with several symptoms of ADHD including inattention, impulsivity, and hyperactivity that are seen in multiple settings, Ryan has also experienced a significant traumatic event: the sudden death of his father when he was 9 years old. After his father's death, additional stressors arose in Ryan's life including the subsequent rapid move away from his friends and support group and his mother's emergent depression. Additionally, even though Ryan has been described as a "highly energetic toddler and preschooler," his attentional and behavioral difficulties as a child did not appear to greatly impact his learning aside from some mild difficulties. In fact, few concerns were raised by his teachers until more recently. Given our discussion on the complexities of differentiating ADHD and trauma (and the overlap between the two), Ryan's presentation can be viewed through the lens of either disorder. Rather than focusing on a singular diagnosis, however, the more helpful action that can be undertaken by teachers and caregivers in his life is understanding that Ryan's symptoms may have multiple causes.

Ryan's teacher and mother have both taken one of the most important steps in beginning the process of improving Ryan's behavioral functioning and well-being: communication with the multiple individuals that interact with him on a daily basis. Open communication is the first step that any teacher, clinician, or parent should take upon recognizing symptoms that represent a change in an adolescent's behavior and/or symptoms that are impairing to everyday functioning in home or at school. Upon talking to each other, Ryan's mother and his teacher have realized that his symptoms of hyperactivity, inattention, and distractibility are persistent across settings. Further consultation with Ryan's pediatrician has shed light on the possibility that symptoms – which initially presented as likely ADHD – may also be the result of a significant trauma and several subsequent changes in location, support, and friendships. Ryan's mother's depression may have also played a significant role in changes in his behavior and emotional well-being, particularly if it was left untreated.

If Ryan's presentation is not that of *just* ADHD or *just* a reaction to an earlier trauma and continued stressors, treatment should include interventions that target both areas. In this case, given the relative recency of Ryan's father's death, treatment for Ryan that first addresses his emotional well-being is likely to be most effective. If symptoms of ADHD persist upon stabilization of Ryan's mood, then they should be addressed accordingly, with behavioral or pharmaceutical interventions (or a combination of the two).

However, as previously mentioned, no one child or adolescent's presentation – or treatment – will be exactly the same. A teenager with more severe ADHD symptomatology may not be able to access treatment targeted to improve emotional well-being until behavioral symptoms are under control [18]. Similarly, a teen who is experiencing chronic or acute depression in relation to death, grief, or another associated trauma may require a stabilization of mood before ADHD symptoms can be assessed or addressed [19]. In order to determine the best treatment trajectory, parents, teachers, and clinicians should be attuned to all symptoms present in their respective settings and should be actively communicating with other caregivers. In addition to being attuned to an adolescent's functioning, caregivers should ensure that they are not prematurely diagnosing ADHD or trauma-related disorders without first gathering a full medical and psychosocial history. In Ryan's case, had his pediatrician not highlighted the possible impact of his family's trauma, she may have intervened by treating his ADHD symptoms rather than referring him for further evaluation and/or therapy. Additionally, if Ryan's trauma history had been viewed as the only cause of his difficulties concentrating in school and at home, his teachers and mother may have not been provided with the appropriate strategies to support his attention and behavioral regulation both at school and at home.

Tips
- It's important to know if the adolescent – with ADHD or ADHD symptoms – has experienced trauma; note that not all adolescents who are exposed to trauma will go on to develop PTSD.
- Perspectives on trauma, like ADHD, vary considerably across cultures and ethnicities. As always, conversations on this topic should be approached with utmost cultural humility.
- The National Child Traumatic Stress Network (https://www.nctsn.org/) provides a range of resources, curricula, and trainings, including a clinician fact sheet "Is it ADHD or Child Traumatic Stress?" (https://www.nctsn.org/resources/it-adhd-or-child-traumatic-stress-guide-clinicians).

Conclusions

Exposure to traumatic life events places adolescents at risk for emotional distress and regulatory difficulties. It is important that caregivers understand that ADHD-like symptoms can be influenced by factors such as trauma. Evaluation of adolescents who present with ADHD-like symptoms, therefore, should always include an assessment of the potential contribution of trauma. When trauma exposure is part of an adolescent's profile, treatment interventions should be multifaceted and target emotional functioning as well as behavioral symptoms. Interventions should be carefully monitored for effectiveness and modified when needed. Importantly, adolescents whose ADHD symptoms are confounded by traumatic occurrences have the potential to be successful and flourish if given the appropriate supports and services.

References

1. Visser SN, Danielson ML, Bitsko RH, Holbrook JR, Kogan MD, Ghandour RM, et al. Trends in the parent-report of health care provider-diagnosed and medicated attention-deficit/hyperactivity disorder: United States, 2003–2011. J Am Acad Child Adolesc Psychiatry. 2014;53(1):34–46. https://doi.org/10.1016/j.jaac.2013.09.001.
2. American Academy of Pediatrics, Subcommittee on Attention-Deficit/Hyperactivity Disorder, Steering Committee on Quality Improvement and Management. ADHD: clinical practice guideline for the diagnosis, evaluation and treatment of attention-deficit/hyperactivity disorder in children and adolescents. Pediatrics. 2011;128(5):1007–22. https://doi.org/10.1542/peds.2011-2654.
3. Brown NM, Brown SN, Briggs RD, German M, Belamarich PF, Oyeku SO. Associations between adverse childhood experiences and ADHD diagnosis and severity. Acad Pediatr. 2017;17(4):349–55. https://doi.org/10.1016/j.acap.2016.08.013.
4. Jimenez ME, Wade R Jr, Schwartz-Soicher O, Lin Y, Reichman NE. Adverse childhood experiences and ADHD diagnosis at age 9 years in a National Urban Sample. Acad Pediatr. 2017;17(4):356–61. https://doi.org/10.1016/j.acap.2016.12.009.
5. About Child Trauma. The National Child Traumatic Stress Network. 2018. http://www.nctsn.org/what-is-child-trauma/about-child-trauma. Accessed 21 Nov 2018.
6. Green BL, Korol M, Grace MC, Vary MG, Leonard AC, Gleser GC, et al. Children and disaster: age, gender, and parental effects on PTSD symptoms. J Am Acad Child Adolesc Psychiatry. 1991;30(6):945–51. https://doi.org/10.1097/00004583-199111000-00012.
7. Diagnostic and statistical manual of mental disorders: DSM-5. Arlington: American Psychiatric Association; 2013.
8. Health Resources and Services Administration, Maternal and Child Health Bureau in collaboration with the U.S. Census Bureau. National survey of children's health. Child and Adolescent Health Measurement Initiative, Data Resource Center for Child and Adolescent Health. 2018. http://www.childhealthdata.org. Accessed 21 Nov 2018.
9. Rinne-Albers MAW, van der Wee NJA, Lamers-Winkelman F, Vermeiren RRJM. Neuroimaging in children, adolescents, and young adults with psychological trauma. Eur Child Adolesc Psychiatry. 2013;22:745–55. https://doi.org/10.1007/s00787-013-0410-1.
10. Passler MA, Issac W, Hynd GW. Neuropsychological development of behavior attributed to frontal lobe functioning in children. Dev Neuropsychol. 1985;4:349–70. https://doi.org/10.1080/87565648509540320.

11. Ghanizadeh A, Mohammadi MR, Moini R. Comorbidity of psychiatric disorders and parental psychiatric disorders in a sample of Iranian children with ADHD. J Atten Disord. 2008;12:149–55. https://doi.org/10.1177/1087054708314601.

12. Cook A, Spinazzola J, Ford J, Lanktre C, Blaustein M, Cloitre M, et al. Complex trauma in children and adolescents. Psychiatr Ann. 2005;35(5):390–8. https://doi.org/10.3928/00485713-20050501-05.

13. Adverse Childhood Experiences Study. Centers for Disease Control and Prevention. 2018. http://www.cdc.gov/violenceprevention/acestudy/about.html. Accessed 21 Nov 2018.

14. Wu NS, Shairer LC, Dellor E, Grella C. Childhood trauma and health outcomes in adults with comorbid substance abuse and mental health disorders. Addict Behav. 2010;35:68–71. https://doi.org/10.1016/j.addbeh.2009.09.00.

15. Famularo R, Kinscherff R, Fenton T. Psychiatric diagnoses of maltreated children: preliminary findings. J Am Acad Child Adolesc Psychiatry. 1992;31(5):863–7.

16. McLeer SV, Callaghan M, Henry D, Wallen J. Psychiatric disorders in sexually abused children. J Am Acad Child Adolesc Psychiatry. 1994;33:313–9.

17. Biederman J, Petty C, Spencer TJ, Woodworth KY, Bhide P, Zhu J, et al. Is ADHD a risk for posttraumatic stress disorder (PTSD)? Results from a large longitudinal study of referred children with and without ADHD. World J Biol Psychiatry. 2013;15:49–55. https://doi.org/10.3109/15622975.2012.756585.

18. Siegfried CB, Blackshear K, National Child Traumatic Stress Network, with assistance from the National Resource Center on ADHD: A Program of Children and Adults with Attention/Deficit Hyperactivity Disorder (CHADD). Is it ADHD or child traumatic stress? A guide for clinicians. Los Angeles, CA & Durham, NC: The National Child Traumatic Stress Network. 2016. Available from: http://www.nctsn.org/resources/it-adhd-or-child-traumatic-stress-guide-clinicians. Accessed 27 Dec 2018.

19. Biederman J, Petty CR, Spencer TJ, Woodworth KY, Bhide P, Zhu J, et al. Examining the nature of the comorbidity between pediatric attention deficit/hyperactivity disorder and post-traumatic stress disorder. Acta Psychiatr Scand. 2013;128(1):78–87. https://doi.org/10.1111/acps.12011.

20. Szymanski K, Sapanski MA, Conway F. Trauma and ADHD – association or diagnostic confusion? A clinical perspective. J Infant Child Adolesc Psychother. 2011;10(1):51–9. https://doi.org/10.1080/15289168.2011.575704.

21. Nigg JT, Carver L. Commentary: ADHD and social disadvantage: an inconvenient truth? A reflection on Russell et al. (2014) and Larsson et al. (2014). J Child Psychol Psychiatry. 2014;55(5):446–7. https://doi.org/10.1111/jcpp.12237.

22. Sanderud K, Murphy S, Elklit A. Child maltreatment and ADHD symptoms in a sample of young adults. Eur J Psychotraumatol. 2016;7(1):32061. https://doi.org/10.3402/ejpt.v7.32061.

23. Ouyang L, Fang X, Mercy J, Perou R, Grosse SD. Attention-deficit/hyperactivity disorder symptoms and child maltreatment: a population-based study. J Pediatr. 2008;153(6):851–6. https://doi.org/10.1016/j.jpeds.2008.06.002.

24. Ruiz R. How childhood trauma could be mistaken for ADHD. The Atlantic. 2014. http://www.theatlantic.com/health/archive/2014/07/how-childhood-trauma-could-be-mistaken-for-adhd/373328/. Accessed 15 Nov 2018.

25. Ford JD. Traumatic victimization in childhood and persistent problems with oppositional-defiance. J Aggress Maltreat Trauma. 2002;6:25–58. https://doi.org/10.1300/J146v06n01_03.

26. Anda RF, Felitti VJ, Bremner JD, Walker JD, Whitfield C, Perry BD, et al. The enduring effects of abuse and related adverse experiences in childhood. Eur Arch Psychiatry Clin Neurosci. 2006;256(3):174–86. https://doi.org/10.1007/s00406-005-0624-4.

27. McLaughlin KA, Sheridan MA, Winter W, Fox NA, Zeanah CH, Nelson CA. Widespread reductions in cortical thickness following severe early-life deprivation: a neurodevelopmental pathway to attention-deficit/hyperactivity disorder. Biol Psychiatry. 2014;76(8):629–38. https://doi.org/10.1016/j.biopsych.2013.08.016.

28. Glod CA, Teicher MH. Relationship between early abuse, posttraumatic stress disorder, and activity levels in prepubertal children. J Am Acad Child Adolesc Psychiatry. 1996;35:1384–93.

29. Shonkoff JP, Garner AS. Committee on psychosocial aspects of child and family health, committee on early childhood adoption, and dependent care, section on developmental and behavioral pediatrics. The lifelong effects of early childhood adversity and toxic stress. Pediatrics. 2012;129(1):232–46. https://doi.org/10.1542/peds.2011-2663.

30. Cuffe SP, McCullough EL, Pumariega AJ. Comorbidity of attention deficit disorder and posttraumatic stress disorder. J Child Fam Stud. 1994;3(3):327–36.

31. Rucklidge JJ, Brown DL, Crawford S, Kaplan BJ. Retrospective reports of childhood trauma in adults with ADHD. J Atten Disord. 2006;9(4):631–41. https://doi.org/10.1177/1087054705283892.

32. Swensen AR, Birnbaum HG, Secnik K, Marynchenko M, Greenberg P, Claxton A. Attention-deficit/hyperactivity disorder: increased costs for patients and their families. J Am Acad Child Adolesc Psychiatry. 2003;42(12):1415–23. https://doi.org/10.1097/00004583-200312000-0008.

33. The ADHD Diagnostic Process. CHADD. 2018. http://chadd.org/for-professionals/the-adhd-diagnostic-process. Accessed 27 Dec 2018.

34. Trauma Guide. American Academy of Pediatrics. 2018. http://www.aap.org/en-us/advocacy-and-policy/aap-health-initiatives/healthy-foster-care-america/Pages/Trauma-Guide.aspx. Accessed 27 Dec 2018.

35. Wilson JP, Tang CS. Cross-cultural assessment of psychological trauma and PTSD. New York: Springer Publishing; 2007.

36. Overview. The National Child Traumatic Stress Network. 2018. http://www.nctsn.org/treatments-and-practices/trauma-treatments/overview. Accessed 27 Dec 2018.

Chapter 14
ADHD and Substance Use

Nicholas Chadi, Leslie Green, and Miriam Schizer

Case Example

Evan is a 17-year-old with long-standing ADHD and increasingly heavy use of marijuana. Treated with stimulant medication in elementary school, adherence diminished in his early adolescence. Marijuana use began when he was 14 years old, and he currently smokes daily to "calm down." He and his mother have been told that he cannot be treated for his ADHD while he continues his current level of substance use. However, he wants to graduate from high school and is struggling to stay focused to complete his work, whether he has been smoking or not. Evan, his parents, and his teachers find that his inattention is preventing him from succeeding in school.

Background

Substance use during adolescence is common and often associated with negative health outcomes [1]. While many of the negative consequences of substance use

N. Chadi (✉)
Division of Adolescent Medicine, Department of Pediatrics, Sainte-Justine University
Hospital Centre, Université de Montreal, Montreal, QC, Canada
e-mail: nicholas.chadi@umontreal.ca

L. Green
Adolescent Substance Use and Addiction Program, Division of Developmental Medicine,
Boston Children's Hospital, Boston, MA, USA
e-mail: leslie.green@childrens.harvard.edu

M. Schizer
Adolescent Substance Use and Addiction Program, Division of Developmental Medicine,
Department of Pediatrics, Boston Children's Hospital, Harvard Medical School,
Boston, MA, USA
e-mail: miriam.schizer@childrens.harvard.edu

© Springer Nature Switzerland AG 2020
A. Schonwald (ed.), *ADHD in Adolescents*,
https://doi.org/10.1007/978-3-030-62393-7_14

occur later in life, more than 95% of individuals who use substances initiate use before the age of 25 [2]. This early substance use initiation has a significant impact on the development of the brain, which continues well into the third decade of life [3].

The relationship between substance use and ADHD is complex and has been at the heart of many research investigations [4]. Youth with ADHD are at higher risk of misusing drugs and alcohol, and youth with substance use disorders (SUDs) are disproportionately affected by ADHD, which in turn may impact treatment and recovery [5]. After a brief discussion of the health effects of substance use in adolescents, we will explore some of the common risk and protective factors that may lead to or prevent SUDs in adolescents with ADHD. We will then review the implications of treated versus untreated ADHD in the development of SUDs and discuss strategies for the effective management of ADHD in the context of substance use.

Substance Use in Adolescence: An Overview

In the past three decades, advances in neuroimaging technology have improved understanding of the process of human brain development. We now know that specific parts of the brain reach maturity before others: this is particularly important when it comes to addictive behaviors [6]. In fact, while the amygdala and nucleus accumbens—two parts of the brain that play a key role in emotional processing and the experience of pleasure and reward, respectively—are fully developed by mid-adolescence, the prefrontal cortex, responsible for higher-level thinking, including planning, impulse control, and decision-making, is not fully developed until the late twenties [7]. This neurodevelopmental difference leads to what is sometimes recognized as a "rational thinking gap," leaving the brain of an adolescent more susceptible to the pleasurable effects and unwanted consequences tied to the use of addictive substances, such as alcohol, nicotine, marijuana, and other drugs, compared to the brain of an adult [8].

> The earlier the onset of substance use, the higher the likelihood of developing a SUD later in life [9].

For instance, if a young person starts using alcohol at the age of 13, the risk of having problematic alcohol use over the life span is approximately 50%, five times the population risk. This pattern of four- to fivefold increase in risk across the life span with early-onset substance use is similar for other substances [10].

The risk of developing SUDs is only one of the numerous health risks linked to early initiation of substance use. Perhaps one of the most concerning risks relates to the impact of alcohol and drug use on the process of brain maturation and development. In fact, exposure during adolescence to the three psychoactive substances most commonly used by adolescents (alcohol, nicotine, and marijuana) has been associated with long-term losses in attention capacity, memory formation, and intellectual abilities [11, 12]. This capacity decline can lead to various impairments at school, at work, or in sports and extracurricular activities [13].

Another important and concerning impact of substance use during adolescent years is the strong association between alcohol and drug use and increased adverse mental health outcomes, like depression and anxiety, and in some cases suicidal ideation, bipolar disease, and psychosis [14]. While alcohol and drugs have not yet been shown to be a direct cause of mental illness, several studies have established a temporal relationship in which substance use often predated mental health symptoms; this was not seen only in youth with pre-established mental health problems. In several cases, substance use can complicate the course of mental health conditions and can represent an important barrier to treatment [15]. Finally, although this is beyond the scope of this chapter, alcohol and drugs have been shown to impact the physical health and well-being of adolescents. Increased risk of high blood pressure, stroke, cancer, and respiratory or liver problems are only some of the multiple risks associated with early onset of alcohol and drug use [16]. These health risks are particularly concerning for adolescents with ADHD who take medications that may have dangerous interactions with alcohol and drugs.

ADHD and Substance Use: Risk and Exacerbating Factors

> Substance use exacerbates coexisting ADHD, and ADHD is a known risk factor for substance use and progression to SUDs [5].

The health risks associated with substance use in adolescence, whether physiological, cognitive, or mental/emotional as outlined above, are of considerable concern for individuals with ADHD given the higher rates of adolescent substance use in those who carry an ADHD diagnosis. The impact is bidirectional. An influential report published in 2011 documented the relationship between ADHD and substance use in 27 longitudinal studies [17]. The authors concluded that compared to children without ADHD, children with ADHD were significantly more likely to use nicotine in their lifetime and were three times more likely to develop nicotine dependence in adolescence or adulthood. Children with ADHD were also more likely to use marijuana and to develop SUDs with marijuana, cocaine, and alcohol in adolescence or adulthood. In general, they reported that individuals with ADHD were more than 2.5 times more likely than peers without ADHD to develop illicit substance abuse or dependence [17–22]. Specific substance use trends seen in adolescents with ADHD are listed below (Table 14.1).

Further, experiencing a higher number of ADHD symptoms is associated with a lower age at nicotine use initiation and vice versa [21]. Youth with ADHD may also

Table 14.1 Substance use trends seen in adolescents with ADHD

Substance use trends seen in adolescents with ADHD
Earlier initiation of use
Less time between use initiation and development of a SUD
Strong association with behavioral disorders
More acute substance use picture when ADHD is not detected, diagnosed, or treated early
Direct relationship with more severe and/or persistent ADHD symptoms [5, 20, 22–24]

be tempted to use substances like marijuana in an attempt to "self-medicate" or decrease symptoms of ADHD [25].

> While "self-medication" of ADHD symptoms with marijuana is commonly reported by adolescents with ADHD and may appear to provide temporary relief of some symptoms of impulsivity or hyperactivity, the use of marijuana is ultimately harmful and counterproductive and carries many more side effects than potential benefits [26].

The heightened risk for substance use and SUDs associated with ADHD extends into adulthood. One study conducted in a large group of adults followed since birth showed that individuals with ADHD who did not develop SUDs in adolescence still had higher rates of drug exposure as adults and were approximately 3.5 times more likely to develop new drug dependence in adulthood compared to individuals without ADHD [27]. This study raised the importance of close monitoring of these individuals for substance-related problems well into adulthood, especially if there is a co-occurring behavior disorder.

Connections Between ADHD and Substance Use

Potential explanations for the higher rates of substance use among adolescents with ADHD include neurobiological, psychiatric, environmental, and social factors. These factors are also known to interact with one another, creating a more complicated and severe health picture for youth who carry multiple risk factors [22]. Thus, it is important to understand these variables and their possible interplay in order to consider best intervention strategies.

Neurobiological Factors

The first set of factors to consider reside in the brain. Brain imaging technology has revealed that individuals with ADHD may experience lower levels of the chemical neurotransmitter dopamine in specific areas of the brain, leading to decreased attention capacity and learning aptitude, as well as lower mood and sense of pleasure [20]. Substance use leads to an increase in dopamine levels, especially in the brain's reward center—the nucleus accumbens—reversing symptoms experienced with the lower dopamine levels associated with ADHD. Thus, one theory postulates that adolescents with ADHD find symptom relief with the use of psychoactive substances, using them as a form of self-medication [5]. This neurobiological vulnerability could account for the higher rates of problematic substance use and SUDs seen in adolescents and adults with ADHD.

Adolescents with ADHD have also been found to initiate use of substances earlier than their peers without ADHD [28]. As has already been discussed, earlier initiation of substance use is correlated with higher likelihood of any substance use escalating to problematic use and ultimately to meeting criteria for a SUD [23]. This correlation is in part due to the stage of brain development occurring during early adolescence, a stage in which the brain is actively identifying pleasurable and aversive environmental stimuli, cueing the individual toward the former and away from the latter [29]. Given the euphoric effects of dopamine the brain receives with substance use, it is "tricked" into believing that substances are essential to survival and will continue to send out signals encouraging substance use whenever possible. This phenomenon could also in part account for the larger numbers of adults with persisting ADHD symptoms who develop SUDs later in life [23]. Of note, some research has shown that there is a shorter time between initiation of use and meeting criteria for a SUD diagnosis for adolescents with ADHD than for their non-ADHD diagnosed peers, though the mechanism leading to this condensed time frame is not well known [22].

> With early initiation of use, adolescents become "hard-wired" to be prompted by their own brain to continue and even increase substance use.

Further, research has shown that substance use in adolescence can reduce attentional, memory, and impulse control capacities, negatively impacting the developing prefrontal cortex. This impact leads to decreased capacity for behavioral regulation, which in turn negatively impacts the course of the ADHD [24]. There is evidence that alcohol use alone hinders the connection between the pleasure center in the temporal lobe of the brain and the prefrontal cortex, where impulse control occurs, meaning that the more an individual consumes alcohol, the weaker their ability to control the impulse to consume alcohol over time [6].

Psychiatric Factors

The next category of factors is those in the psychiatric domain. There are several psychiatric disorders that are common in both adolescents with ADHD and adolescents with substance use. Behavioral disorders specifically have been found to be not only common in individuals with ADHD but also a strong predictor of more severe clinical symptomatology, more severe functional impairments, higher persistence of ADHD into adulthood, and worse long-term outcomes related to ADHD disorder [23]. Epidemiological study findings show prevalence rates of oppositional defiant disorder/conduct disorder (ODD/CD) of at least 25% among teens with ADHD, with many studies showing even higher percentages [23, 30]. CD, which can blossom into antisocial personality disorder (ASP) in adults, is strongly linked with combined ADHD and substance use. This behavioral disorder is defined by deviance that can include aggression toward people or animals, lying, stealing, running away, skipping classes, and property destruction [31]. A number of studies have suggested that the increased risk for SUDs in adolescents with ADHD is actually attributable to the increased prevalence of CD in this population [17]. The association between ADHD and behavioral disorders tends to be stronger in teens with a predominance of hyperactivity/impulse control symptoms of ADHD, as compared to teens with more predominant inattentive-type symptoms [32]. This tendency makes it more likely for boys to be diagnosed with concurrent ADHD and SUDs, as girls with ADHD tend to display fewer of these hyperactivity/impulse control symptoms than their male counterparts.

> With co-occurring ADHD and CD, SUDs are four times more frequent than in adolescents with neither of these diagnoses [2].

Depression and anxiety are two other mental health conditions strongly associated with both substance use and ADHD [33]. These two conditions share several of the psychosocial risk factors that are often seen in adolescents with ADHD, like poor peer relations and academic failure. Further, the symptoms of these disorders, such as low mood, sleep difficulties, physical agitation, chronic worry, muscle tension, difficulty concentrating, and decreased appetite [31], can exacerbate and/or mimic ADHD symptoms [34], increasing the risk of substance use as a means of symptom alleviation [19] and/or of managing emotional processes surrounding difficult psychosocial factors.

Environmental and Social Factors

This final set of factors connecting ADHD and substance use in adolescents includes psychosocial issues faced both at home and in the community. Home life for teens with ADHD can present several risk factors for exacerbated ADHD symptoms and substance use. Research has shown higher stress levels within families of children with ADHD, primarily when combined with ODD/CD, leading to greater frequency of conflict in parent-child relationships and decompensated family functioning [35]. More negative communication patterns between adolescents and parents that more commonly include anger and aggressive conflict patterns have also been described [36]. Such communication and conflict patterns can both break down healthy communication and create a perception in adolescents of uncaring parents, both of which are associated with higher rates of substance use in teens [37]. These family dynamics can be even more impactful for families in which a parent also carries an active ADHD diagnosis. Adults whose ADHD symptoms persist beyond adolescence, more commonly seen in those with comorbid ODD/CD, are at increased risk for more severe functional impairments and resulting comorbidities such as affective disorders and problematic substance use [23]. All of these conditions lend themselves to the conflictual family dynamics detailed above, with parental substance use a commonly known risk factor for substance use in their offspring [17]. Finally, prenatal exposure to nicotine or alcohol is linked to greater risk of ADHD across the life span [22].

Community stressors, including academic and social challenges, faced by many adolescents with ADHD, can leave these teens feeling marginalized and/or experiencing internalizing problems such as depression and anxiety. Further, with less capacity for self-regulation, teens with ADHD may show their emotions through externalizing behaviors, such as anger outbursts or defiance [21], leading to further marginalization and ensuing low self-esteem. As they age, these teens may become comfortable relating to other marginalized peers who are more likely to have aberrant behaviors including substance use [38].

Impact of ADHD Treatment on Substance Use Disorders

ADHD and substance use not only are highly correlated but also, when found together, lead to worse clinical outcomes for each diagnosis with a higher number of comorbidities. Thus, it is imperative to consider the implications of treatment of ADHD and how various interventions can positively impact both ADHD symptom manifestation and substance use behaviors. When ADHD is left untreated, individuals most commonly experience worse long-term outcomes in multiple domains of functioning, including academic, antisocial behavior, driving, nonmedical drug use/addictive behavior, obesity, occupation, services use, self-esteem, and social function outcomes [23]. These findings point to the necessity of treating ADHD and treating it early.

> Recent studies find decreased incidence of SUDs in adolescents who were given pharmacological treatment for their ADHD as children [39].

Psychostimulant medications are often considered first-line treatment of ADHD. Whereas early research prompted concerns that treatment of childhood ADHD with stimulants might increase the risk of later substance use, more recent studies show that pharmacological treatment of ADHD does not predispose to substance use, but rather is protective against it. It is unclear whether this effect persists into adulthood if medication is discontinued.

Adolescents will at times present for diagnosis and treatment with untreated ADHD and an active SUD. Although both disorders should be recognized and treated, for example, using behavioral interventions such as cognitive behavioral therapy, research suggests that pharmacotherapy for ADHD in this context is not as effective in treating either the ADHD symptoms or the SUD. Results are better if the adolescent can achieve a transient period of abstinence from substances before pharmacotherapy is initiated [40]; however, this intervention progression cannot always be achieved, especially if substance use is chronic. In this case, using a harm reduction approach, with the primary objective of decreasing use broadly and the frequency of use in high-risk situations more specifically, could be appropriate.

Treatment Strategies in Adolescents with Concurrent Substance Use and ADHD

There are several ways to prevent or address substance use in adolescents with or without ADHD. The American Academy of Pediatrics now recommends annual Screening, Brief Intervention, and Referral to Treatment (SBIRT) for alcohol and drug use in primary care for all adolescents [41]. This can be done using short, evidenced-based screening tools such as Screening to Brief Intervention (S2BI) [42] or Car, Relax, Alone, Forget, Friends, Trouble (CRAFFT) [43]. In some states, like Massachusetts, where screening for alcohol and substance use by a school staff member is mandatory in all middle school and high schools, SBIRT has become a common practice in various healthcare settings including primary care offices and emergency rooms, as well as in school-based health centers. In the case of a positive screen, or a high clinical suspicion for a SUD, adolescents should undergo a thorough evaluation, and when possible, treatment for SUDs should be initiated before treatment for ADHD [40]. Adolescents can be referred to a specialized outpatient substance use program, an intensive outpatient program, or partial hospitalization program or a medium- to long-term residential treatment program [44]. In some cases, when substance use is very severe or in the case of a drug or alcohol overdose, acute stabilization in hospital or medical detoxification may be required.

Substance use may mimic many of the manifestations of untreated ADHD and prolong the course or make the management of ADHD symptoms more challenging. Inversely, ADHD symptoms may greatly improve if substance use is decreased or interrupted. In a policy statement specifically addressing co-occurring substance use and ADHD, the American Academy of Pediatrics recommends that youth should ideally be assessed for ADHD when not under the influence of alcohol or drugs; however, in some cases, especially when there is strong addiction to alcohol or drugs or when there is long-standing history of substance use, this ideal may not be possible [5]. In these cases, if there is a suspicion that ADHD symptoms are not exclusively related to substance use, it is reasonable and encouraged to initiate careful treatment for ADHD before or while addressing substance use problems.

Health providers may hesitate to prescribe psychostimulant medication to individuals with known substance use problems and a new diagnosis of ADHD [45]. In fact, misuse and diversion of ADHD medication, especially psychostimulants such as methylphenidate (Ritalin) or amphetamines (Adderall), are common among adolescents, affecting up to 10% of high school and college students [46]. Adolescents may be tempted to take doses of medication that are higher than prescribed or crush the medication in order to inhale or inject it, to get "high" or get a stronger, more intense stimulating effect [47]. Prescription stimulants may also be combined with other substances, which increases the likelihood of severe side effects, including cardiac and neurological complications as severe as seizures or cardiac arrest [48]. Diversion and misuse of psychostimulant medications by parents and other household members are also common and reported in as many as 16% of parents of children and adolescents with ADHD [49].

There are several ways to reduce the risk of stimulant diversion and misuse among youth with ADHD. The first, and perhaps most important strategy, is to ensure a proper diagnosis of ADHD and to rule out other co-occurring conditions which, if left unaddressed, may worsen or mimic symptoms of ADHD [5]. Examples may include hearing or visual difficulties, untreated mental health issues such as depression or anxiety, and learning disabilities. Another important step, especially when substance use is known or suspected, is to maximize non-pharmacological treatment options, which may prove effective in reducing many of the most prominent symptoms of ADHD [50, 51].

Once non-pharmacological treatments have been explored, medication treatment should be considered but with careful consideration of risks and benefits. While psychostimulant treatments are often considered first-line treatment, their higher effectiveness needs to be balanced against diversion or misuse potential [25]. We provide below a list of the most commonly prescribed ADHD medications along with their suspected misuse/abuse potential (Table 14.2).

A useful strategy when initiating medication treatment for ADHD in adolescents with known substance use problems is to consider non-psychostimulant medications in the categories of alpha-agonists (i.e., clonidine or guanfacine) and selective norepinephrine reuptake inhibitors (i.e., atomoxetine, sold under the brand name Strattera). These medications, while not as effective as psychostimulant medications, have a lower misuse potential than other approved treatments for ADHD and have been shown to provide some symptom improvement in adolescents [52]. They can be used alone or in combination with other non-medication strategies and ADHD medications.

Table 14.2 List of most commonly used medications for ADHD with suspected relative abuse potential

Stimulant status	Medication type	US trade name	Suspected relative abuse potential[b]
Stimulants			
Short acting/immediate release	Methylphenidate	Ritalin[a]	High
		Methylin[a]	High
	Dexmethylphenidate	Focalin[a]	High
	Amphetamine-dextroamphetamine	Adderall[a]	High
	Dextroamphetamine	Dexedrine	High
		Dextrostat[a]	High
		Procentra	High
Long acting/extended release	Methylphenidate	Metadate CD	Medium
		Metadate ER[a]	Medium
		Ritalin LA[a]	Medium
		Ritalin SR[a]	Medium
		Methylin ER	Medium
		Daytrana Patch	Low
		Concerta[a]	Low
		Quillivant XR	Low
	Dexmethylphenidate	Focalin XR[a]	Low
	Dextroamphetamine	Dexedrine Spansule[a]	Medium
	Amphetamine-dextroamphetamine	Adderall XR[a]	Medium
	Lisdexamfetamine	Vyvanse	Low
Nonstimulants			
α2-Adrenergic agonists	Guanfacine	Intuniv[a]	Low
	Clonidine	Kapvay[a]	Low
Selective norepinephrine reuptake inhibitor	Atomoxetine	Strattera	Low

CR controlled release, *ER* extended release, *LA* long acting, *SR* sustained release, *XR* extended release
Note: (a) Indicates that generic formulation is available. (b) Indicates relative abuse potential is suspected based on length of action and formulation of medication. Reproduced with permission from Harstad et al. [5] by the AAP

When nonstimulant options have been exhausted, the use of an amphetamine precursor (or prodrug; a molecule that needs to be metabolized before it becomes active) such as lisdexamfetamine (sold under the brand name Vyvanse) is thought to carry lower misuse potential among psychostimulants [53]. If amphetamine salts (sold under the brand name Adderall) or methylphenidate (sold under the brand names Ritalin, Concerta, and Biphentin) is selected, the use of longer-acting formulations instead of shorter-acting or immediate-release formulations, either in patch or oral form, should be preferred as they are less likely to be misused [54].

Once a medication has been selected, there are several ways for providers to help reduce the risk of medication misuse [5]. When there is evidence of substance use or prior diversion of prescription medication, providers can consider using a written contract with patients to discuss clear expectations around substance use, adherence to medication, medical follow-up visits, and consequences in the case of medication misuse. Providers should also consider writing shorter prescriptions with frequent refills and frequent follow-up visits, which can be used to monitor response to medication and potential misuse. Initially, it would be reasonable for physicians to schedule weekly or biweekly visits until a steady dose of medication is achieved. Adolescents should be asked at every visit about medication adherence and medication misuse. In some cases, clinic or home urine drug testing can be a helpful tool, which may help assess use of other substances and confirm that the medication is actually being taken [55].

Finally, parents or guardians can play an important role in decreasing misuse potential around ADHD medications. A responsible adult should be instructed to keep a teen's ADHD medication locked up, to minimize risk of patient misuse and, in some cases, misuse by siblings or other youth who may be visiting the home. Parents should also consider dispensing the medication themselves daily under direct observation, especially when there is ongoing substance use. Finally, when daytime medication doses are required, parents can collaborate with teachers or school health providers so that medication is stored in a safe space at school and taken under supervision. While in school, students should not carry bottles of ADHD medications which could be lost, stolen, diverted, or misused. Finally, families should be informed about the risk of medication misuse and diversion. Health providers can provide informational materials in print form or direct patients and families to sources curated by reliable organizations such as the American Academy of Pediatrics and Canadian ADHD Resource Alliance.

Overall, parents, families, and communities can play a key role in substance use prevention and treatment, whether specifically around ADHD medication diversion or substance use in general [56]. In addition, after-school programs, recovery support services such as Alcoholics Anonymous (AA), and other peer and family support groups often offer an important complement to behavioral and medical approaches [58]. Thus, when ADHD and substance use present together in an adolescent's diagnostic picture, the "village" of caregivers, whether at home, school, or medical office, needs to pull together in a collaborative effort of bridging the teen from ADHD and substance use turbulence to finding greater stability and steps toward a successful adulthood.

Family involvement in substance use treatment is associated with more favorable outcomes and sustained recovery for all substances [57].

Case Revisited

Evan's diagnostic profile should be carefully reconsidered, to determine if ADHD remains a problem and if additional disorders have emerged (depression, anxiety). If referral to a substance use program is not available or accessible, his pediatrician can provide psychoeducation about substance use and ADHD. Like many teens, Evan may experience his ADHD symptoms as temporarily improved when he uses marijuana. Using a harm reduction approach, with the primary objective of decreasing use broadly and the frequency of use in high-risk situations more specifically, his pediatrician may educate Evan about the harms caused by substance use, which outweigh the temporary subjective benefits. He is at increased risk of additional substance use into adulthood, and he faces greater legal implications if impaired judgment results in lawbreaking. Evan should also understand that ADHD treatment is less effective for a person with an active substance use disorder. Treatment might start with a nonstimulant medication. Should stimulant medication be indicated, longer-acting formulations are preferred, and careful medication monitoring is essential.

Conclusions

As highlighted throughout this chapter, ADHD and substance use often co-occur and, together, can lead to worsened ADHD and substance use symptom presentation, decreased sense of self, and increased behavioral concerns. There are several distinct opportunities for parents, healthcare providers, and school staff to help prevent, identify, and treat substance-use-related issues in the context of ADHD. Below are some key tips to consider when thinking about how and when to intervene.

Tips
- Screening:

  - Medication and non-medication treatment of ADHD during childhood are protective against later substance use in adolescence. Early intervention should be encouraged, and families hesitant to use medications should be provided information about increased risk of substance use problems when ADHD symptoms are poorly controlled.
  - As adolescents with ADHD tend to initiate substance use earlier than their non-diagnosed peers, universal screening for substance use should be implemented in early adolescence (i.e., by age 12–13).

- Behavioral concerns

  - Early behavioral issues with or without ODD/CD are often found in children with an ADHD subtype that is either mixed or predominantly hyperactive (vs inattentive) and are strongly correlated with substance use in adolescence. Children with symptoms of hyperactivity should be monitored closely as they enter adolescence for poor behavioral choices, including early substance use.

- Girls

  - Because girls less frequently display hyperactivity and behavioral aspects of ADHD, their attentional issues may remain undetected and untreated until sometime during the adolescent years. This can lead to anxiety and depression which are risk factors for substance use in adolescence. ADHD should be considered with early signs of academic difficulties to ensure early diagnosis and treatment.

- Alcohol, marijuana, and nicotine

  - Alcohol, marijuana, and nicotine are by far the most commonly used substances during adolescence. Exposure to each of these substances has negative impacts on brain development and affects the brain's capacity for attention, memory, and executive functioning, further complicating ADHD symptom trajectory. Teens and families should be informed about these important long-term health risks.

- For parents and other caregivers

  - By keeping an open line of communication with school staff and health providers about signs of ADHD and evidence of substance use, families can support diagnosis and treatment of ADHD and possibly prevent substance-use-related problems.
  - In addition, parents and caregivers can play an important supporting role in keeping and dispensing ADHD medication and by monitoring adolescents for ADHD medication effectiveness and adherence.

- For teachers and school staff

  - Teachers and school staff should stay informed about their students' ADHD medications and their potential for being misused. School staff can also help keep ADHD medication in a safe place and dispense it under supervision.
  - Teachers can help recognize symptoms of ADHD in youth with substance use problems and signal to parents any suspected substance use in children known to have ADHD.

- For health providers

  - Providers should screen all adolescent patients with ADHD for substance use using a validated screening tool (e.g. CRAFFT, S2BI).

- Providers should maximize the use of non-pharmacological strategies for the management of ADHD symptoms and consider using nonstimulant medications; if prescribing psychostimulants, longer-acting formulations with lesser misuse potential are usually preferred.
- Providers should frequently monitor adolescent patients for medication effectiveness and medication misuse or diversion; they should opt for short prescription duration and frequent follow-up visits and consider using medication contracts and urine drug screens to monitor adherence in patients with known substance use problems.
- Providers should counsel patients and parents about the risks of misuse and diversion associated with stimulant ADHD medications.
- Providers *should not* withhold ADHD treatment for youth with co-occurring ADHD and substance use; rather, they should address both problems concurrently and take additional precautions for safe and effective treatment.

References

1. Chadi N, Bagley SM, Hadland SE. Addressing adolescents' and young adults' substance use disorders. Med Clin North Am. 2018;102(4):603–20.
2. Substance Abuse and Mental Health Services Administration, Center for Behavioral Health Statistics and Quality. The TEDS report: age of substance use initiation among treatment admissions aged 18 to 30 (Internet). Rockville; 2017 (cited 2017 Nov 10). Available from: https://www.samhsa.gov/data/sites/default/files/WebFiles_TEDS_SR142_AgeatInit_07-10-14/TEDS-SR142-AgeatInit-2014.pdf.
3. Winters KC, Arria A. Adolescent brain development and drugs. Prev Res. 2011;18(2):21–4. Available from: https://www.ncbi.nlm.nih.gov/pubmed/22822298
4. Zaso MJ, Park A, Antshel KM. Treatments for adolescents with comorbid ADHD and substance use disorder. J Atten Disord (Internet). 2015 Feb 5 (cited 2019 Jan 23);108705471556928. Available from: http://journals.sagepub.com/doi/10.1177/1087054715569280.
5. Harstad E, Levy S, Committee on Substance Abuse COS. Attention-deficit/hyperactivity disorder and substance abuse. Pediatrics (Internet). 2014 July 1 (cited 2019 Jan 11);134(1):e293–301. Available from: http://www.ncbi.nlm.nih.gov/pubmed/24982106.
6. Squeglia LM, Gray KM. Alcohol and drug use and the developing brain. Curr Psychiatry Rep. 2016;18(5):46.
7. Blakemore S-J. Imaging brain development: the adolescent brain. Neuroimage (Internet). 2012 June 1 (cited 2019 Jan 23);61(2):397–406. Available from: https://www.sciencedirect.com/science/article/pii/S1053811911013620.
8. Casey BJ, Jones RM. Neurobiology of the adolescent brain and behavior: implications for substance use disorders. J Am Acad Child Adolesc Psychiatry (Internet). 2010;49(12):1189–201. Available from: http://www.sciencedirect.com/science/article/pii/S0890856710006702.
9. Moss HB, Chen CM, Yi H. Early adolescent patterns of alcohol, cigarettes, and marijuana polysubstance use and young adult substance use outcomes in a nationally representative sample. Drug Alcohol Depend. 2014;136:51–62.

10. Hingson RW, Heeren T, Winter MR. Age at drinking onset and alcohol dependence. Arch Pediatr Adolesc Med (Internet). 2006 July 1 (cited 2018 Dec 18);160(7):739. Available from: http://www.ncbi.nlm.nih.gov/pubmed/16818840.

11. Jackson NJ, Isen JD, Khoddam R, Irons D, Tuvblad C, Iacono WG, et al. Impact of adolescent marijuana use on intelligence: results from two longitudinal twin studies. Proc Natl Acad Sci. 2016;113(5):E500–8.

12. Goriounova NA, Mansvelder HD. Short- and long-term consequences of nicotine exposure during adolescence for prefrontal cortex neuronal network function. Cold Spring Harb Perspect Med (Internet). 2012;2(12):a012120. Available from: http://www.ncbi.nlm.nih.gov/pubmed/22983224.

13. Volkow ND, Swanson JM, Evins AE, DeLisi LE, Meier MH, Gonzalez R, et al. Effects of cannabis use on human behavior, including cognition, motivation, and psychosis: a review. JAMA Psychiatry (Internet). 2016;73(3):292–7. Available from: http://www.ncbi.nlm.nih.gov/pubmed/26842658.

14. Conway KP, Green VR, Kasza KA, Silveira ML, Borek N, Kimmel HL, et al. Co-occurrence of tobacco product use, substance use, and mental health problems among youth: findings from wave 1 (2013–2014) of the population assessment of tobacco and health (PATH) study. Addict Behav (Internet). 2018 Jan (cited 2018 Dec 17);76:208–17. Available from: http://www.ncbi.nlm.nih.gov/pubmed/28846942.

15. Priester MA, Browne T, Iachini A, Clone S, DeHart D, Seay KD. Treatment access barriers and disparities among individuals with co-occurring mental health and substance use disorders: an integrative literature review. J Subst Abuse Treat (Internet). 2016 Feb (cited 2019 Jan 23);61:47–59. Available from: http://www.ncbi.nlm.nih.gov/pubmed/26531892.

16. Newmeyer MN, Swortwood MJ, Abulseoud OA, Huestis MA. Subjective and physiological effects, and expired carbon monoxide concentrations in frequent and occasional cannabis smokers following smoked, vaporized, and oral cannabis administration. Drug Alcohol Depend (Internet). 2017 June 1 (cited 2019 Jan 23);175:67–76. Available from: http://www.ncbi.nlm.nih.gov/pubmed/28407543.

17. Lee SS, Humphreys KL, Flory K, Liu R, Glass K. Prospective association of childhood attention-deficit/hyperactivity disorder (ADHD) and substance use and abuse/dependence: a meta-analytic review. Clin Psychol Rev (Internet). 2011 Apr (cited 2019 Feb 11);31(3):328–41. Available from: http://www.ncbi.nlm.nih.gov/pubmed/21382538.

18. Chan Y-F, Dennis ML, Funk RR. Prevalence and comorbidity of major internalizing and externalizing problems among adolescents and adults presenting to substance abuse treatment. J Subst Abuse Treat (Internet). 2008 Jan (cited 2019 Feb 11);34(1):14–24. Available from: https://linkinghub.elsevier.com/retrieve/pii/S0740547207000918.

19. Gudjonsson GH, Sigurdsson JF, Sigfusdottir ID, Young S. An epidemiological study of ADHD symptoms among young persons and the relationship with cigarette smoking, alcohol consumption and illicit drug use. J Child Psychol Psychiatry (Internet). 2012 Mar (cited 2019 Feb 11);53(3):304–12. Available from: http://www.ncbi.nlm.nih.gov/pubmed/22066497.

20. Martinez-Raga J, Szerman N, Knecht C, de Alvaro R. Attention deficit hyperactivity disorder and dual disorders. Educational needs for an underdiagnosed condition. Int J Adolesc Med Health (Internet). 2013 Jan 1 (cited 2019 Feb 11);25(3):231–43. Available from: http://www.ncbi.nlm.nih.gov/pubmed/23846135.

21. Vitulano ML, Fite PJ, Hopko DR, Lochman J, Wells K, Asif I. Evaluation of underlying mechanisms in the link between childhood ADHD symptoms and risk for early initiation of substance use. Psychol Addict Behav (Internet). 2014 Sep (cited 2019 Feb 11);28(3):816–27. Available from: http://doi.apa.org/getdoi.cfm?doi=10.1037/a0037504.

22. Zulauf CA, Sprich SE, Safren SA, Wilens TE. The Complicated Relationship Between Attention Deficit/Hyperactivity Disorder and Substance Use Disorders. Curr Psychiatry Rep (Internet). 2014 Mar 15 (cited 2019 Feb 11);16(3):436. Available from: http://www.ncbi.nlm.nih.gov/pubmed/24526271.

23. Franke B, Michelini G, Asherson P, Banaschewski T, Bilbow A, Buitelaar JK, et al. Live fast, die young? A review on the developmental trajectories of ADHD across the lifespan. Eur Neuropsychopharmacol (Internet). 2018 Oct (cited 2019 Feb 11);28(10):1059–88. Available from: http://www.ncbi.nlm.nih.gov/pubmed/30195575.
24. Ilbegi S, Groenman AP, Schellekens A, Hartman CA, Hoekstra PJ, Franke B, et al. Substance use and nicotine dependence in persistent, remittent, and late-onset ADHD: a 10-year longitudinal study from childhood to young adulthood. J Neurodev Disord (Internet). 2018 Dec 27 (cited 2019 Feb 11);10(1):42. Available from: https://jneurodevdisorders.biomedcentral.com/articles/10.1186/s11689-018-9260-y.
25. Harstad E, Wisk LE, Ziemnik R, Huang Q, Salimian P, Weitzman ER, et al. Substance use among adolescents with attention-deficit/hyperactivity disorder: reasons for use, knowledge of risks, and provider messaging/education. J Dev Behav Pediatr (Internet). 2017 (cited 2019 Feb 11);38(6):417–23. Available from: http://insights.ovid.com/crossref?an=00004703-201707000-00009.
26. Wilens TE, Adamson J, Sgambati S, Whitley J, Santry A, Monuteaux MC, et al. Do individuals with ADHD self-medicate with cigarettes and substances of abuse? Results from a controlled family study of ADHD. Am J Addict (Internet). 2007 Jan (cited 2019 Jan 11);16(s1):14–23. Available from: http://www.ncbi.nlm.nih.gov/pubmed/17453603.
27. Levy S, Katusic SK, Colligan RC, Weaver AL, Killian JM, Voigt RG, et al. Childhood ADHD and risk for substance dependence in adulthood: a longitudinal, population-based study. Skoulakis EMC, editor. PLoS One (Internet). 2014 Aug 27 (cited 2019 Feb 11);9(8):e105640. Available from: http://dx.plos.org/10.1371/journal.pone.0105640.
28. Chang Z, Lichtenstein P, Larsson H. The effects of childhood ADHD symptoms on early-onset substance use: a Swedish Twin Study. J Abnorm Child Psychol (Internet). 2012 Apr 27 (cited 2019 Feb 12);40(3):425–35. Available from: http://www.ncbi.nlm.nih.gov/pubmed/21947618.
29. Volman SF, Lammel S, Margolis EB, Kim Y, Richard JM, Roitman MF, et al. New insights into the specificity and plasticity of reward and aversion encoding in the mesolimbic system. J Neurosci (Internet). 2013 Nov 6 (cited 2019 Feb 12);33(45):17569–76. Available from: http://www.jneurosci.org/cgi/doi/10.1523/JNEUROSCI.3250-13.2013.
30. Ercan ES, Kandulu R, Uslu E, Ardic UA, Yazici KU, Basay BK, et al. Prevalence and diagnostic stability of ADHD and ODD in Turkish children: a 4-year longitudinal study. Child Adolesc Psychiatry Ment Health (Internet). 2013 Aug 7 (cited 2019 Feb 12);7(1):30. Available from: http://www.ncbi.nlm.nih.gov/pubmed/23919416.
31. American Psychiatric Association. Diagnostic and statistical manual of mental disorders (Internet). 5th edn. Arlington, VA: American Psychiatric Association; 2013 (cited 2018 Dec 20). Available from: https://psychiatryonline.org/doi/book/10.1176/appi.books.9780890425596.
32. Elkins IJ, McGue M, Iacono WG. Prospective effects of attention-deficit/hyperactivity disorder, conduct disorder, and sex on adolescent substance use and abuse. Arch Gen Psychiatry (Internet). 2007 Oct 1 (cited 2019 Feb 12);64(10):1145. Available from: http://www.ncbi.nlm.nih.gov/pubmed/17909126.
33. Tong L, Shi H-J, Zhang Z, Yuan Y, Xia Z-J, Jiang X-X, et al. Mediating effect of anxiety and depression on the relationship between Attention-deficit/hyperactivity disorder symptoms and smoking/drinking. Sci Rep (Internet). 2016 Apr 29 (cited 2019 Feb 12);6(1):21609. Available from: http://www.ncbi.nlm.nih.gov/pubmed/26923609.
34. Skirrow C, McLoughlin G, Kuntsi J, Asherson P. Behavioral, neurocognitive and treatment overlap between attention-deficit/hyperactivity disorder and mood instability. Expert Rev Neurother (Internet). 2009 Apr 9 (cited 2019 Jan 23);9(4):489–503. Available from: http://www.tandfonline.com/doi/full/10.1586/ern.09.2.
35. Deault LC. A systematic review of parenting in relation to the development of comorbidities and functional impairments in children with attention-deficit/hyperactivity disorder (ADHD). Child Psychiatry Hum Dev (Internet). 2010 Apr 19 (cited 2019 Feb 12);41(2):168–92. Available from: http://www.ncbi.nlm.nih.gov/pubmed/19768532.

36. Edwards G, Barkley RA, Laneri M, Fletcher K, Metevia L. Parent-adolescent conflict in teenagers with ADHD and ODD. J Abnorm Child Psychol (Internet). 2001 Dec (cited 2019 Feb 12);29(6):557–72. Available from: http://www.ncbi.nlm.nih.gov/pubmed/11761288.
37. Ackard DM, Neumark-Sztainer D, Story M, Perry C. Parent–child connectedness and behavioral and emotional health among adolescents. Am J Prev Med (Internet). 2006 Jan (cited 2019 Feb 12);30(1):59–66. Available from: http://www.ncbi.nlm.nih.gov/pubmed/16414425.
38. Savolainen J, Hurtig TM, Ebeling HE, Moilanen IK, Hughes LA, Taanila AM. Attention deficit hyperactivity disorder (ADHD) and criminal behaviour: the role of adolescent marginalization. Eur J Criminol (Internet). 2010 Nov 21 (cited 2019 Jan 23);7(6):442–59. Available from: http://journals.sagepub.com/doi/10.1177/1477370810376568.
39. Quinn PD, Chang Z, Hur K, Gibbons RD, Lahey BB, Rickert ME, et al. ADHD medication and substance-related problems. Am J Psychiatry (Internet). 2017 Sep 29 (cited 2019 Jan 27);174(9):877–85. Available from: http://ajp.psychiatryonline.org/doi/10.1176/appi.ajp.2017.16060686.
40. Wilens TE, Morrison NR. Substance-use disorders in adolescents and adults with ADHD: focus on treatment. Neuropsychiatry (London) (Internet). 2012 Aug (cited 2019 Feb 12);2(4):301–12. Available from: http://www.ncbi.nlm.nih.gov/pubmed/23105949.
41. Levy SJ, Williams JF. Substance use screening, brief intervention, and referral to treatment. Pediatrics (Internet). 2016/06/20. 2016;138(1). Available from: https://www.ncbi.nlm.nih.gov/pubmed/27325634.
42. Levy S, Shrier L. Adolescent screening, brief intervention, and referral for treatment for alcohol and other drug use - toolkit for providers (Internet). Boston, MA; 2015 (cited 2017 Oct 9). Available from: https://www.mcpap.com/pdf/S2BI%20Toolkit.pdf.
43. Knight JR, Sherritt L, Harris SK, Gates EC, Chang G. Validity of brief alcohol screening tests among adolescents: a comparison of the AUDIT, POSIT, CAGE, and CRAFFT. Alcohol Clin Exp Res (Internet). 2003;27(1):67–73. Available from: https://doi.org/10.1111/j.1530-0277.2003.tb02723.x.
44. American Society for Addiction Medicine. An introduction to the ASAM criteria for patients and families (Internet). 2015 (cited 2019 Jan 23). Available from: http://www.asam.org/for-the-public/definition-of-addiction.
45. Matthys F, Soyez V, van den Brink W, Joostens P, Tremmery S, Sabbe B. Barriers to Implementation of treatment guidelines for ADHD in adults with substance use disorder. J Dual Diagn (Internet). 2014 July 3 (cited 2019 Jan 11);10(3):130–8. Available from: http://www.ncbi.nlm.nih.gov/pubmed/25392286.
46. Johnston LD, Miech RA, O'malley PM, Bachman JG, Schulenberg JE, Patrick ME. Monitoring the future national survey results on drug use, 1975–2018: Overview, key findings on adolescent drug use (Internet). Ann Arbor; 2019 (cited 2019 Feb 11). Available from: http://www.monitoringthefuture.org/pubs/monographs/mtf-overview2018.pdf.
47. Stevens JR, Wilens TE, Stern TA. Using stimulants for attention-deficit/hyperactivity disorder: clinical approaches and challenges. Prim care companion CNS Disord (Internet). 2013 (cited 2019 Jan 11);15(2). Available from: http://www.ncbi.nlm.nih.gov/pubmed/23930227.
48. Cairns R, Daniels B, Wood DA, Brett J. ADHD medication overdose and misuse: the NSW Poisons Information Centre experience, 2004–2014. Med J Aust (Internet). 2016 Mar 7 (cited 2019 Jan 11);204(4):154. Available from: http://www.ncbi.nlm.nih.gov/pubmed/26937669.
49. Pham T, Milanaik R, Kaplan A, Papaioannou H, Adesman A. Household diversion of prescription stimulants: medication misuse by parents of children with attention-deficit/hyperactivity disorder. J Child Adolesc Psychopharmacol (Internet). 2017 Oct (cited 2019 Jan 11);27(8):741–6. Available from: http://www.ncbi.nlm.nih.gov/pubmed/28686059.
50. Feldman ME, Charach A, Bélanger SA. ADHD in children and youth: Part 2—Treatment. Paediatr Child Health (Internet). 2018 Oct 24 (cited 2019 Jan 11);23(7):462–72. Available from: https://academic.oup.com/pch/article/23/7/462/5142945.

51. Non-pharmacological interventions for Attention Deficit Hyperactivity Disorder (Internet). Canadian Pediatric Society. 2018 (cited 2019 Jan 11). p. 2. Available from: https://www.cps.ca/en/tools-outils/.
52. Chan E, Fogler JM, Hammerness PG. Treatment of attention-deficit/hyperactivity disorder in adolescents. JAMA (Internet). 2016 May 10 (cited 2019 Jan 11);315(18):1997. Available from: http://www.ncbi.nlm.nih.gov/pubmed/27163988.
53. Faraone S V, Upadhyaya HP. The effect of stimulant treatment for ADHD on later substance abuse and the potential for medication misuse, abuse, and diversion. J Clin Psychiatry (Internet). 2007 Nov (cited 2019 Jan 11);68(11):e28. Available from: http://www.ncbi.nlm.nih.gov/pubmed/18052554.
54. Colaneri N, Keim S, Adesman A. Physician practices to prevent ADHD stimulant diversion and misuse. J Subst Abuse Treat (Internet). 2017 Mar (cited 2019 Jan 11);74:26–34. Available from: http://www.ncbi.nlm.nih.gov/pubmed/28132697.
55. Hadland SE, Levy S. Objective testing: urine and other drug tests. Child Adolesc Psychiatr Clin N Am (Internet). 2016 (cited 2019 Jan 11);25(3):549–65. Available from: http://www.ncbi.nlm.nih.gov/pubmed/27338974.
56. Hernandez L, Rodriguez AM, Spirito A. Brief family-based intervention for substance abusing adolescents. Child Adolesc Psychiatr Clin N Am (Internet). 2015 July (cited 2018 Apr 22);24(3):585–99. Available from: http://www.ncbi.nlm.nih.gov/pubmed/26092741.
57. Baldwin SA, Christian S, Berkeljon A, Shadish WR. The effects of family therapies for adolescent delinquency and substance abuse: a meta-analysis. J Marital Fam Ther (Internet). 2012 Jan 1 (cited 2019 Jan 23);38(1):281–304. Available from: http://doi.wiley.com/10.1111/j.1752-0606.2011.00248.x.
58. Dunne T, Bishop L, Avery S, Darcy S. A review of effective youth engagement strategies for mental health and substance use interventions. J Adolesc Health. 2017;60(5):487–512.

Chapter 15
ADHD, Gaming Disorder, and Beyond

Michael Tsappis, Michael Rich, and Jill R. Kavanaugh

Case Example

Renee is a 16-year-old tenth grader in high school. She has ADHD and has been treated successfully with a long-acting methylphenidate for many years. She and her father enjoy playing video games together, but she now plays with others after he goes to sleep. She is awake until 3–4 AM, hard to wake for school, and falling asleep in school. She refuses to stop earlier, indicating that she has friends online and "needs the downtime." Her parents are reluctant to remove her devices, as she needs them for school and socialization. They do not want to turn off the wireless connection or cellular service during the night so that her older sister in college can call if she needs anything. Her parents don't know what to do.

M. Tsappis (✉)
Clinic for Interactive Media and Internet Disorders (CIMAID), Division of Adolescent Medicine and Department of Psychiatry, Boston Children's Hospital,
Harvard Medical School, Boston, MA, USA
e-mail: michael.tsappis@childrens.harvard.edu

M. Rich
Harvard Medical School, Boston, MA, USA

Center on Media and Child Health (CMCH) and Clinic for Interactive Media and Internet Disorders (CIMAID), Boston Children's Hospital, Boston, MA, USA

Harvard T.H. Chan School of Public Health, Boston, MA, USA
e-mail: Michael.rich@childrens.harvard.edu

J. R. Kavanaugh
Center on Media and Child Health (CMCH) and Clinic for Interactive Media and Internet Disorders (CIMAID), Boston Children's Hospital, Boston, MA, USA
e-mail: Jill.kavanaugh@childrens.harvard.edu

© Springer Nature Switzerland AG 2020
A. Schonwald (ed.), *ADHD in Adolescents*,
https://doi.org/10.1007/978-3-030-62393-7_15

Background

Adolescence is not what it used to be. Today's youth grow up in an increasingly engaging and efficient technological environment. Nearly limitless access to ideas, information, and tools for creativity and interaction can be held in the palm of one's hand, resulting in new approaches to education, social connection, and entertainment. Eight- to 12-year-old tweens spend nearly 6 hours per day, and teens aged 13 to 18 spend almost 9 hours a day engaging with electronic screen media [1]. The family television in a shared living space has been superseded by each family member having access to multiple screens, many of them mobile. Not only are adolescents spending significant time in front of a screen, but also they are often spending that time in front of more than one screen simultaneously [2]. Alone in their rooms, adolescents can be found doing homework on a laptop on which a music video is playing, while their cell phones are alternating between group chats and posts on social media. For the adolescent with attention-deficit/hyperactivity disorder (ADHD), the quantity and complexity of easily available screen media make focusing thoughts, controlling impulses, and completing tasks even more difficult.

Disorders of Problematic Interactive Media Use

During the 1950s, television rapidly penetrated American homes, becoming a part of and shaping our daily activities. As television viewing increased, displacing physical activities and public events, clinicians and researchers began to consider the effects on children's health and development of increasing amounts of time spent using screens [3]. The rising popularity of video games in the 1980s raised concerns about some children losing control of their interactive media use [4]. Psychodynamic formulations involving social alienation and attempts to control aggression were proposed, with associations made to obsessive-compulsive disorder [5]. By the 1990s, uncontrolled use of Internet and video games came to be formulated as a behavioral addiction [6, 7]. Subsequent research and commentary referred to electronic media use problems with a variety of names, frequently including terms like "compulsive" or "addiction." However, controversy surrounds how best to categorize uncontrolled media use [8]. As uses of the Internet broadened, so did the ways in which some individuals lost the ability to regulate their use of interactive media. In addition to disordered console and Internet-based video game use, forms of problematic media use described in research literature have included social media use disorders [9], dysregulated online pornography use [10], binge-watching of streaming video [11], and smartphone dependence [12].

The Diagnostic and Statistical Manual of Mental Disorders (DSM) is the primary reference in the United States for behavioral health problems [13]. Rapid development in personal media technology occurring during the decade between publication of the fourth and fifth editions of the DSM led to dramatic increases in interactive media use. In response to rising clinical concerns about uncontrolled use leading to psychological and social impairment, the *Conditions for Further Study* section of the DSM-5 contains proposed diagnostic criteria for "Internet gaming disorder" (see the proposed diagnostic criteria in Table 15.1) [14]. In 2018, the World Health Organization added "gaming disorder" to the International Classification of Diseases, Eleventh Edition (ICD-11) (see criteria in Table 15.2) [15]. The DSM-5 characterizes Internet gaming disorder as a form of behavioral addiction, and in the ICD-11, gaming disorder is grouped under a parent section titled "Disorders due to substance use or addictive behaviors." Official recognition by the medical community of dysfunctional interactive media use represents an important step in furthering our understanding of these new types of behavior problems. However, both descriptions are limited as they reinforce the questionable concept of addiction and they neglect to recognize and describe dysfunctional social media, pornography, information-bingeing, and other problems beyond video

Table 15.1   Proposed diagnostic criteria for Internet gaming disorder (DSM-5)

Persistent and recurrent use of the Internet to engage in games, often with other players, leading to clinically significant impairment or distress as indicated by five (or more) of the following in a 12-month period:
1. Preoccupation with Internet games. (The individual thinks about previous gaming activity or anticipates playing the next game; Internet gaming becomes the dominant activity in daily life.) *Note*: This disorder is distinct from Internet gambling, which is included under gambling disorder
2. Withdrawal symptoms when Internet gaming is taken away. (These symptoms are typically described as irritability, anxiety, or sadness, but there are no physical signs of pharmacological withdrawal.)
3. Tolerance—the need to spend increasing amounts of time engaged in Internet games
4. Unsuccessful attempts to control the participation in Internet games
5. Loss of interests in previous hobbies and entertainment as a result of, and with the exception of, Internet games
6. Continued excessive use of Internet games despite knowledge of psychosocial problems
7. Has deceived family members, therapists, or others regarding the amount of Internet gaming
8. Use of Internet games to escape or relieve a negative mood (e.g., feelings of helplessness, guilt, anxiety)
9. Has jeopardized or lost a significant relationship, job, or educational or career opportunity because of participation in Internet games
Note: Only nongambling Internet games are included in this disorder. Use of the Internet for required activities in a business or profession is not included nor is the disorder intended to include other recreational or social Internet use. Similarly, sexual Internet sites are excluded
Specify current severity:
Internet gaming disorder can be mild, moderate, or severe depending on the degree of disruption of normal activities. Individuals with less severe Internet gaming disorder may exhibit fewer symptoms and less disruption of their lives. Those with severe Internet gaming disorder will have more hours spent on the computer and more severe loss of relationships or career or school opportunities

Table 15.2 6C51 Gaming disorder (ICD-11)

Description
Gaming disorder is characterized by a pattern of persistent or recurrent gaming behavior ("digital gaming" or "video gaming"), which may be online (i.e., over the Internet) or offline, manifested by the following:
1. Impaired control over gaming (e.g., onset, frequency, intensity, duration, termination, context)
2. Increasing priority given to gaming to the extent that gaming takes precedence over other life interests and daily activities
3. Continuation or escalation of gaming despite the occurrence of negative consequences
The behavior pattern is of sufficient severity to result in significant impairment in personal, family, social, educational, occupational, or other important areas of functioning. The pattern of gaming behavior may be continuous or episodic and recurrent. The gaming behavior and other features are normally evident over a period of at least 12 months in order for a diagnosis to be assigned, although the required duration may be shortened if all diagnostic requirements are met and symptoms are severe
Exclusions
• Hazardous gaming (QE22)
• Bipolar type I disorder (6A60)
• Bipolar type II disorder (6A61)

Reproduced from the World Health Organization [15]

gaming. To accurately and comprehensively reflect empirical evidence from the clinic, we use the nomenclature problematic interactive media use (PIMU), as it is inclusive of the various presentations and focuses concern on problematic interactive behavior rather than the device or operation. Recognizing associations of dysfunctional interactive media use with known pathologies will help characterize PIMU as a diagnosis, multiple diagnoses, or a syndrome of known pathologies, enhancing efforts to develop effective, evidence-based treatments for these problems in their current and potential future forms.

PIMU and Attention-Deficit/Hyperactivity Disorder

A consistent finding of studies from the United States, Europe, Southwest Asia, and East Asia is an increased prevalence of PIMU among children and adolescents with ADHD [16–23].

Individuals with more severe ADHD symptoms are likely to experience more severe problems related to interactive media use; this "dose-response" relationship appears most notable in the relation between hyperactive-impulsive symptoms of ADHD and disordered media use [24, 25]. Increased prevalence of PIMU has been found among individuals with impulsivity, or inhibitory control weakness [26, 27], and those with relative deficits in working memory [28] as dimensional traits isolated from diagnosed ADHD. Prospective longitudinal research has found that individuals with diagnosed ADHD were more likely to develop problematic gaming [29] and Internet addiction (IA) [30] but that those with these forms of PIMU were not more likely than those without PIMU to develop ADHD. However, recent research found that 15- and 16-year-old high-frequency social media users with no symptoms of ADHD at baseline were more likely to develop ADHD symptoms over the next 24 months [31].

As children with ADHD develop into and through adolescence, they begin to accrue a burden of multiple experiences of under-functioning, negative consequences, and alienation. Untreated ADHD increases one's risks for academic underachievement, impairments in family and social functioning, underemployment, imprisonment, motor vehicle accidents, criminality, and substance use disorders [32]. Youth with ADHD suffer disproportionately when struggling to negotiate social expectations established for stronger attention and impulse control capabilities. For example, youth with ADHD experience less reward and more punishment for their frequent late arrivals, not completing tasks, or saying the wrong thing because their impulsivity outpaces their ability to stop and think.

Development of PIMU occurs over time. Interactive computer software has long been used by educators as an effective means of engaging and maintaining the attention of students with ADHD because it limits distractions and reinforces focus on educational material [33, 34]. For different types of learners, electronic screen media provide an opportunity to deliver information in engaging formats using written and spoken words, images, video, sound, and music, potentially lessening boredom typical of ADHD [35]. Similarly, these technologies offer new ways to create and produce. A person with ADHD may struggle to write an essay but be more successful recording a podcast or shooting a video that demonstrates understanding of the material. Advances in interactive technology have created a digital environment that offers educational "work-arounds" for those with ADHD but simultaneously placed them at increased risk for impaired functioning if they cannot extricate themselves from engagement.

> Children and adolescents with ADHD thrive in this immersive environment, and their mastery of it results in feelings of competence.

Interactive electronic games provide distraction and entertainment. When youth with ADHD are able to isolate with their devices, relief comes in a virtual space where a stimulating interface paired with high enjoyment engages, activates, and measurably improves their brain attentional functions [36]. Their impulsivity, in the form of rapid, reflexive response to stimuli, is rewarded. They find freedom from the confusion and discomfort experienced in the more complex, chaotic physical world. The variable rewards of gaming and social media continuously draw them in, increasing use builds greater skill, and enhanced performance is rewarded in an ongoing cycle. "Locked in" gamers become disinhibited, achieving a soothing flow state. When parents ask these gamers to shut down to do homework or sleep, it is experienced as an intrusion, a noxious separation from their domain of mastery to the discomfort of real-life demands. Their reaction, unimpeded by inhibitory control, is angry and aggressive and can become physically violent.

PIMU Comorbidities

With broader knowledge of mental conditions that have been associated with PIMU, we can develop a more nuanced understanding of the pathways to developing PIMU and identify prevention and intervention opportunities. While PIMU is prevalent among youth with ADHD, other psychiatric disorders also manifest themselves as dysfunctional interactive media behavior. Negative emotions, in the form of both anxiety and depressed mood, are consistently shown to be associated with PIMU [16, 24, 37]. Specifically, social anxiety, along with social difficulties such as loneliness and social isolation, is diagnosed more frequently among those who present with dysregulated media use [38–40]. One prospective research study found that social phobia predicted subsequent development of PIMU [30]. Relational problems among problematic interactive media users are not isolated to interactions with peers; those struggling with PIMU experience increased problems with connectedness and engagement with family and supports as well [41, 42]. Increased aggression toward others has been found among problematic interactive media users [43], particularly among males who play "first-person shooters" and other violent interactive games [44–46]. Suicide represents the second leading cause of death among adolescents [47]. Adolescents struggling with PIMU are more likely to endorse suicidal thinking [20], including planning for suicide [48] and suicide attempts [49].

> Most concerning is the strong association of PIMU with serious safety risks.

Treatment

Many parents believe that their children are spending too much time with interactive media. Their children explain that everyone else is doing the same. The difficulty is determining which young people need clinical intervention. Frequently, the first sign that a young person's interactive media use has impaired them is excessive daytime sleepiness, poor sleep quantity or quality, or indirect effects of sleep disruption or deprivation such as academic deterioration [50, 51]. PIMU can decrease effective sleep through one or more mechanisms:

- Intentional delay of sleep to pursue interactive media activities [52]
- Prolonged sleep latency due to arousal from screen content and melatonin suppression resulting from exposure to blue light [53]
- Increased frequency of early morning awakening and sleep disturbances such as nightmares or sleepwalking [54]

The strong association between ADHD and PIMU provides an initial basis on which to develop treatment strategies for those struggling with these conditions. Children with diagnosed ADHD and PIMU treated with methylphenidate, a central nervous system stimulant, have shown improvements in both ADHD and disordered media use symptoms [55]. Improvement in ADHD and PIMU was also achieved in adolescents treated with either methylphenidate or atomoxetine, a non-stimulant medication approved for the treatment of ADHD [56]. When both conditions are identified in the same person, treatment planning and determination of response to treatment should include consideration of changes in media use, such as reducing maladaptive nighttime media use habits for a person treated for ADHD with stimulant medications.

The risks presented by negative emotion can also be an appropriate target for medical treatment. Selective serotonin reuptake inhibitors (SSRIs) are first-line medication interventions for clinical depression and anxiety. Medication trials of the SSRI escitalopram showed reductions in PIMU [57, 58]. Bupropion, an atypical antidepressant, has been shown to improve symptoms of ADHD [59]. A well-designed, blinded, placebo-controlled study of bupropion for male patients suffering from both depression and PIMU resulted in improvements in both conditions [60].

Research and development of best approaches to psychological therapy for media use disorders is ongoing. Cognitive behavioral therapy (CBT) is an active, structured psychotherapy involving therapist guidance toward the development of skills needed to improve functioning. Specifically, CBT aims to improve awareness of the self and surrounding circumstances, consciousness of one's feelings and thoughts that occur in response to those circumstances, and ultimately acquisition of skills needed to achieve control over unpleasant thoughts, feelings, and resultant behaviors [61]. CBT interventions for PIMU have shown to be effective at reducing problematic media use behaviors that exist in formal trials [62, 63].

> The entire family is affected when a child or adolescent struggles with PIMU.

Treatment strategies frequently include changing the family environment, including the locations of devices, device-free zones like bedrooms and eating areas, durations and times of day for interactive media use, and sibling and parental media use behaviors. Family therapy can address intrafamily relationships and modeling of dysregulated media use, develop effective communication and problem-solving strategies, and repair and support adolescent-parent relationships. Improvement has been demonstrated in adolescents with PIMU treated with family therapy [64–67].

The most effective approach to prevention of and intervention on PIMU is for parents and caregivers to recognize the importance of children's interactive screen media use for education, communication, or entertainment and have limiting, rather than restrictive or permissive, expectations for media use. The rapid penetration of electronic technology into every aspect of our daily lives has outpaced efforts to establish standard guidance for parents, educators, and other caregivers. Proactively establishing rules surrounding media use with clear limits, including when and where electronic media may be accessed, is an actionable step in support of adaptive media use patterns [68, 69]. For all young people, but especially those with ADHD whose educational adaptations use interactive media, the goal is not to abstain from or blindly restrict interactive media, but to optimize outcomes through mindful and focused use.

Case Revisited

Renee's intentional delay of sleep to pursue interactive media activities is a common sign of impairment caused by interactive media. Ideally, she and her family would have received proactive psychoeducation regarding the increased risk for PIMU in those with ADHD, so that household rules and expectations for interactive media use were established. At this point, Renee should be screened for anxiety and depression, comorbidities of both ADHD and PIMU, and other social challenges or stressors. She would benefit from a referral for CBT to improve awareness of her circumstances, of her own feelings, and of the thoughts that occur in response. During CBT, she can ultimately acquire skills needed to achieve control over unpleasant thoughts. Concomitant SSRI treatment is appropriate for moderate to severe levels of anxiety or depression. Her family dynamics and modeled dysregulated media use should be explored, as family therapy may be a useful addition to her treatment plan.

Conclusions

As interactive screen media have rapidly been incorporated into every aspect of our lives, some children, adolescents, and adults are suffering from dysregulated use of these powerful technologies. While much is being learned about media use disorders, the clinical community has yet to determine whether PIMU is a distinct new diagnosis or a syndrome, the signs and symptoms of known diagnoses that are manifesting themselves in the interactive media environment. Anticipating that newer, faster, and more engaging technologies are yet to come, we must maintain a dynamic, rapidly adapting approach to investigation, identification, and intervention.

Understanding the increased risk of individuals with ADHD to develop PIMU helps to recognize and treat children and adolescents suffering from disordered media use. A prior diagnosis of ADHD should be a cue to screen for PIMU, but PIMU may also be the first presentation of previously unrecognized ADHD. Whether comorbid with ADHD or not, anxiety and depression associated with PIMU must be addressed. Optimal treatment of mood and anxiety disorders may reduce maladaptive media use and promote the child's ability to succeed in real-life activities, which, in turn, can improve mood and anxiety.

As in all aspects of child health, prevention of PIMU and other media-related disorders is the ideal. It is most effective to establish—proactively—household rules and expectations for interactive media use. Establishment of clear expectations reduces temptation for the parent and child to negotiate norms or values at the moment of attempted limit setting. The American Academy of Pediatrics provides a Family Media Use Plan [70] that parents can customize to their own lifestyles, circumstances, and values. Media use limits and expectations can, and should, be modified from time to time as the child or adolescent proceeds through development. In families with multiple children, this can require different rules for children of different ages, needs, and developmental capabilities, making equity more complicated and oversight more difficult. Media use disorders are experienced, and resolved, by all members of a household. With effective anticipatory guidance, prevention, and treatment as needed, we can promote healthy family relationships and communication; nurture development of the skills needed for mindful, self-regulated use of interactive media; and support children to be healthy, productive, and happy in the digital age.

Tips
- Screen all adolescents, especially those with ADHD, for problematic interactive media use.
- Psychoeducation should include explanation of how "locked in" gamers become disinhibited, achieve a soothing flow state, and experience interruptions as a noxious separation from their domain of mastery to the discomfort of real-life demands.
- Look hard for co-occurring ADHD, anxiety, and/or depression in adolescents with problematic interactive media use.

References

1. Rideout V. (2015) The Common Sense census: media use by tweens and teens. Common Sense Media. https://www.commonsensemedia.org/sites/default/files/uploads/research/census_researchreport.pdf. Accessed Jan 1 2019.
2. Felt LJ, Robb MB. Technology addiction: Concern, controversy, and finding balance. Common Sense Media. 2016. https://www.commonsensemedia.org/sites/default/files/uploads/research/csm_2016_technology_addiction_research_brief_0.pdf. Accessed Jan 1 2019:10.
3. Television and the child. Lancet. 1959;273(7065):186–8.
4. Ross DR, Finestone DH, Lavin GK. Space invaders obsession. JAMA. 1982;248(10):1177.
5. Harry B. Obsessive video-game users. JAMA. 1983;249(4):473.
6. Fisher S. Identifying video game addiction in children and adolescents. Addict Behav. 1994;19(5):545–53.
7. Young KS. Internet addiction: the emergence of a new clinical disorder. Cyberpsychol Behav. 1998;1(3):237–44.
8. Király O, Griffiths MD, Demetrovics Z. Internet gaming disorder and the DSM-5: conceptualization, debates, and controversies. Curr Addict Rep. 2015;2(3):254–62.
9. Kuss DJ, Griffiths MD. Online social networking and addiction – a review of the psychological literature. Int J Environ Res Public Health. 2011;8(9):3528–52.

10. Bostwick JM, Bucci JA. Internet sex addiction treated with naltrexone. Mayo Clin Proc. 2008;83(2):226–30.
11. Walton-Pattison E, Dombrowski SU, Presseau J. 'Just one more episode': frequency and theoretical correlates of television binge watching. J Health Psychol. 2018;23(1):17–24.
12. Cheever NA, Moreno MA, Rosen LD. When does internet and smartphone use become a problem? In: Moreno MA, Radovic A, editors. Technology and adolescent mental health. Cham: Springer International Publishing; 2018. p. 121–31.
13. Regier DA, Kuhl EA, Kupfer DJ. The DSM-5: classification and criteria changes. World Psychiatry. 2013;12(2):92–8.
14. American Psychiatric Association. Conditions for further study. In: Diagnostic and statistical manual of mental disorders. 5th ed. Arlington: American Psychiatric Publishing; 2013.
15. World Health Organization. 6C51 Gaming disorder. 2018. http://id.who.int/icd/entity/1448597234. Accessed Jan 13 2019.
16. Bozkurt H, Coskun M, Ayaydin H, Adak I, Zoroglu SS. Prevalence and patterns of psychiatric disorders in referred adolescents with internet addiction. Psychiatry Clin Neurosci. 2013;67(5):352–9.
17. Carli V, Durkee T, Wasserman D, Hadlaczky G, Despalins R, Kramarz E, Wasserman C, Sarchiapone M, Hoven CW, Brunner R, Kaess M. The association between pathological internet use and comorbid psychopathology: a systematic review. Psychopathology. 2013;46(1):1–13.
18. Chan PA, Rabinowitz T. A cross-sectional analysis of video games and attention deficit hyperactivity disorder symptoms in adolescents. Ann General Psychiatry. 2006;5(1):16.
19. Evren B, Evren C, Dalbudak E, Topcu M, Kutlu N. Relationship of internet addiction severity with probable ADHD and difficulties in emotion regulation among young adults. Psychiatry Res. 2018;269:494–500.
20. Kaess M, Durkee T, Brunner R, Carli V, Parzer P, Wasserman C, Sarchiapone M, Hoven C, Apter A, Balazs J, Balint M, Bobes J, Cohen R, Cosman D, Cotter P, Fischer G, Floderus B, Iosue M, Haring C, Kahn JP, Musa GJ, Nemes B, Postuvan V, Resch F, Saiz PA, Sisask M, Snir A, Varnik A, Ziberna J, Wasserman D. Pathological internet use among European adolescents: psychopathology and self-destructive behaviours. Eur Child Adolesc Psychiatry. 2014;23(11):1093–102.
21. Kahraman O, Demirci EO. Internet addiction and attention-deficit-hyperactivity disorder: effects of anxiety, depression and self-esteem. Pediatr Int. 2018;60(6):529–34.
22. Yen JY, Ko CH, Yen CF, Wu HY, Yang MJ. The comorbid psychiatric symptoms of internet addiction: attention deficit and hyperactivity disorder (ADHD), depression, social phobia, and hostility. J Adolesc Health. 2007;41(1):93–8.
23. Yoo HJ, Cho SC, Ha J, Yune SK, Kim SJ, Hwang J, Chung A, Sung YH, Lyoo IK. Attention deficit hyperactivity symptoms and internet addiction. Psychiatry Clin Neurosci. 2004;58(5):487–94.
24. Dalbudak E, Evren C. The relationship of internet addiction severity with attention deficit hyperactivity disorder symptoms in Turkish university students; impact of personality traits, depression and anxiety. Compr Psychiatry. 2014;55(3):497–503.
25. Gunes H, Tanidir C, Adaletli H, Kilicoglu AG, Mutlu C, Bahali MK, Topal M, Bolat N, Uneri OS. Oppositional defiant disorder/conduct disorder co-occurrence increases the risk of internet addiction in adolescents with attention-deficit hyperactivity disorder. J Behav Addict. 2018;7(2):284–91.
26. Cao F, Su L, Liu T, Gao X. The relationship between impulsivity and internet addiction in a sample of Chinese adolescents. Eur Psychiatry. 2007;22(7):466–71.
27. Walther B, Morgenstern M, Hanewinkel R. Co-occurrence of addictive behaviours: personality factors related to substance use, gambling and computer gaming. Eur Addict Res. 2012;18(4):167–74.
28. Nie J, Zhang W, Chen J, Li W. Impaired inhibition and working memory in response to internet-related words among adolescents with internet addiction: a comparison with attention-deficit/hyperactivity disorder. Psychiatry Res. 2016;236:28–34.

29. Ferguson CJ, Ceranoglu TA. Attention problems and pathological gaming: resolving the 'chicken and egg' in a prospective analysis. Psychiatry Q. 2014;85(1):103–10.
30. Ko CH, Yen JY, Chen CS, Yeh YC, Yen CF. Predictive values of psychiatric symptoms for internet addiction in adolescents: a 2-year prospective study. Arch Pediatr Adolesc Med. 2009;163(10):937–43.
31. Ra CK, Cho J, Stone MD, De La Cerda J, Goldenson NI, Moroney E, Tung I, Lee SS, Leventhal AM. Association of digital media use with subsequent symptoms of attention-deficit/hyperactivity disorder among adolescents. JAMA. 2018;320(3):255–63.
32. Hamed AM, Kauer AJ, Stevens HE. Why the diagnosis of attention deficit hyperactivity disorder matters. Front Psych. 2015;6:168.
33. Sonne T, Obel C, Gr K, #248, nb, #230. Designing real time assistive technologies: a study of children with ADHD. Paper presented at the Proceedings of the annual meeting of the Australian special interest group for computer human interaction, Parkville, 2015.
34. Lewandowski L, Wood W, Miller LA. Technological applications for individuals with learning disabilities and ADHD. In: Luiselli JK, Fischer AJ, editors. Computer-assisted and web-based innovations in psychology, special education, and health. San Diego: Academic Press; 2016. p. 61–93.
35. Chou W-J, Chang Y-P, Yen C-F. Boredom proneness and its correlation with internet addiction and internet activities in adolescents with attention-deficit/hyperactivity disorder. Kaohsiung J Med Sci. 2018;34(8):467–74.
36. Green CS, Bavelier D. Action video game modifies visual selective attention. Nature. 2003;423:534.
37. Dalbudak E, Evren C, Aldemir S, Coskun KS, Ugurlu H, Yildirim FG. Relationship of internet addiction severity with depression, anxiety, and alexithymia, temperament and character in university students. Cyberpsychol Behav Soc Netw. 2013;16(4):272–8.
38. Chak K, Leung L. Shyness and locus of control as predictors of internet addiction and internet use. Cyberpsychol Behav. 2004;7(5):559–70.
39. Weinstein A, Dorani D, Elhadif R, Bukovza Y, Yarmulnik A, Dannon P. Internet addiction is associated with social anxiety in young adults. Ann Clin Psychiatry. 2015;27(1):4–9.
40. Kamal NN, Mosallem FAE-H. Determinants of problematic internet use among el-minia high school students, Egypt. Int J Prev Med. 2013;4(12):1429–37.
41. Gunuc S, Dogan A. The relationships between Turkish adolescents' internet addiction, their perceived social support and family activities. Comput Hum Behav. 2013;29(6):2197–207.
42. Chang FC, Chiu CH, Miao NF, Chen PH, Lee CM, Chiang JT, Pan YC. The relationship between parental mediation and internet addiction among adolescents, and the association with cyberbullying and depression. Compr Psychiatry. 2015;57:21–8.
43. Ko CH, Yen JY, Liu SC, Huang CF, Yen CF. The associations between aggressive behaviors and internet addiction and online activities in adolescents. J Adolesc Health. 2009;44(6):598–605.
44. Anderson CA, Sakamoto A, Gentile DA, Ihori N, Shibuya A, Yukawa S, Naito M, Kobayashi K. Longitudinal effects of violent video games on aggression in Japan and the United States. Pediatrics. 2008;122(5):e1067–72.
45. Gentile DA, Lynch PJ, Linder JR, Walsh DA. The effects of violent video game habits on adolescent hostility, aggressive behaviors, and school performance. J Adolesc. 2004;27(1):5–22.
46. Willoughby T, Adachi PJ, Good M. A longitudinal study of the association between violent video game play and aggression among adolescents. Dev Psychol. 2012;48(4):1044–57.
47. Heron M. Deaths: leading causes for 2016. National Center for Health Statistics. 2018. https://www.cdc.gov/nchs/data/nvsr/nvsr67/nvsr67_06.pdf. Accessed Jan 1 2019.
48. Messias E, Castro J, Saini A, Usman M, Peeples D. Sadness, suicide, and their association with video game and internet overuse among teens: results from the youth risk behavior survey 2007 and 2009. Suicide Life Threat Behav. 2011;41(3):307–15.
49. Lin IH, Ko CH, Chang YP, Liu TL, Wang PW, Lin HC, Huang MF, Yeh YC, Chou WJ, Yen CF. The association between suicidality and internet addiction and activities in Taiwanese adolescents. Compr Psychiatry. 2014;55(3):504–10.

50. Poulain T, Vogel M, Buzek T, Genuneit J, Hiemisch A, Kiess W. Reciprocal longitudinal associations between adolescents' media consumption and sleep. Behav Sleep Med. 2018:1–15.
51. Twenge JM, Krizan Z, Hisler G. Decreases in self-reported sleep duration among U.S. adolescents 2009-2015 and association with new media screen time. Sleep Med. 2017;39:47–53.
52. Hale L, Guan S. Screen time and sleep among school-aged children and adolescents: a systematic literature review. Sleep Med Rev. 2015;21:50–8.
53. Chang AM, Aeschbach D, Duffy JF, Czeisler CA. Evening use of light-emitting ereaders negatively affects sleep, circadian timing, and next-morning alertness. Proc Natl Acad Sci U S A. 2015;112(4):1232–7.
54. Arora T, Broglia E, Thomas GN, Taheri S. Associations between specific technologies and adolescent sleep quantity, sleep quality, and parasomnias. Sleep Med. 2014;15(2):240–7.
55. Han DH, Lee YS, Na C, Ahn JY, Chung US, Daniels MA, Haws CA, Renshaw PF. The effect of methylphenidate on internet video game play in children with attention-deficit/hyperactivity disorder. Compr Psychiatry. 2009;50(3):251–6.
56. Park JH, Lee YS, Sohn JH, Han DH. Effectiveness of atomoxetine and methylphenidate for problematic online gaming in adolescents with attention deficit hyperactivity disorder. Hum Psychopharmacol. 2016;31(6):427–32.
57. Atmaca M. A case of problematic internet use successfully treated with an SSRI-antipsychotic combination. Prog Neuro-Psychopharmacol Biol Psychiatry. 2007;31(4):961–2.
58. Dell'Osso B, Altamura A, Hadley SJ, Debeer B, Hollander E. An open-label trial of escitalopram in the treatment of impulsive-compulsive internet usage disorder. Eur Neuropsychopharmacol. 2006;16:S82–3.
59. Ng QX. A systematic review of the use of bupropion for attention-deficit/hyperactivity disorder in children and adolescents. J Child Adolesc Psychopharmacol. 2017;27(2):112–6.
60. Han DH, Renshaw PF. Bupropion in the treatment of problematic online game play in patients with major depressive disorder. J Psychopharmacol. 2012;26(5):689–96.
61. Oar EL, Johnco C, Ollendick TH. Cognitive behavioral therapy for anxiety and depression in children and adolescents. Psychiatr Clin North Am. 2017;40(4):661–74.
62. Stevens MWR, King DL, Dorstyn D, Delfabbro PH. Cognitive-behavioral therapy for internet gaming disorder: a systematic review and meta-analysis. Clin Psychol Psychother. 2019;26(2):191–203.
63. Winkler A, Dorsing B, Rief W, Shen Y, Glombiewski JA. Treatment of internet addiction: a meta-analysis. Clin Psychol Rev. 2013;33(2):317–29.
64. Liu QX, Fang XY, Yan N, Zhou ZK, Yuan XJ, Lan J, Liu CY. Multi-family group therapy for adolescent internet addiction: exploring the underlying mechanisms. Addict Behav. 2015;42:1–8.
65. Shek DT, Tang VM, Lo CY. Evaluation of an internet addiction treatment program for Chinese adolescents in Hong Kong. Adolescence. 2009;44(174):359–73.
66. Zhong X, Zu S, Sha S, Tao R, Zhao C, Yang F, Li M, Sha P. The effect of a family-based intervention model on internet-addicted Chinese adolescents. Soc Behav Pers. 2011;39(8):1021–34.
67. Han DH, Kim SM, Lee YS, Renshaw PF. The effect of family therapy on the changes in the severity of on-line game play and brain activity in adolescents with on-line game addiction. Psychiatry Res. 2012;202(2):126–31.
68. Chng GS, Li D, Liau AK, Khoo A. Moderating effects of the family environment for parental mediation and pathological internet use in youths. Cyberpsychol Behav Soc Netw. 2015;18(1):30–6.
69. Ramirez ER, Norman GJ, Rosenberg DE, Kerr J, Saelens BE, Durant N, Sallis JF. Adolescent screen time and rules to limit screen time in the home. J Adolesc Health. 2011;48(4):379–85.
70. American Academy of Pediatrics Family media plan. https://www.healthychildren.org/English/media/Pages/default.aspx. Accessed Jan 1 2019.

Part III
ADHD: Critical Truths

Chapter 16
Race, Culture, and Ethnicity in ADHD

Joanna E. Perdomo, Clement J. Bottino, Sabrina Sargado, and Natalie Cerda

Case Example

Alexander is a 13-year-old boy repeating sixth grade. He was diagnosed with ADHD by his primary care doctor in second grade. Alexander's mother subsequently sought multiple alternative medical explanations for his behavior. She reports significant stigma associated with mental health conditions in her home country of Cape Verde. Yet, she felt pressured by Alexander's educational team and pediatrician to start medication treatment for ADHD.

Background

Although there is significant variability in the prevalence rate of ADHD in different parts of the world, variations may be more attributable to methodological differences in studies rather than true variability in prevalence [1]. Despite worldwide recognition of ADHD, the degree to which symptoms are viewed as pathologic or impairing is context-dependent [2] and can vary depending on factors such as

J. E. Perdomo (✉)
Division of General Pediatrics, Boston Children's Hospital,
Harvard Medical School, Boston, MA, USA
e-mail: joanna.perdomo@childrens.harvard.edu

C. J. Bottino
Division of General Pediatrics, Boston Children's Hospital, Harvard Medical School,
Boston, MA, USA
e-mail: clement.bottino@childrens.harvard.edu

S. Sargado · N. Cerda
Division of Developmental Medicine, Boston Children's Hospital, Boston, MA, USA
e-mail: sabrina.sargado@childrens.harvard.edu; Natalie.Cerda@childrens.harvard.edu

© Springer Nature Switzerland AG 2020   219
A. Schonwald (ed.), *ADHD in Adolescents*,
https://doi.org/10.1007/978-3-030-62393-7_16

geography, race, ethnicity, culture, religion, and family values. Furthermore, these factors can drive inequities in diagnosis and treatment.

Racial and ethnic disparities exist in the diagnosis and treatment of ADHD for adolescents. A 2016 study by Coker et al. [3] showed that fifth, seventh, and tenth grade African American children as compared to White and Latino children had *higher* rates of parent-reported symptoms of ADHD. However, African American and Latino children were *less* likely than White children to have ever received a diagnosis of ADHD. Additionally, the same study found African American and Latino children with ADHD symptoms or diagnosis had lower parent-reported rates of medication treatment for ADHD compared to their White counterparts, suggesting ADHD is underdiagnosed and undertreated in African American and Latino children, rather than overdiagnosed and overtreated in White children. This corroborated findings of other studies that demonstrate lower rates of diagnosis [4, 5], medication use [5, 6], and more fragmented care of ADHD for minority youth [7], even when accounting for confounding factors such as maternal age, insurance status, language, and birth weight [8].

The factors driving diagnostic and therapeutic racial inequities are complex and manifold. They include language barriers, health insurance status, neighborhood safety, and unequal school supports [4, 9]. In this chapter, we use cultural humility and racial justice lenses to explore these inequities and learn how, as clinicians, educators, parents, and communities, we can start to address these factors to provide the best care to *all* adolescents.

Expectations in Adolescence

ADHD is diagnosed in a clinical setting, but the majority of the time, concerns are first raised at home and in schools [10]. Therefore, understanding what families and teachers expect of adolescents and what factors drive these expectations is important in order to appreciate why—or why not—concerns for ADHD may be raised in adolescents.

Adolescence is defined as the period following the onset of puberty in which a child develops into an adult [11]. The concept of adolescence has been described for centuries, and a circumscribed period akin to adolescence is seen in most cultures and parts of the world [12]. The universality of adolescence is further reinforced by findings of neurological changes that occur during this period [13]. However, the duration, influences, and reactions that map onto these brain changes are dependent on social and cultural contexts, which, in turn, can lead to variability in expectations set forth in adolescence [12, 14, 15].

For example, the view of adolescence as a time of "storm and stress"— increased peer influences, parental conflict, mood disruptions, and risk-taking behavior—was a notion first popularized in 1904 by G. Stanley Hall [16].

Hall was an American psychologist whose views on adolescence were shaped by evolutionary theory and the Western, industrialized world in which he lived [14, 17]. Although this view still characterizes Western conceptions of adolescence, the degree of turmoil described does not hold true in all parts of the world [16].

Another schema for understanding differences in expectations in adolescence stem from the concepts of collectivism and individualism. Western cultures are thought of as individualist, emphasizing the attainment of independence and individual expression. In contrast, Eastern cultures are viewed as collectivist, emphasizing conformity and the good of the whole over that of the individual [18]. A study by Qu et al. [19] asked American and Chinese youth about their concepts of adolescence. American, more than Chinese, adolescents viewed adolescence as a time of decreased familial responsibility, increased peer relatedness, and increased individuation from parents. These findings align with individualist cultures in the United States in contrast to more collectivist cultures in China. However, these two schema are not mutually exclusive. For example, a combination of valuing both collectivism and individualism in adolescence is described in India, with importance placed on both commitment to family and to seeking competitiveness and autonomy [12].

Expectations for the adolescent's role in school and work vary across the world: in most developed countries, adolescents are expected to attend school through high school; in developing countries, many adolescents leave school and enter the workforce earlier to contribute to their family's income.

A multitude of other factors contribute to varying views of adolescence. Additional attitudes affecting views on adolescent development include those regarding gender, sexuality, and religious beliefs [12].

Lastly, attitudes about race play a role in shaping expectations of adolescents. While explicit racism, such as using derogatory labels, has become less acceptable in society, implicit biases—unconscious stereotypes and prejudices that exist within everyone and affect all forms of interpersonal interaction—are ubiquitous. Underlying all of this is structural racism: the ways in which institutions, policies, and practices perpetuate racial inequities. These forces shape the environment in which expectations of adolescents are set and in which consequences are delivered [20].

In medical systems, implicit biases have been shown to have profoundly adverse effects on clinicians, educators, and parents' views and contribute to inequities in treatment and care [21–25]. In school systems, racial biases have been demonstrated in teachers' perceptions and expectations of adolescents' behavior and academic success. Furthermore, Black students who were exposed to more Black teachers had lower rates of suspension [26]. In a study of over 8000 tenth grade public school students across the United States, White and non-Black teachers as compared to Black teachers were significantly more likely to expect that Black students would not graduate high school and less likely to expect that they would attain a college degree [27]. Awareness of pervasive racial biases and the ways in which they can unknowingly exist and perpetuate structural inequities is key in order to begin to dismantle them.

> In a study of 20,000 students from kindergarten to eighth grade, White teachers were significantly more likely than Black teachers to see the same Black student's behavior as more disruptive, impulsive, and argumentative [26].

Assessment of Cultural Differences During ADHD Diagnosis

The American Psychiatric Association (APA) and the DSM-5 Cross-Cultural Issues Subgroup (DCCIS) jointly developed a tool to assist clinicians in making person-centered cultural assessments to inform diagnosis and treatment planning: the Cultural Formulation Interview (CFI) [28]. Using this set of 16 questions, clinicians may obtain information during a mental health assessment about the impact of culture on key aspects of an individual's clinical presentation and care [29]. Per the APA, the CFI can be reproduced without permission by researchers and by clinicians for use with their patients [30]. Best practice highlights for treating diverse patient populations are also available at the APA website [31].

Trust, mutual respect, and a deep understanding of one's values are integral building blocks to forming a strong and effective partnership between educators, medical care providers, and families. Strong partnerships bridge cultural divides, allowing for each party to widen their perspective. This can lead to improved quality of care and is a step toward ensuring healthcare equity.

Parent Perspectives

According to the US Surgeon General's report assessing racial and ethnic disparities in mental health, "communication and trust are particularly critical in treatment" [32]. This report highlights that barriers to care such as mistrust, fear, discrimination, and language differences carry particular significance for minority populations accessing mental health treatments.

Factors that may influence decision-making among minority populations regarding healthcare treatments include actual or perceived negative experiences in healthcare settings [32]. A grave history of maltreatment of minority populations in medical and school systems perpetuates mistrust, which can lead to hesitancy for people of color to seek medical and school systems for help [32, 33]. Clinicians and educators are encouraged to address discrimination experienced by youth and their families by asking questions, listening empathetically, and showing support regarding this source of unjust stress.

Educator and Healthcare Professional Perspectives

> By validating the significant inequality of discrimination and its impact on all aspects of well-being, clinicians and educators have an opportunity to align themselves with affected families, to form mutually respectful and trusting relationships, and to move toward just and equitable education and care.

Healthcare professionals and educators should be aware of current racial and ethnic disparities in the diagnosis and management of ADHD. In an effort to reduce these disparities, professionals need to pay particular attention to concerns raised by minority parents regarding their child's learning and behavior in a culturally sensitive manner [8]. Disparities in ADHD care occur by kindergarten; in order to effectively work toward equity, it is imperative that efforts from healthcare and school-based professionals begin early and remain steady throughout every child's life course [8]. Understanding one's personal biases and stereotypes regarding race, culture, and ethnicity may help to decrease the impact of implicit bias on medical decision-making, thereby leading to increased equity across important health outcomes [24]. The influence of implicit bias on clinical management is modifiable.

> To reduce the potential impact that implicit bias may have on decision-making regarding ADHD care, healthcare professionals and educators are encouraged to adhere to clinical guidelines with the use of objective decision tools such as parent- and teacher-report measures.

Encouraging and fostering communication are fundamental as ethnic and cultural differences are considered. Healthcare and education professionals can work toward acknowledging and becoming aware of their own biases and stereotypes. A self-assessment is available on the Project Implicit Web servers at the Harvard University [34].

Working with Families

Expectations of adolescence vary for a variety of reasons, many of which were explored in this chapter. In an ever-globalizing world, it is important to acknowledge and honor that no one adolescent, family, provider, or educator fits neatly into a box; understanding the many contexts that shape one's life is paramount. Shifts away from a *cultural competency* approach have made way for a *cultural*

Table 16.1 Interview questions for adolescent patients and their families

	Interview questions for adolescent patients and their families
1	What were your parents' experiences of adolescence, and how have these shaped your expectations of adolescence?
2	Are you expected to fulfill caretaking or financial responsibilities for your family (e.g., care for younger siblings or older relatives, hold a job)?
3	What education level do you hope to attain?
4	What stressors do you and your family face?
5	What is your gender identity and sexuality? How do you feel about it? How does your family feel about it?
6	Do you or your family encounter any challenges based on language barriers?
7	What are your religious beliefs? Are they similar or different from those of your family? How do they shape your views of adolescence?

humility approach, in which humility, flexibility, and self-reflection are employed to understand aspects of a person's identity that are important to them while mitigating personally held biases [35]. Through cultural humility, we learn about the diverse aspects of identity and the views that an individual or family holds, which fosters trust, understanding, and mutual respect. Therefore, to conclude this chapter, we provide questions that honor many facets of identity to consider and utilize when understanding a patient and family's views on adolescence (Table 16.1). These are stated as if speaking to an adolescent confidentially but, with the adolescent's permission, can open a shared conversation with their family.

Case Revisited

The relationships between Alexander's family and school and his family and pediatrician both need repair. A point person on his school team could meet with Alexander's mother and learn, with authentic curiosity, about her family's journey and their values and beliefs. Including the school nurse, guidance counselor, or adjustment counselor may help the team hear this family's story from different perspectives. During these conversations, the great value his family places on education could serve as a bridge, fostering trust, communication, and a therapeutic alliance across the cultural divide. Similarly, his pediatrician might arrange a longer appointment time for a deeper conversation with Alexander and his mother. Understanding her experiences with the medical and school systems, the family's belief system, their priorities, and their expectations of him will start a more mutually respectful and collaborative relationship in service of optimizing Alexander's care.

Conclusions

In the last decade, there have been increasing rates of ADHD diagnosis among adults, yet rates of detection among major racial and ethnic subgroups are substantially lower than in their counterparts. It has been suggested that there should be an increased focus on careful, unbiased, structured screening and documentation of symptoms across development, especially as the field attempts to further delineate the temporal precedence of ADHD, patterns of comorbidity, and its consequences.

Greater consideration must be placed on the historical and present-day influences on healthcare seeking and delivery, along with an increased understanding of how these vary for families of different races/ethnicities, as well as culturally sensitive approaches to identify and treat ADHD equitably across the total population [3, 9].

Giving patients and families the opportunity to communicate often proves key in fostering relationships with school and clinical teams. Understanding a family's values, expectations of a student's performance and behavior, and historical experiences can shed new light for educators and clinicians.

Tips
- Clinical practitioners should proactively and universally elicit goals, address concerns, identify strengths, and focus on aspects of the problem that matter most to the adolescent and family [3].
- Lead with cultural humility, acknowledging the adolescent's family as the expert of their child, culture, values, goals, and beliefs.
- Provide care and information in the family's preferred language.
- Connect families with community resources when possible.
- Clarify barriers to care in the context of cultural concerns. Elicit potential concerns about the clinician-patient relationship, including experiences with racism/discrimination, language barriers, or cultural differences that may impede communication and quality of care.

References

1. Polanczyk G, de Lima MS, Horta BL, Biederman J, Rohde LA. The worldwide prevalence of ADHD: a systematic review and metaregression analysis. Am J Psychiatry. 2007;164(6):942–8.
2. Smith M. Hyperactive around the world? The history of ADHD in global perspective. Soc Hist Med. 2017;30(4):767–87.
3. Coker TR, Elliott MN, Toomey SL, et al. Racial and ethnic disparities in ADHD diagnosis and treatment. Pediatrics. 2016;138(3):e20160407.
4. Collins KP, Cleary SD. Racial and ethnic disparities in parent-reported diagnosis of ADHD: National Survey of Children's Health (2003, 2007, and 2011). J Clin Psychiatry. 2016;77(1):52–9.

5. Rowland AS, Umbach DM, Stallone L, Naftel AJ, Bohlig EM, Sandler DP. Prevalence of medication treatment for attention deficit-hyperactivity disorder among elementary school children in Johnston County, North Carolina. Am J Public Health. 2002;92(2):231–4.
6. Hoagwood K, Jensen PS, Feil M, Vitiello B, Bhatara VS. Medication management of stimulants in pediatric practice settings: a national perspective. J Dev Behav Pediatr. 2000;21(5):322–31.
7. Guevara JP, Feudtner C, Romer D, et al. Fragmented care for inner-city minority children with attention-deficit/hyperactivity disorder. Pediatrics. 2005;116(4):e512–7.
8. Morgan PL, Staff J, Hillemeier MM, Farkas G, Maczuga S. Racial and ethnic disparities in ADHD diagnosis from kindergarten to eighth grade. Pediatrics. 2013;132(1):85–93.
9. Alegria M, Green JG, McLaughlin KA, Loder S. Disparities in child and adolescent mental health and mental health services in the U.S. William T. Grant Foundation Inequality Report. 2015. https://www.massgeneral.org/mongan-institute/centers/dru/research/publications.
10. Sax L, Kautz KJ. Who first suggests the diagnosis of attention-deficit/hyperactivity disorder? Ann Fam Med. 2003;1(3):171–4.
11. OxfordDictionaries.com. https://en.oxforddictionaries.com/definition/adolescence (Accessed 8/18/20).
12. Arnett JJ. Adolescent Psychology Around the World. 2007. Available from: http://www.psypress.com/adolescent-psychology-around-the-world-9781848728899.
13. Blakemore SJ, Choudhury S. Development of the adolescent brain: implications for executive function and social cognition. J Child Psychol Psychiatry. 2006;47(3–4):296–312.
14. Choudhury S. Culturing the adolescent brain: what can neuroscience learn from anthropology? Soc Cogn Affect Neurosci. 2010;5(2–3):159–67.
15. Crockett LJ. Cultural, historical, and subcultural contexts of adolescence: implications for health and development. In: Schulenberg J, Maggs JL, Hurrelmann K, editors. Health risks and developmental transitions during adolescence. Cambridge: Cambridge University Press; 1997. p. 23–53.
16. Arnett JJ. Adolescent storm and stress, reconsidered. Am Psychol. 1999;54(5):317–26.
17. Arnett JJ. G. Stanley Hall's adolescence: brilliance and nonsense. Hist Psychol. 2006;9(3):186–97.
18. Trommsdorff G. Parent-adolescent relations in changing societies: a cross-cultural study. In: Noack P, et al., editors. Psychological responses to social change: human development in changing environments. Berlin: de Gruyter; 1995. p. 189–218.
19. Qu Y, Pomerantz EM, Wang M, Cheung C, Cimpian A. Conceptions of adolescence: implications for differences in engagement in school over early adolescence in the United States and China. J Youth Adolesc. 2016;45(7):1512–26.
20. Kendall J, Hatton D. Racism as a source of health disparity in families with children with attention deficit hyperactivity disorder. ANS Adv Nurs Sci. 2002;25(2):22–39.
21. Blair IV, Fairclough DL, Price DW, Wright LA. Clinicians ' implicit ethnic/racial bias and perceptions of care among Black and Latino patients. Ann Fam Med. 2013;11:43–52.
22. Cooper LA, Roter DL, Carson KA, et al. The associations of clinicians' implicit attitudes about race with medical visit communication and patient ratings of interpersonal care. Am J Public Health. 2012;102(5):979–87.
23. Dovidio JF, Penner LA, Albrecht TL, Norton WE, Gaertner SL, Shelton JN. Disparities and distrust: the implications of psychological processes for understanding racial disparities in health and health care. Soc Sci Med. 2008;67(3):478–86.
24. Sabin JA, Greenwald AG. The influence of implicit bias on treatment recommendations for 4 common pediatric conditions: pain, urinary tract infection, attention deficit hyperactivity disorder, and asthma. Am J Public Health. 2012;102(5):988–95.
25. Sabin JA, Rivara FP, Greenwald AG. Physician implicit attitudes and stereotypes about race and quality of medical care. Med Care. 2008;46(7):678–85.
26. Wright AC. Teachers' perceptions of students' disruptive behavior: the effect of racial congruence and consequences for school suspension. 2015. Available from: https://aefpweb.org/

sites/default/files/webform/41/Race%20Match,%20Disruptive%20Behavior,%20and%20
School%20Suspension.pdf.
27. Gershenson S, Holt SB, Papageorge N, Papageorge NW. Who believes in me? The effect of
    student-teacher demographic match on teacher expectations who believes in me? The Effect
    of Student-Teacher Demographic Match on Teacher Expectations Upjohn Institute Working
    Paper 15–231. 2015. Available from: https://doi.org/10.17848/wp15-231.
28. https://www.psychiatrictimes.com/view/dsm-5-cultural-formulation-interview-and-evolution-
    cultural-assessment-psychiatry.
29. https://blog.pdresources.org/culturally-competent-cultural-formulation-interview/.
30. https://www.psychiatry.org/File%20Library/Psychiatrists/Practice/DSM/APA_DSM5_
    Cultural-Formulation-Interview.pdf.
31. https://www.psychiatry.org/psychiatrists/cultural-competency/education/
    best-practice-highlights.
32. Gilbert C. Unequal treatment: confronting racial and ethnic disparities in health care [Internet].
    J Natl Med Assoc. 2005;97:303 p. Available from: http://www.nap.edu/catalog/10260/
    unequal-treatment-confronting-racial-and-ethnic-disparities-in-health-care.
33. U.S. Department of Health and Human Services. Mental health: culture, race, and ethnicity – a
    supplement to mental health: a report of the Surgeon General. US Dep Heal Hum Serv Subst
    Abus Ment Heal Serv Adm Cent Ment Heal Serv. 2001:1–204.
34. https://implicit.harvard.edu/implicit/takeatest.html (Accessed 8/18/20).
35. Tervalon M, Murray-Garcia J. Cultural humility versus cultural competence: a critical distinc-
    tion in definitions. J Health Care Poor Underserved. 1998;9(2):117.

Chapter 17
Relationships, Sexuality, and Sexual Behavior in Adolescents with ADHD

Frinny Polanco Walters and Joshua Borus

Case Example

Desta is a 17-year-old high school senior with ADHD, inattentive subtype, and learning disabilities. She plans to attend the local community college to study criminal justice. She has had a few boyfriends in the past and a handful of additional sexual encounters. Recently, Desta broke up with a boyfriend and was feeling excluded by their group of friends. She spent time with a different group from her neighborhood and felt pressured to have sexual intercourse with someone she doesn't know well, despite not wanting to. She presents to the school health center with lower abdominal pain and is found to have a sexually transmitted infection.

Background

All teens are in danger of making unsafe decisions about sex, exposing them to higher risk of pregnancy, sexually transmitted infections, and sexual violence, necessitating fact-based counseling and access to contraception. The current data demonstrates this is *more pronounced* for teens with ADHD for whom impulse control is even more limited, due to underdeveloped executive function. In this chapter, we discuss the role ADHD symptoms can play in friendship and romantic relationship dysfunction, involvement in risky sexual behavior, and both violence victimization and perpetration. We also discuss current literature explaining the pathophysiology behind these deficits, along with evidence-based interventions

F. P. Walters (✉) · J. Borus
Division of Adolescent/Young Adult Medicine, Boston Children's Hospital,
Boston, MA, USA
e-mail: Frinny.PolancoWalters@childrens.harvard.edu; Joshua.Borus@childrens.harvard.edu

© Springer Nature Switzerland AG 2020   229
A. Schonwald (ed.), *ADHD in Adolescents*,
https://doi.org/10.1007/978-3-030-62393-7_17

demonstrated to be effective. This chapter will guide clinicians, parents, and teachers as they assist teens with ADHD to learn to manage intimate and sexual relationships responsibly, by reviewing the known data about sexual behaviors of adolescents with ADHD.

Friendships

Friendships are important and are valued by almost all children and adolescents regardless of ADHD status. High-quality friendships are composed of positive features including intimacy, support, and validation, whereas poor-quality friendships are characterized by conflict, criticism, and aggression. All of these poor friendship traits may jeopardize academic, behavioral, and socio-emotional functioning [1]. What we know from the literature is familiar to most working with this group of teens:

1. Children with ADHD often have trouble starting and maintaining friendships [2], and their friendships are shorter in duration than those in typically developing children [3].
2. Similarly, adolescents with ADHD have fewer friends than their peers without ADHD [1].
3. Compared with typically developing youth, adolescents and young adults with ADHD are perceived as less sociable and less likeable by peers and experience more negative interactions with peers [4].
4. They are also more likely to exhibit specific social skills deficits that contribute to peer rejection and bullying which in turn may contribute to future negative outcomes, including school dropout, substance abuse, and psychopathology [5].

Youth with ADHD may be aware of their maladaptive behaviors (interrupting, breaking rules, failing to attend to others), but they lack the self-control to modify them [4]. Additionally, they often prioritize certain characteristics in friendships—such as being fun and entertaining—over those valued by typically developing peers (such as intimacy, perspective taking, and active engagement in games suited for two children) [6]. This may lead to decreased likelihood of developing mutually satisfying friendships and increased likelihood of experiencing rejection [1, 6].

Parents and teachers of youth with ADHD report that adolescents with more symptoms of ADHD are ignored or rejected by many of their peers [7]. Such findings are consistent with those reported by Gardner et al. from their research examining peer relationships and friendships in children and adolescents diagnosed with ADHD which found that adolescents with ADHD were more likely to experience rejection than typically developing adolescents [5].

The association between experiencing peer rejection and having a diagnosis of ADHD during childhood or adolescence has been researched extensively. In a study investigating the quality of both same-sex and other-sex friendships in adolescents with and without ADHD:

1. Older adolescents with ADHD perceived their friendships to be less supportive compared to the friendships of their typically developing counterparts.
2. Ratings of friendship social support diminished across age in youth with ADHD and increased for typically developing peers [1].

Why do those with ADHD find less support in friendships as they age? Maybe friendships were always problematic—as youth with ADHD age, they experience social dysfunction which is not adequately addressed, only to become more apparent with time. Alternatively, as youth age, their relationships become more complex; those with ADHD may not have adequate skills to manage these changes. Supporting this second theory are the findings of a research study evaluating students in a small liberal arts college: those with greater ADHD symptoms reported both greater difficulty providing emotional support and managing interpersonal conflict than their peers experiencing fewer ADHD symptoms [8]. Authors of this study further report that the students' friends reported providing more nurturance than they received from students with ADHD and more difficulty engaging in behaviors of high-quality relationships.

More recently, researchers have focused on examining friendship quality among youth with ADHD. For instance, a study done in a small community in the United States by Glass et al. explored whether the symptoms of ADHD were related to close friendship quality as reported by both the adolescents with ADHD and their same-sex friends. Encouragingly, they found that the adolescents with high levels of ADHD symptoms reported having close and positive friendships [7]. However, the authors of this study did not measure the levels of ADHD symptoms of the same-sex friends, which is a potential confounder as adolescents with ADHD have reported higher-quality friendship behaviors from friends who match their ADHD symptom severity [7].

Caregivers and teachers should be mindful that ADHD inhibits adolescents' understanding of social cues needed to realize they are bothersome to others.

Adolescents with ADHD should receive social skills training that focuses on enhancing positive qualities in order to promote positive interactions with peers. Parents and teachers should be aware of the adolescents' social skills deficits and assist them in developing better self-regulation and address the maladaptive behaviors. Delineating the specific actions that are drawing negative attention and creating a plan that addresses these actions may prove beneficial. Limit setting is important while also remembering that adolescence is a time of establishing character and independence. Involving clinicians as part of a supportive team is also important to help teens develop the strengths that will lead them to build strong friendships. Ideally, adolescents prepared with the right tools will experience less rejection from peers, and if they do, they will respond appropriately. Finally, adolescents with ADHD struggling to establish friendships should be motivated to practice cooperation, empathy, and enhancement of social skills that would allow them to build durable friendships. While no data explicitly supports the impact of appropriate medication in improving friendship quality, it is logical that mitigating the impulsivity and difficulty of self-regulation—which may alienate friends—could lead to improved outcomes in this area.

Romantic Relationships

Romantic relationship initiation and maintenance may be an area of weakness for individuals with ADHD given impairments in social functioning and seem to be impacted by the subtype of ADHD experienced.

Social networks typically evolve as children enter adolescence and begin to include members of the opposite sex and romantic partners. Problematic self-regulation impacts the ability to manage fluctuating emotions and worsens dysfunctional communication patterns. This results in unfavorable outcomes such as relational dissolution [4]. For instance, romantic satisfaction has been negatively correlated with inattentive presentation [9]. Young adults with inattention tend to reach dating milestones at a later age, have lower number of steady dating relationships, feel less comfortable or assertive in particular situations, use fewer relational problem-solving techniques, spend less time on their relationships, and express love and affection less than individuals with fewer inattentive symptoms [10]. Marsh and colleagues examined the role of sexual anxiety and fear of intimacy in American college students with ADHD and compared them to Chinese college students with ADHD to see if they exhibited similar patterns. Their results suggest that those with more ADHD symptoms, particularly inattention, regard intimate situations as more frightening and report more concern about intimacy when reflecting on past relationships [11]. Since sexuality and ADHD are viewed differently in both cultures, similarities in the relationship between ADHD symptomatology and sexuality among students from the different countries suggest these findings are universal and not cultural.

Hyperactive-impulsive symptoms of ADHD are associated with different relationship difficulties than those experienced by individuals with more inattentive symptoms. Research has shown greater difficulty in developing and maintaining serious romantic relationships. The romantic behavior of those with combined-type ADHD includes greater assertiveness and earlier and more frequent sexual experiences in contrast to the passivity, disinterest, and inexperience of the inattentive population [4]. A Canadian study compared romantic involvement, relationship content, and relationship quality of adolescents with ADHD to that of typically developing adolescents. Adolescents with ADHD reported having more romantic relationships than their typically developing peers, which was credited to the attributes of individuals with ADHD: more forgetful, disorganized, distracted, failing to meet their responsibilities, impulsive, explosive, and more likely to engage in verbal and physical outbursts than their peers without ADHD [12].

The relationship between difficulty establishing intimate relationships and ADHD has also been studied among young adults across the United States. We should consider that findings derived from work on adolescents and young adults with ADHD who are in college are not reflective of all adolescents with ADHD. By virtue of gaining college entry, this group reflects a skewed population. Many studies have corroborated the finding that presence of hyperactive-impulsive symptoms is a small yet statistically significant predictor of the use of aggressive tactics during relationship conflict. One study done in a moderate-sized university in the northeast examined the role of inattention and hyperactivity-impulsivity in relationship maintenance of undergraduate college students involved in romantic relationships. Specifically, they investigated whether:

- ADHD symptoms among undergraduate college students who were involved in romantic relationships of at least 6 months were associated with problems in relationship functioning and which mechanisms lead to problems.
- Different symptoms produce different patterns of difficulty.

They found that both inattention and hyperactivity-impulsivity symptoms play a role in romantic relationship dissolution in both those with and without ADHD [10].

Another study of undergraduate students investigated the differences in conflict resolution behavior and satisfaction in long-term, young adult, heterosexual couples with a partner, either with or without inattentive or combined-type ADHD. They found that overall couples in which one partner had combined-type ADHD exhibited more negative conflict resolution and less satisfaction compared to couples with a predominantly inattentive partner or a partner without a diagnosis of ADHD [4]. In a comprehensive review, Barkley et al. explain that if not addressed, these issues persist through adulthood and may have an impact on marital satisfaction and family functioning [13].

Parents and clinicians can provide support to adolescents with a diagnosis of ADHD by discussing expectations about romantic relationships. Discussions should occur before the adolescent starts dating. Topics of conversation to discuss with teens should include expectations about having different opinions from their significant others and prepare them to address these challenges. Furthermore, they should be provided with skills to develop the vocabulary necessary to clearly explain how they feel and to provide their partners with opportunities to also express themselves. Social skills training may help promote good listening skills, essential for the well-being of romantic relationships. Parents should pay close attention to their child's specific deficits and collaborate with clinicians to provide solutions to support their teen's self-confidence, a necessary ingredient for every healthy relationship.

Adolescents with ADHD should understand that having a different opinion from a loved one is part of any relationship. Managing conflicts in a respectful and positive way can strengthen the relationship.

Table 17.1 Unsafe sexual behaviors more common in adolescents with ADHD

Unsafe sexual behaviors more common in adolescents with ADHD
Increased number of partners
Higher rates of sexually transmitted infections
Teenage pregnancy
Sexual abuse victimization
Sexual abuse perpetration

Risky Sexual Behavior, Sexually Transmitted Infections, and Teen Parenting

Adolescents with ADHD are at increased risk of engaging in unsafe sexual behavior; examples are listed in Table 17.1.

Not surprisingly, impulsivity has been associated with risky sexual behavior among adolescents and young adults with ADHD [14]. For instance, US college students with more ADHD symptoms, particularly symptoms of hyperactivity/impulsivity, engage in more risky sexual behavior including less contraceptive use, more alcohol use before sex, more intercourse with uncommitted partners, impulsive sex, and more risky anal sex [11]. Independent of hyperactivity/impulsivity symptoms, the link between inattention symptoms and risky sexual behavior among adolescents with ADHD is significantly increased as well [15]. In addition to the core symptoms of ADHD which are inattention and hyperactivity/impulsivity, comorbidities are also associated with increased susceptibility to risky sexual behaviors [16]. Specifically, conduct problems and problematic substance use have been examined among high-risk youth with ADHD involved in the juvenile justice system and found to mediate the relationship with risky sexual behavior [17]. Risk for increase in number of lifetime sexual partners has been correlated with high baseline ADHD symptom severity and increased parental marital problems, while positive parenting was associated with decrease in total sexual partners [18]. This leads to consideration of other counseling interventions which may target youth with ADHD.

> These data demonstrate the impact of parenting interventions for teens, suggesting some malleability in the relationship between ADHD and sexual practices.

In addition to STIs, higher ADHD symptom severity has been associated with a younger age of sexual debut leading to unplanned pregnancies and teenage childbearing and parenting [1, 18, 19]. Since we know that ADHD increases the risk of unsafe sexual behavior, Danish researchers investigated whether ADHD is a risk factor for teen parenting. Using Denmark's national registry, which includes data from millions of Danes, researchers found that individuals with ADHD were significantly more likely to become parents between the ages of 12–16 and 17–19 and, if they became parents, to have more children than peers without ADHD [20]. However, those with ADHD were significantly less likely to become parents after 25 years of age and to become parents at all compared to non-ADHD peers, which is consistent with research showing that mental health disorders are associated with a decreased likelihood of having children [20]. This was the first time that the relationship between having ADHD and the age at parenthood has been examined. Most of the research studies focus on investigating the association of early parenthood with offspring ADHD. This also follows logically what we see with data about romantic relationships. Most pregnancies during the 12–19 years are not desired or with probable lifetime partners, but over 25, where most sex occurs within the confines of long-term romantic relationships, pregnancies are less likely to develop if the ADHD cohort is less prone to being in long-term relationships.

> Children born to teenage parents have more than twice the risk of being diagnosed with ADHD compared to children born to parents between the ages of 26 and 30 years [21].

Is this increased risk due to susceptibility passed down from parents with ADHD, or is it connected to environmental factors associated with young parents? A group of other cohort studies from Europe posits answers. A Finnish study examined whether low parental age is associated with ADHD and found that ADHD was associated with young fathers or mothers at the time of birth [22]. In this study, offspring with both parents younger than 20 years of age had a higher risk of being diagnosed with ADHD than those having only one young parent. Authors attribute this susceptibility to ADHD in the offspring to the following:

- Young parents having a history of hyperactivity symptoms although not quite severe enough to warrant a diagnosis of ADHD
- Impulsivity symptoms which can contribute to early sexual behaviors
- Negative parenting behaviors (including depression, marital conflict, family disruption, maternal substance use including cannabis and alcohol during pregnancy)
- Little or no prenatal care (associated with adverse outcomes and in turn associated with increased risk of ADHD) [22]

Using data from Swedish national registries, researchers established that the association between early maternal age and offspring ADHD is mainly explained by genetic confounding rather than environmental risk factors, denoting that teenage childbearing is likely a marker of genetic predisposition [23]. Epidemiological studies show that ADHD is one of the psychiatric disorders with the strongest genetic basis [24] and adolescents with ADHD are at higher risk of teenage childbearing due to ADHD symptoms they inherited from their progenitors. It is possible that the combination of these genetic risk factors and environmental variables may have an additive effect.

Youth with ADHD, like their neurotypical peers, should receive comprehensive education about human sexuality and reproductive health from trusted adults such as parents, clinicians, and teachers. Lessons should include sexual expression, contraceptive strategies, and rights and responsibilities of sexual behavior. Ideally, youth with an individualized education program (IEP) should receive this information from staff trained in sexual health education content and relevant skill development. Clinicians should also follow recommendations of the Centers for Disease Control and Prevention (CDC) and American Academy of Pediatrics (AAP) and screen sexually active adolescents and young adults for STIs at least annually given their increased risk to acquire STIs. Teens with ADHD should be educated about substance use and its general negative consequences but also as they relate to risky sexual behavior. Environmental factors should also be addressed, and psychosocial interventions such as parent training that addresses family problems should be instituted to promote healthy and mutually respectful behavior.

Violence Victimization and Perpetration

Findings suggest that impulsivity and attention switching deficits are more characteristic of intimate partner violence (IPV) perpetrators than nonviolent participants; this suggests that ADHD symptoms may be more prevalent in violent populations [25].

Does ADHD correlate with physical, psychological, or sexual violence as either perpetrator or victim? Unlike other facets of interpersonal relations explored in this chapter which show mixed data and are not always clearly interpretable (such as the data about ADHD and romantic relationships), the preponderance of data in this area clearly points to increased risks. Ngo and colleagues studied peer-to-peer sexual violence among middle and high school students in southeastern Michigan and found that those who reported clinically significant level of ADHD via the Youth Self Report (YSR/11–18) had both higher odds of peer-to-peer sexual violence victimization and engagement in sexual perpetration during the past year [26].

While ADHD has been seen as more prevalent in males, it has negative long-term implications for young women's relationships in adulthood. Ohlsson et al. examined the association between parent-reported ADHD symptoms in childhood and self-reports of coercive sexual victimization at age 18 and found that the effect of sexual victimization was not specific to ADHD [27]. This Swedish study found that while ADHD was associated with a doubled increased risk of coercive sexual victimization in females, this was thought to be moderated by general neurodevelopmental disorder rather than by ADHD itself. However, further effects of ADHD and its role on sexual victimization of women were examined by Snyder et al. who explored ADHD as a risk factor in the prediction of sexual victimization including unwanted sexual touching and rape in college women. They found that overall, women with ADHD experienced sexual victimization at significantly higher rates than women without ADHD [2].

In line with prior research, a study of young women with childhood ADHD who were followed longitudinally showed that they experienced five times more physical IPV victimization between 17 and 24 years of age compared to females without childhood ADHD [28]. This coheres logically with findings that females with ADHD are at higher risk of victimization for bullying and other forms of aggression. Women with ADHD may be more vulnerable to sexual offenders due to associated social deficits. Academic achievement has been demonstrated to be a significant mediator of the relationship between childhood ADHD symptomatology and physical IPV victimization, mirroring a trend with neurotypical peers that higher levels of female academic achievement are protective against IPV [28].

As reported by Guendelman et al., participants with persistent ADHD were twice

> Greater ADHD symptom severity has also been associated with increased risk for IPV victimization.

as likely to experience IPV relative to those with transient diagnoses and nine times more likely to experience IPV than those without any history of ADHD diagnosis [28]. Wymbs and colleagues also investigated the degree to which ADHD symptoms were associated with risk of college students perpetrating or being victims of intimate partner violence [29]. They found that college students reporting greater ADHD symptom severity endorsed higher rates of psychological and physical IPV perpetration as well as higher rates of psychological IPV victimization. Additionally, a review of multiple studies on childhood and adult ADHD and its link to IPV and domestic violence identified hyperactive, impulsive, and inattentive symptoms as risk factors for adult IPV. This relationship was mediated by comorbid psychiatric disorders including conduct disorder and antisocial personality disorder [30]. Using a population-based sample, Fang et al. investigated whether the link between childhood ADHD and young adult IPV perpetration may be attributed to inattention or hyperactivity/impulsivity. Interestingly, in their findings, inattention independently predicted young adult IPV perpetration without injury, while hyperactivity/impulsivity independently predicted IPV perpetration resulting in injury even when controlling for conduct disorder [31].

Mechanisms

Oxytocin is a hormone often referred to as the "love hormone" as it has been recognized for its role in strengthening social bonding especially during hugging and sex.

The exact mechanism underlying the disordered physiological processes associated with the social and communication difficulties linked to ADHD is unknown. However, interesting research involving oxytocin merits further exploration. Oxytocin, a hormone released from the brain commonly associated with childbirth, breastfeeding, and maternal bonding, has been recently studied to better understand whether it is implicated in the social functioning skills of children and adolescents with ADHD. First, it was discovered that oxytocin-related genes influenced social cognition in various disorders that are characterized by impairment in social communication [32]. Recently, an association of oxytocin-related genes and ADHD was found [33]. Sasaki and colleagues were the first to report decreased serum oxytocin levels in children and adolescents with ADHD compared to age- and sex-matched neurotypical controls suggesting that decreased levels of oxytocin may play a role in the functional changes associated with ADHD [34]. Such findings are consistent with those reported by Demirci and colleagues who examined the relationship between aggression, empathy, and oxytocin levels in male children and adolescents aged 7–18 years with ADHD without comorbidity. Their findings also suggest that decreased levels of this hormone may play a role in the social limitations, aggression, and empathy skills that affect social situations among youth with ADHD. Specifically, there was a negative correlation between oxytocin levels and aggression scores and positive correlation between oxytocin levels and empathy scores in patients with ADHD [35]. Additionally, serum levels of oxytocin have been shown to be significantly higher in medicated ADHD patients than in drug-naïve counterparts [34]. This is not surprising given that we know that reducing the ADHD symptoms, which often interfere with relationship building, may lead to improved social skills and strengthen friendships and romantic relationships.

Medication and Psychological Treatment

Stimulants are the first-line treatment for ADHD as evidenced by clinical trials which have acknowledged reduction of core symptoms of ADHD with these medications. There is vast literature showing significant improvement in symptoms of inattention, impulsiveness, and hyperactivity when children and adolescents are treated with medications. However, the evidence base for the effect of medications on outcomes including quality of friendships and romantic relationships and rates of risky sexual behavior leading to unwanted teenage pregnancy is scarce. Among males with ADHD, both short-term and long-term medication use have been associated with a lower risk of subsequent STIs [16]. This makes sense since the underlying symptoms of ADHD put adolescents and young adults at increased risk for such negative outcomes. Once they receive treatment with medication, symptoms improve, and risk-taking behavior diminishes.

Unfortunately, discontinuation of medication is common in adolescence and

> Pharmacological treatments have been proven to reduce the probability of contracting an STI in youth with ADHD [36].

young adulthood [37]. Medication adherence among adolescents with ADHD diminishes or stops due to improvement of ADHD symptoms or dislike of the way the medication makes them feel. A British study showed that prevalence of prescribing medications including methylphenidate, dexamphetamine, and atomoxetine to adolescents and young adults with ADHD in primary care drops significantly from age 15 to 21 years despite persistence of symptoms [37]. Regardless of the age of patients, if they are exhibiting symptoms of ADHD, clinicians should provide adequate treatment because by helping with symptoms of inattention, impulsiveness, and hyperactivity, it may lower the risk of engaging in unsafe sexual behaviors. As many clinicians worry about misuse of stimulants in young adulthood, it is recommended for clinicians to monitor stimulant prescriptions closely to prevent abuse, misuse, and diversion. Clinicians should also counsel adolescents with ADHD about misuse, as those who are prescribed stimulant medications and divert their medications are at increased risk of peer victimization compared to youth without ADHD [38].

Psychotropic medications can provide improvements in cognitive functioning and, when combined with psychotherapeutic interventions, result in improved concentration, organization, and coping [39]. Psychosocial treatments include classroom-, family-, and youth-focused interventions. The goal is to train caregivers and teachers to implement contingencies to shape behavior, setting them up with the tools to teach children the skills needed to compensate for ADHD deficits. Treatments include behavioral parent training, behavioral classroom management, and behavioral peer interventions [40]. Some research studies suggest that adolescents who comply with psychosocial treatment, such as interpersonal skills training, experience significant improvements in social functioning [41]. Conversely, other research studies argue that these interventions work best in childhood and lack a robust response in adolescents with ADHD. Favorable outcomes have been demonstrated with the use of cognitive behavior therapy (CBT) in this population, especially when combined with medical therapy [42]. CBT intervention alone has been widely researched among adults with ADHD and demonstrated to be effective in improving core symptoms of ADHD and functioning [43]. In addition to CBT, clinicians should consider using some of the strategies that are fundamental of dialectical behavioral therapy (DBT) such as distress tolerance, interpersonal effectiveness, and emotional regulation to successfully establish coping mechanisms and empower adolescents with ADHD and establish healthy relationships.

Case Revisited

Desta's situation is complicated. Her ADHD, inattentive subtype, may diminish her ability to sustain friendships during her breakup. Like other teens with ADHD, she may misperceive her friendships to be less supportive than someone without ADHD might. Working with a counselor can help her develop tools to strengthen her peer relationships. Unfortunately, adolescents with ADHD are at increased risk of sexual victimization, likely impacted by social deficits. Comorbid psychiatric disorders also impact this risk, and so Desta should be screened carefully. Ideally, Desta would have been armed with confidence, social skills, and knowledge about victimization risk and empowered and skilled to make safer choices. Ideally, her family would be involved and supportive, with a long-standing practice of open and honest, nonjudgmental conversation. At this point, her medical needs (and risk for pregnancy) should be addressed. Though mental health screening may identify urgent referral needs, she should be provided with psychosocial treatment regardless; treatment should include interpersonal skills training and components of DBT (distress tolerance, interpersonal effectiveness, and emotional regulation). Finally, efficacy of and adherence to ADHD medication should also be explored, given the high rates of nonadherence in the adolescent population and the expected improvement in decision-making with treated ADHD symptoms.

Conclusions

In summary, research demonstrates that adolescents and young adults with ADHD experience difficulties with relationships. They are at increased risk for unsafe sexual behavior leading to negative sexual and reproductive health outcomes. These findings provide support for the need to continue evidence-based services for adolescents with ADHD that equips them with skills to build healthy relationships. Emphasizing positive close friendships and romantic relationships while teaching teens how to provide emotional support and sympathy may be an effective way to intervene socially and to avoid peer exclusion and rejection, which may contribute to negative outcomes that persist into adulthood. Community and educational programs should support adolescents and young adults with ADHD by providing them with information to help them understand how their behaviors may be interpreted during their interactions with others and social skills training to improve the ability to provide emotional support and manage conflict in friendships. Peer functioning interventions should be made part of standard treatment recommendations in community and clinic settings. All adolescents and young adults, in particular females, should be provided with the skills to decrease the risk of being sexually victimized by controlling impulsivity and learning how to discern danger signs. Teaching individuals with ADHD to focus on the good qualities of their friends and partners—and to forego the impulsive desire to act aggressively—may lead them to be more successful in maintaining all relationships.

Tips
- It is essential for adolescents with ADHD to be supported with effective interventions that manage the core symptoms of ADHD as early as possible.
- Individual therapy may help youth with ADHD to have better control over their impulsivity and emotions.
- Clinicians should prioritize counseling regarding violence victimization and perpetration during clinic visits.
- Comorbidities—especially psychiatric disorders—should be taken into consideration and managed appropriately in an effort to prevent behavior dysregulation that leads to violence.
- Teachers can support all adolescents, particularly females, with ADHD by focusing on enhancing academic skills through educational support.

References

1. Rokeach A, Wiener J. Friendship quality in adolescents with ADHD. J Atten Disord (Internet). 2017;108705471773538. Available from: http://journals.sagepub.com/doi/10.1177/1087054717735380.
2. Snyder JA. The link between ADHD and the risk of sexual victimization among college women: expanding the lifestyles/routine activities framework. Violence Against Women. 2015;21(11):1364–84.
3. Marton I, Wiener J, Rogers M, Moore C. Friendship characteristics of children with ADHD. J Atten Disord. 2015;19(10):872–81.
4. Canu WH, Tabor LS, Michael KD, Bazzini DG, Elmore AL. Young adult romantic couples' conflict resolution and satisfaction varies with partner's attention-deficit/hyperactivity disorder type. J Marital Fam Ther. 2014;40(4):509–24.
5. Gardner DM, Gerdes AC. A review of peer relationships and friendships in youth with ADHD. J Atten Disord. 2015;19(10):844–55.
6. Mikami AY. The importance of friendship for youth with attention-deficit/hyperactivity disorder. Clin Child Fam Psychol Rev. 2010;13(2):181–98.
7. Glass K, Flory K, Hankin BL. Symptoms of ADHD and close friendships in adolescence. J Atten Disord. 2012;16(5):406–17.
8. McKee TE. Peer relationships in undergraduates with ADHD symptomatology: selection and quality of friendships. J Atten Disord. 2017;21(12):1020–9.
9. Overbey GA, Snell WE, Callis KE. Subclinical ADHD, stress, and coping in romantic relationships of university students. Artic J Atten Disord. 2011;15(1):67–78.

10. VanderDrift LE, Antshel KM, Olszewski AK. Inattention and hyperactivity-impulsivity: their detrimental effect on romantic relationship maintenance. J Atten Disord. 2019;23(9):985–94.
11. Norvilitis JM, Marsh LE, Ingersoll TS, Li B, Norvilitis JM, Ingersoll TS, et al. ADHD symptomatology, fear of intimacy, and sexual anxiety and behavior among college students in China and the United States. J Atten Disord. 2015;19(3):211–21.
12. Rokeach A, Wiener J. The romantic relationships of adolescents with ADHD. J Atten Disord. 2018;22(1):35–45.
13. Barkley RA, Murphy KR, Fischer M. ADHD in adults: what the science says. New York: Guilford Press; 2008.
14. Dir AL, Coskunpinar A, Cyders MA. A meta-analytic review of the relationship between adolescent risky sexual behavior and impulsivity across gender, age, and race. Clin Psychol Rev. 2014;34:551–62.
15. Isaksson J, Stickley A, Koposov R, Ruchkin V. The danger of being inattentive - ADHD symptoms and risky sexual behaviour in Russian adolescents. Eur Psychiatry. 2018;47:42–8.
16. Chen M-H, Hsu J-W, Huang K-L, Bai Y-M, Ko N-Y, Su T-P, et al. Sexually transmitted infection among adolescents and young adults with attention-deficit/hyperactivity disorder: a nationwide longitudinal study. J Am Acad Child Adolesc Psychiatry. 2018;57(1):48–53.
17. Sarver DE, McCart MR, Sheidow AJ, Letourneau EJ. ADHD and risky sexual behavior in adolescents: conduct problems and substance use as mediators of risk. J Child Psychol Psychiatry. 2014;55(12):1345–53.
18. Roy A, Hechtman L, Arnold LE, Swanson JM, Molina BSG, Sibley MH, et al. Childhood predictors of adult functional outcomes in the multimodal treatment study of attention-deficit/hyperactivity disorder (MTA). J Am Acad Child Adolesc Psychiatry. 2017;56(8):687–95.
19. Hechtman L, Swanson JM, Sibley MH, Stehli A, Owens EB, Mitchell JT, et al. Functional adult outcomes 16 years after childhood diagnosis of attention-deficit/hyperactivity disorder: MTA results. J Am Acad Child Adolesc Psychiatry. 2016;55(11):945–52.
20. Østergaard SD, Dalsgaard SS, Faraone SV, Munk-Olsen T, Laursen TM, Ostergaard SD, et al. Teenage parenthood and birth rates for individuals with and without attention-deficit/hyperactivity disorder: a nationwide cohort study. J Am Acad Child Adolesc Psychiatry. 2017;56(7):578–84.
21. Mikkelsen SH, Olsen J, Bech BH, Obel C. Parental age and attention-deficit/hyperactivity disorder (ADHD). Int J Epidemiol. 2017;46(2):409–20.
22. Chudal R, Joelsson P, Gyllenberg D, Lehti V, Leivonen S, Hinkka-Yli-Salomaki S, et al. Parental age and the risk of attention-deficit/hyperactivity disorder: a nationwide, population-based cohort study. J Am Acad Child Adolesc Psychiatry. 2015;54(6):487–94.
23. Chang Z, Lichtenstein P, D'onofrio BM, Almqvist C, Kuja-Halkola R, Sjö Lander A, et al. Maternal age at childbirth and risk for ADHD in offspring: a population-based cohort study. Int J Epidemiol. 2014;43(6):1815–24.
24. Grimm O, Kittel-Schneider S, Reif A. Recent developments in the genetics of attention-deficit hyperactivity disorder. Psychiatry Clin Neurosci. 2018;72(9):654–72.
25. Romero-Martínez Á, Lila M, Moya-Albiol L. The importance of impulsivity and attention switching deficits in perpetrators convicted for intimate partner violence. Aggress Behav. 2019;45:129–38.
26. Ngo QM, Veliz PT, Kusunoki Y, Stein SF, Boyd CJ. Adolescent sexual violence: prevalence, adolescent risks, and violence characteristics. Prev Med (Baltim). 2018;116:68–74.
27. Ohlsson Gotby V, Lichtenstein P, Langstrom N, Pettersson E, Långström N, Pettersson E. Childhood neurodevelopmental disorders and risk of coercive sexual victimization in childhood and adolescence - a population-based prospective twin study. J Child Psychol Psychiatry. 2018;59(9):957–65.
28. Guendelman MD, Ahmad S, Meza JI, Owens EB, Hinshaw SP. Childhood attention-deficit/hyperactivity disorder predicts intimate partner victimization in young women. J Abnorm Child Psychol. 2016;44(1):155–66.

29. Wymbs BT, Dawson AE, Suhr JA, Bunford N, Gidycz CA. ADHD symptoms as risk factors for intimate partner violence perpetration and victimization. J Interpers Violence. 2017;32(5):659–81.
30. Buitelaar NJL, Posthumus JA, Buitelaar JK. ADHD in childhood and/or adulthood as a risk factor for domestic violence or intimate partner violence: a systematic review. J Atten Disord. 2015:1–12.
31. Fang X, Massetti GM, Ouyang L, Grosse SD, Mercy JA. Attention-deficit/hyperactivity disorder, conduct disorder, and young adult intimate partner violence. Arch Gen Psychiatry. 2010;67(11):1179–86.
32. Park J, Willmott M, Vetuz G, Toye C, Kirley A, Hawi Z, et al. Evidence that genetic variation in the oxytocin receptor (OXTR) gene influences social cognition in ADHD. Prog Neuro-Psychopharmacol Biol Psychiatry. 2010;34(4):697–702.
33. Kalyoncu T, Özbaran B, Köse S, Onay H. Variation in the oxytocin receptor gene is associated with social cognition and ADHD. J Atten Disord. 2019;23(7):702–71.
34. Sasaki T, Hashimoto K, Oda Y, Ishima T, Kurata T, Takahashi J, et al. Decreased levels of serum oxytocin in pediatric patients with attention deficit/hyperactivity disorder. Psychiatry Res. 2015;228(3):746–51.
35. Demirci E, Ozmen S, Kilic E, Oztop DB. The relationship between aggression, empathy skills and serum oxytocin levels in male children and adolescents with attention deficit and hyperactivity disorder. Behav Pharmacol. 2016;27(8):681–8.
36. Chorniy A, Kitashima L. Sex, drugs, and ADHD: the effects of ADHD pharmacological treatment on teens' risky behaviors. Labour Econ. 2016;43:87–105.
37. Lichtenstein P, Halldner L, Zetterqvist J, Sjölander A, Serlachius E, Fazel S, et al. Medication for attention deficit-hyperactivity disorder and criminality. N Engl J Med. 2012;367(21):2006–20.
38. Epstein-Ngo QM, McCabe SE, Veliz PT, Stoddard SA, Austic EA, Boyd CJ. Diversion of ADHD stimulants and victimization among adolescents. J Pediatr Psychol. 2016;41(7):786–98.
39. Katzman DK. Neinstein's adolescent and young adult health care: a practical guide. In: Callahan T, Gordon CM, Joffe A, Rickert VL, editors. Philadelphia Wolters Kluwer Health; 2016. 1812 p.
40. Schoenfelder EN, Sasser T. Skills versus pills: psychosocial treatments for ADHD in childhood and adolescence. Pediatr Ann. 2016;45(10):e367–72.
41. Schultz BK, Evans SW, Langberg JM, Schoemann AM. Outcomes for adolescents who comply with long-term psychosocial treatment for ADHD. J Consult Clin Psychol. 2017;85(3):250–61.
42. Modesto-Lowe V, Charbonneau V, Farahmand P. Psychotherapy for adolescents with attention-deficit hyperactivity disorder: a pediatrician's guide. Clin Pediatr (Phila). 2017;56(7):667–74.
43. Weiss M, Murray C, Wasdell M, Greenfield B, Giles L, Hechtman L. A randomized controlled trial of CBT therapy for adults with ADHD with and without medication. BMC Psychiatry. 2012;12:30.

Part IV
ADHD: Nuts and Bolts of the Teenage Years

Chapter 18
Parenting Adolescents with ADHD

Kate Linnea, Dasha Solomon, and Carrie Mauras

Case Example

James is a 17-year-old male who is an 11th grade student. Most mornings, James has difficulty waking up to his alarm and hits the snooze button several times. His mother typically is forced to wake him up in order for him to be able to get ready for school; as you can imagine, this is not a pleasant experience for James or his mother and often results in mother and son yelling at one another and feeling frustrated. With little time to prepare for his day, James must rush out of his house in the morning, and one of his parents has to drive him to school, often resulting in being late to work. James also is often late to school, and he sometimes forgets to take his stimulant medication as he rushes out the door. James does not only forget to take his medication but also sometimes forgets to pack his folders with completed homework and his flute, which he needs for band practices and performances. As a result, his father often finds himself leaving work to bring James his flute. When he is unable to do so, James cannot perform, and he lets his bandmates down. Understandably, James feels bad when his father has to leave work, when he disappoints his band members, and when he forgets the homework that he completed at home. Further impacting his self-esteem is that he struggles to focus and sometimes gets in trouble on the days that he misses his medication. James looks forward to the weekends, when he can spend time with his friends. James's parents dread the occasional weekends when they both have to travel for work and worry the entire time they are gone.

K. Linnea (✉) · D. Solomon
Division of Developmental Medicine, Boston Children's Hospital, Boston, MA, USA
e-mail: Kate.linnea@childrens.harvard.edu; Dasha.solomon@childrens.harvard.edu

C. Mauras
Department of Psychiatry, Cambridge Health Alliance, Touchstone Neurodevelopmental Center, Woburn, MA, USA
e-mail: Cmauras@touchstonema.com

© Springer Nature Switzerland AG 2020
A. Schonwald (ed.), *ADHD in Adolescents*,
https://doi.org/10.1007/978-3-030-62393-7_18

Background

"I can't wait for my child to become a teenager!" said no parent ever. While they welcome the relief from the physical exhaustion of parenting a younger child, many parents worry about the changing demands and associated stress of parenting an adolescent. In this transitional period from childhood to adulthood, adolescents experience physical, neurodevelopmental, intellectual, social, and psychological changes. Issues of independence, identity, sexuality, and risk-taking abound. For these reasons and more, parenting a teenager can be particularly stressful. Parenting a teenager with attention-deficit/hyperactivity disorder (ADHD) may be even more stressful as the increased risks for teenagers with ADHD are indisputable.

Academic and Executive Functioning and the Role of Parents

It is no secret that youth with ADHD often experience academic impairment, and this domain has arguably received the most attention in the literature. As academic performance during adolescence can have significant implications for employment and higher education opportunities, the impairments experienced by teenagers with ADHD are particularly concerning. Such impairments can be seen in academic achievement, specifically, as well as in behavior relevant to academic success. Regarding the latter, youth with ADHD have higher rates of suspension, tardiness, absenteeism, and school dropout [1–3]. Academically, high school students with ADHD have lower class placement and GPAs than their non-ADHD peers [2, 3]. Perhaps not surprisingly, teachers have been shown to rate teenagers with ADHD as completing and handing in fewer assignments relative to students without ADHD and as not performing to their potential [2].

Greater independence as youth move through school, coupled with increased executive functioning demands, is thought to contribute to academic failures experienced by teenagers with ADHD [4]. Indeed, as students move through middle school and into high school, they become increasingly responsible for managing their own schedules, tracking and completing homework assignments and projects, and even getting themselves to school in the morning. Such responsibilities require planning, organization, and time management, skills that are sometimes lacking in youth with ADHD [5, 6]. For example, in a study of teenagers with ADHD, parents and teachers rated youth as experiencing significant difficulties in task planning and management of materials, which were significant predictors of school grades [5]. Childhood executive functioning predicts academic achievement in adolescents [6], and individuals with ADHD and executive functioning impairment are particularly worse off academically. More specifically, children with ADHD and executive functioning impairments experience lower academic achievement than youth with ADHD without executive dysfunction, as well as their non-ADHD peers [7].

In theory, the role of the parent should lessen as children move through school and become more independent. While this is true for parents of teens with ADHD, their involvement remains critical to support the academic success of their adolescents given the previously mentioned skill deficits.

Thankfully, interventions with parenting components are emerging with promising results. The Supporting Teens' Academic Needs Daily-Group (STAND-G) is a structured program to guide parents in collaborating with their teen with ADHD. Utilizing a behavioral parent-training model within a group format [8], STAND-G involves direct teaching of skills to teens as well as parent coaching related to academic monitoring and use of an academic contract. Results examining STAND-G indicated high rates of parent satisfaction and compliance with intervention procedures, even following the completion of the program. Following the STAND-G intervention, parents rated improvements in their teens'

- organization
- time management
- academic habits
- home behavior

These improvements inconsistently translated to meaningful gains in GPA, but improvements in GPA could be appreciated when implemented in a middle school cohort in an individual format [9]. When considering demographic variables and treatment outcomes across studies, the authors speculate that younger adolescents may require more intensive intervention that is often achieved in individual format but that there may be an important benefit to conducting STAND using a group-based format for older teens [8].

Social Functioning and the Role of Parents

Youth with ADHD experience social impairment [10]. They are often rejected by their peers and are less likely to have close dyadic friendships [11]. Research in this area has consistently highlighted the behaviors that are characteristic of ADHD as contributing to such impairment. It is easy to understand how symptoms of hyperactivity, impulsivity, and inattention hinder a teen's ability to make and maintain friendships. For example, interrupting and talking excessively may interfere with appropriate social interactions and are likely aversive to peers. Symptoms of inattention may reduce the likelihood that an individual notices and thus responds to social cues. Inattention in adolescents, when youth are relatively more responsible for their own schedule, may result in missed social obligations, which also is likely to be upsetting or annoying to peers. Indeed, while symptoms of hyperactivity and impulsivity may be most socially impairing in childhood, inattention has been found to be particularly problematic for teens in the social domain [12].

Unfortunately, reducing ADHD symptoms and associated problematic behaviors through the use of evidence-based treatments does little to normalize peer relationships in youth with ADHD [13]. In fact, social difficulties persist in adolescents who no longer meet diagnostic criteria for ADHD but who were diagnosed as children [14]. One reason for the persistence of social challenges – regardless of ADHD symptom presentation – may be that a child's negative reputation among their peers is thought to be firmly established at an early age, and it is challenging to change these negative views [15].

> Teenagers with ADHD seem to be the target of various forms of victimization (i.e., relational, reputational, physical).

Youth with ADHD often end up socializing with other rejected peers, thus further limiting opportunities to learn from prosocial peers [16] and increasing the likelihood of engaging in dangerous or problematic behavior. Perhaps because of the limited choices available to them [17], adolescents with ADHD tend to gravitate toward deviant or nonconventional peer groups [18]. This is particularly important, as deviant peer group affiliation is thought to play a significant role in adolescent substance use, and this is especially the case for youth with ADHD. For example, one study found that deviant peer group affiliation either partially or fully mediated the relation between childhood ADHD and substance use in adolescents [18]. Parents seem to be aware of this phenomenon, as one study revealed that almost half of parents of youth with a history of ADHD reported that their teenager's friends were a bad influence, versus only 28% of parents of adolescents without ADHD [14]. In a study of youth with ADHD, 57% reported being the target of victimization at a rate of at least once per week, and such victimization was associated with increased rates of depression and anxiety [19].

As briefly illustrated above, peer rejection and social difficulties are associated with a host of negative outcomes, particularly for adolescents with ADHD. The evidence also suggests that social difficulties experienced by youth with ADHD should be addressed early in a child's life. Perhaps fittingly, the work that has examined the role of the parent in the social functioning of youth with ADHD has largely been conducted in preschool and school-aged children and has focused on parenting characteristics. For example, maternal warmth and responsiveness are associated with teacher-rated acceptance and positive social behavior in preschoolers with hyperactivity [20], and authoritative parenting beliefs predict greater social standing in youth with ADHD [21]. Importantly, though, research reveals that the role of the parent is complex. In a study examining the impact of parental warmth and power assertion on the social status and behavior of boys with ADHD, parent sex and child-perceived loneliness within the context of the family were revealed as pertinent variables [22]. More specifically, the significant associations between parental warmth and social status and behavior (in the expected directions), as well as power assertion and social status (again in the expected direction), were only significant when considering fathers, not mothers, and moderated by child-perceived loneliness within the family.

Theoretically, parents can have a significant impact on the social functioning of their child. Not only do parents provide a context for their child to learn appropriate social behaviors, but also they are responsible for initiating or following through on social events (e.g., sport participation, extracurricular activities), especially at a young age when appropriate social development and competency are crucial.

In a recent study examining potential protective factors, parent involvement emerged as a significant buffer to social impairment in teens with ADHD [23], highlighting the role of the parent and providing clues that parent competency is important. In a study that implemented an intervention targeting social functioning of youth with ADHD by working exclusively with the parents, improvements in youth's social skills and friendship quality as rated by parents were demonstrated, and teachers indicated greater peer acceptance and less peer rejection for youth in the intervention group [24]. Importantly, while this study yielded promising results, the authors highlight that improvements should be interpreted at the friendship level and are not thought to have normalized social status and acceptance.

While peer challenges in youth with ADHD are well established, we know little about how to normalize social functioning in these children and adolescents. Only recently have studies begun to examine the role of the parent in the social functioning of youth with ADHD, particularly the ways in which parents may be part of intervention.

> Research suggests that parenting characteristics including warmth, social behaviors, and involvement in the initiation of prosocial activities can play an important role in the social domain for youth with ADHD. Furthermore, as patterns of behavior and peer relationships are established before adolescence, earlier intervention is recommended.

Risk-Taking Behavior and the Role of Parents

Adolescence is a time of greater independence and increased responsibility. It is during this time that youth obtain a driver's license, attend social gatherings without parents, and are likely to be exposed to alcohol and drugs. All parents become concerned about safety as they watch their children emerge into teenagers, but the feelings are magnified for parents of youth with ADHD. Given decreased inhibition and increased impulsivity, teens with ADHD are at greater risk for poor decision-making in situations that are challenging for any teenager to navigate. Youth with ADHD may be less likely to think through all options when presented with a challenging scenario (e.g., offered a ride home by someone who has been drinking alcohol), as well as to remember the consequences of previous actions/poor decisions. Teenagers with ADHD are more likely than their non-ADHD counterparts to engage in risky behaviors including reckless driving, substance use, and risky sexual behavior.

Driving

Motor vehicle accidents are a leading cause of death for teens in the United States [25]. In 2016, young drivers were involved in 9% of all fatal crashes, despite making up only 5.4% of the total driving population [26]. Driving with teen passengers, being male, and being a newly licensed driver are all risk factors for motor vehicle accidents in young drivers [27]. Unfortunately, ADHD also appears to put teens at greater driving risk. Specifically, studies have found that youth with ADHD are more likely than those without ADHD to drive without a license, to have had their license suspended or revoked, to receive speeding citations, and to have been involved in and at fault for automobile accidents [1, 28–30]. Teens with attention problems also have been found to be significantly more likely to drive under the influence of alcohol [31], further exacerbating driving risk and potential fatal outcomes.

> One study in youth with and without ADHD found not only a higher rate of crashes or near crashes in young drivers with ADHD but also that these drivers were more likely than controls to be texting or interacting with passengers right before such events [30].

Interestingly, a study examining the behavior of parents of youth with ADHD during supervised driving found that parents failed to engage in parenting practices thought to be most effective for teens with ADHD. Such practices include praising desired behavior and offering frequent corrective feedback on performance. Rather, only one instance of praise was observed, and rates of instruction/feedback on driving performance were quite low [32].

> Parenting behaviors outside of the vehicle also have been consistently highlighted as critical in the safety of teenage drivers.

For example, parent monitoring and restrictions have been linked to driving safety in adolescents [33]. For parents of teenagers with ADHD, monitoring requires more than obtaining teenagers' self-reports on their driving practices, as individuals with ADHD can demonstrate poor insight and accuracy when rating their own driving problems/behaviors [34]. Teenagers with ADHD tend to overestimate their driving competency generally and in specific domains [35].

The Supporting a Teen's Effective Entry to the Roadway (STEER) program was specifically created for parents/families of young drivers with ADHD; parent behavior management training, teen communication training, the use of a monitoring device, simulated driving, and parent coaching were components of this program [36]. The wealth of critical components included in this intervention is promising, as are the high satisfaction and attendance rates of parents and teens who have participated in the STEER program [37]. Despite this, a clinical trial comparing STEER to community intervention yielded mixed results with respect to parent and driving outcomes. More specifically, while parents in the STEER program used relatively fewer negative parenting strategies, this finding was not maintained at 12-month follow-up, and there was no difference in the use of positive parenting strategies between groups. While teens in the STEER program reported a significant reduction in risky driving relative to those in the community group, there was no difference between groups in observed risky driving behaviors. Importantly, several methodological limitations may have contributed to these findings, and there is certainly not enough evidence to dismiss the potential positive impact of the STEER intervention.

> Based on what we do know about driving behaviors in typically developing teens and the intervention needs of adolescents with ADHD, factors including parental monitoring, limit setting, and the use of monitoring devices are likely all important for promoting safe driving behaviors in youth with ADHD.

Substances and Risky Sexual Behavior

Though results have been somewhat mixed and the relationship is complex, overall, research indicates that youth with ADHD are at an increased risk for substance use. Relative to controls, teenagers with ADHD have reported higher levels of alcohol, tobacco, and illicit drug use [38]. Childhood ADHD also is associated with earlier use of illicit drugs and first use of cigarettes [38], and relative to their non-ADHD peers, adolescents with ADHD are more likely to initiate alcohol use at an early age [8]. Findings related to the timing of initial exposure to substances are important, as early substance use is a well-established predictor of substance use disorder [39].

Substance use also has been linked to risky sexual behavior in youth with ADHD, with one study finding that problematic alcohol and marijuana use accounted for the association between ADHD symptoms and risky sexual behavior [40]. While more research is needed, for youth with ADHD, there is emerging evidence that risky sexual behavior may take place regardless of substance use [41]. In a study of young adults, childhood ADHD was associated with earlier onset of sexual activity and intercourse, more sexual partners, less use of birth control, and greater rates of partner pregnancy [42]. In a study examining romantic relationships in teens with and without ADHD, males with ADHD reported age of first sexual intercourse to be almost 2 years earlier than their typically developing peers, and youth with ADHD had nearly twice as many lifetime sexual partners [43].

Parents play a role in their teenager's risky decision-making and safety, and parental influence may be particularly pronounced for youth with ADHD. In a study examining parenting variables in adolescents with and without ADHD, a significant association between parental knowledge and substance use emerged across groups. Importantly, this association was strongest for parents of teens with ADHD [44]. Feeling supported by a parent also is associated with a decrease in cigarette use in adolescents with a history of childhood ADHD [45]; notably, in this sample, ADHD symptoms were associated with reduced parent social support. Of the studies examining traits and behaviors of parents that have a positive impact on substance use in teens, ADHD symptoms are typically associated with lower rates of these parenting variables. For example, a study demonstrating that low paternal warmth predicted substance use disorder in youth with ADHD also revealed that ADHD status was associated with lower levels of this same variable [46]. In terms of intervention, youth with ADHD who were randomized to intensive behavioral treatment, which included parent training, reported less substance use at 24-month follow-up than those randomized to other treatment conditions without a parent component [47].

In a study demonstrating significantly higher rates of unfamiliar sexual partners in college students with ADHD relative to those without, mother-child closeness predicted fewer unfamiliar sexual partners for individuals with ADHD only [48].

Research examining the role of the parent in adolescent risky sexual behavior in youth with ADHD is even scarcer than that dealing with substance use. This is particularly problematic as similar to the substance use domain parent characteristics may play an even greater role in youth risky sexual behavior for individuals with versus without ADHD.

While we await research focused specifically on understanding and reducing sexual risk-taking behaviors in adolescents with ADHD, parents and providers are directed toward the general literature on reducing sexual risk-taking in adolescence. Specifically, parental monitoring has emerged as a highly important variable. In a large-scale review, Dittus and colleagues (2015) [49] found higher levels of parental monitoring were associated with lower likelihood of adolescents ever having engaged in sexual intercourse and greater likelihood of using both condoms and contraceptives. Global monitoring (e.g., parents' knowledge of teens' whereabouts, friends, activities) and sexual-behavior-specific monitoring (e.g., enforcement of rules regarding friends and dating) are important in reducing risk behavior. The positive effects of parental monitoring on reducing risk behavior were robust across age, gender, and sexual experience.

Parental monitoring and limit setting in the context of a warm parent-child relationship are recommended to counteract the increased risk-taking behaviors of adolescents with ADHD. Parents and providers are encouraged to establish open lines of communication early and to clearly convey expectations as well as consequences and to actively monitor youth behavior through the teenage years.

How Parent Factors and Family Stress Impact Teens with ADHD

As illustrated above, parenting teens with ADHD can be particularly challenging and requires a greater level of involvement and skill than may be necessary for teens without ADHD. Furthermore, parents are encouraged to lend their own executive functioning skills to their children with ADHD, while they help them to learn these skills [50].

> ADHD treatments often task parents with "steering the ship," as they are responsible for administering medication, delivering behavioral intervention in the home, and advocating for such intervention in the schools.

Complicating matters is that these same parents experience higher rates of mental health diagnoses than the average population [51]. For example, higher rates of maternal depression and paternal substance abuse have been found in parents of youth with ADHD compared to parents of youth without ADHD [52]. ADHD also is common among parents of children with ADHD [53], which is not particularly surprising given the significant heritability of the disorder [54]. In fact, 25%–50% of parents of youth with ADHD are estimated to also have ADHD [55].

Fortunately, research on youth with ADHD and parenting has begun to account for parental ADHD status. This is particularly important as ADHD symptoms in parents impact not only their own response to treatment but also the response of the child. More specifically, parental ADHD is associated with reduced response to behavioral intervention in youth, and elevated parental ADHD symptoms are associated with relatively less improvement in negative parenting following behavioral parent training [56].

Differences in parenting styles and level of conflict also emerge when parental ADHD is introduced. In a study of teenagers with ADHD and their parents, mothers with ADHD demonstrated less adaptive parenting and had higher levels of parent-adolescent conflict than mothers without ADHD [57]. Interestingly, though, the potential impact of parental ADHD symptoms on a child may vary depending on the child's own diagnostic status. For example, maternal inattention was found to be associated with less negative parent-child interaction in youth with ADHD, but this was not found for comparison children [58].

To examine the possibility that parents and children who share diagnostic status may actually do better together relative to mismatched diagnostic dyads, frequency and intensity of conflict among teens with and without ADHD and their parents with varying levels of ADHD symptoms were studied [59]. Interestingly, evidence emerged supporting a "similarity misfit" for mothers and adolescents with high levels of inattentive symptoms but a "similarity fit" for fathers and their adolescents. More specifically, while the greatest levels of conflict were observed when mothers *and* their adolescents demonstrated high levels of inattention, this was not the case for fathers. Rather, fathers with the greatest levels of inattention had the least amount of conflict with their highly inattentive adolescents [59].

Not surprisingly, the relationship between parents often suffers, and discord between parents of youth with ADHD is not uncommon [60]. In a study examining communication between parents of youth with and without ADHD, parents communicated less positively and more negatively before and after interacting with a confederate child demonstrating disruptive behavior; the impact of such disruptive behavior on negative interparental communication was most pronounced for parents of children with, versus without, ADHD [61]. Parents of youth with externalizing presentations, including ADHD, report less marital satisfaction and fight more often than parents of youth without ADHD [62, 63]. While not consistently revealed across studies, when examined in a cohort from birth to young adulthood, parents of children with ADHD were not only more likely to divorce but also quicker to divorce relative to parents of children without ADHD [60].

> While there may be a host of contributing factors, mothers and fathers of teenagers with ADHD report significantly more parenting stress than parents of teenagers without ADHD [64].

Higher levels of parent-teen conflict, social isolation, and feelings of guilt and incompetence also have been reported by mothers of adolescents with ADHD [57, 64]. Nevertheless, parents of children with ADHD are not doomed. Instead, armed with this knowledge, parents, as well as providers who support parents, are encouraged to underscore the importance of parents' mental health treatment. Furthermore, understanding the negative impact of parenting a child with ADHD on marital health, efforts directed toward buffering relationships and social supports are encouraged.

Evidence-Based Intervention for Adolescents with ADHD

Although the literature focuses primarily on interventions for young children with ADHD, it is critical to note that the importance of intervention does not diminish with age. Without appropriate treatment, children diagnosed with ADHD are more likely to experience a variety of negative outcomes as they move into adolescence and adulthood [65]. As such, important stakeholders in the field advocate for continued intervention into the adolescent and adult years [66].

To date, there have been far fewer studies looking at intervention for adolescents with ADHD than for young children [65]. For example, the success of traditional parent-training programs, which are highly successful for managing behavior problems with children, is not as well studied in adolescents. While research indicates that medication management continues to be the first line of treatment for adolescents with ADHD [67], there is also a great need for intervention to address the specific psychosocial needs of adolescents and their families given the unique vulnerabilities they experience.

We end this chapter by highlighting interventions and parent management strategies to help teens effectively manage the increased demands of adolescence, minimize risky behaviors, and navigate other common challenges that often co-occur with ADHD. Ultimately, the goal is to help adolescents achieve academic success, foster positive peer relationships, develop strategies to promote positive self-esteem, and establish tools to manage executive function demands in adolescents and into adulthood. Although adolescence is a time for increased independence, parents and caretakers remain crucial to successful intervention and serve as the primary influence over their teen's behavior [68, 69]. Multimodal treatment including medication management, school advocacy, and individual and family therapy with an emphasis on collaborative problem-solving are likely to be even more important as a child with ADHD transitions into adolescence [8].

Specific evidence-based techniques are outlined below. It is critically important to remember that intervention will be most successful when an adolescent's individual strengths, interests, and personality are incorporated and their specific areas of need are targeted. In other words, while the principles will remain the same, treatment must always be tailored to the individual.

Therapeutic Interventions

Working with a mental health professional for both individual and family therapy is recommended when treating teens with ADHD. Such intervention is useful in the following:

- Providing psychoeducation regarding ADHD
- Strengthening communication between adolescents and their parents
- Reducing conflict
- Establishing goals to improve executive functions and behaviors

In turn, psychoeducation is an important treatment variable, as an understanding of ADHD as a neurobiological disorder is an important predictor of treatment adherence [70]. Families may also benefit from education about ADHD in order to correct misguided assumptions about the disorder. For example, it is especially important to clarify that ADHD is not due to a lack of willpower and that children and adolescents with ADHD will need ongoing support and treatment [71].

Cognitive-behavioral treatment approaches, parent-teen collaborative problem-solving, and motivational interviewing techniques are effective interventions to address behavior problems and family conflict among adolescents with ADHD [72, 73]. Collaborative behavioral therapies aim to establish clear behavioral expectations, determine mutually agreed upon goals between parents and adolescents, and help adolescents achieve those goals while promoting more independence [8].

Another promising intervention for adolescents with ADHD and their families is mindfulness-based cognitive therapy (MBCT). Haydicky and colleagues (2015) [74] evaluated the efficacy of an 8-week parallel parent/adolescent MBCT group. Immediately following the completion of the group, parents reported reductions in adolescents' inattention, conduct problems, and peer relationship problems. Furthermore, parents reported reductions in their parenting stress and increases in mindful parenting. Improvements in adolescent symptomatology and mindful parenting were maintained through 6-week follow-up, as were reductions in parenting stress. Of note, adolescents did not report improvement on any variables during the intervention period; however, they reported reduced internalizing problems at follow-up.

Adolescent-directed interventions, including programs delivered in peer settings during the summer (e.g., Summer Treatment Program-Adolescent; STP-A) that target improvements in daily functioning, may be more motivating to adolescents than traditional outpatient care [8, 75]. Recently, several researchers have utilized technology including web-based grade portals [9], computerized driving monitoring devices [76], and video feedback [77] to enhance motivation of tech-savvy adolescents to participate in behavioral therapy approaches [9].

Other therapies may be necessary depending on co-occurring challenges. For example, if an adolescent is abusing alcohol or substances, a referral to a substance abuse program should be the first step [78]. Co-occurring disorders including anxiety or depression may also require specific interventions, including individual therapy and targeted medications. Other modalities of psychoeducation and therapeutic intervention can be provided through books, websites, videos, executive functioning coaches, or local support groups.

Psychopharmacologic Intervention and Adherence

Pharmacotherapy, specifically the use of stimulant medication, is an evidence-based treatment for ADHD in youth [67, 79]. The symptom reduction provided by medication may position an adolescent and the family to be more successful in implementing behavioral interventions. Despite the potential benefits of pharmacological intervention, studies reveal low adherence rates by teens, with some research citing that up to 90% of adolescents who were prescribed stimulant medication refused to take it [80, 81]. A more recent systematic review of ADHD treatment for adolescents additionally noted premature treatment cessation of stimulant medication despite continued symptoms of ADHD [79]. As such, it is important that we investigate ways to improve medication adherence in teens and highlight that buy-in on the part of the teen is critical. For now, parents are encouraged to gradually increase their adolescents' understanding of why they are prescribed medication, what the medication is, how it works, what makes it effective, and what they have to do to manage their own medication. Regarding the latter, apparent noncompliance may sometimes merely reflect the absence of a system that sets the teen up for success in terms of taking their medication.

Parents are advised to set up a clear routine that outlines the time the medication is to be taken, where the medication will be stored, and that provides any necessary reminders (e.g., automatic reminder/alarm on a smart phone or watch, or note on the bathroom mirror) is often necessary. As teens get older and prepare to move out of the house (e.g., to attend college), it will be important that they have learned the skills to manage medical appointments and refills. As parents will not be able to manage their teens' medication forever, transfer of the responsibility from the parent to the adolescent is critical for long-term medication adherence.

School Advocacy and Communication

Despite adolescents' increasing need for independence, they still require the support and advocacy of their parents or caregivers. Families should work as a team to educate the school about the teenager's specific needs, including both strengths and weaknesses. Parents play an important role in advocating for the teenager with regard to implementing a 504 Accommodation Plan or pursuing appropriate testing to determine whether or not there is a need for special education services and an individualized education program (IEP). If an independent neuropsychological or psychological evaluation has been completed outside of the school setting, parents will need to bring the report to the appropriate coordinator at school and work together with the school to develop an educational plan. Ongoing communication between school personnel, parents, and the adolescent, as well as monitoring of the effectiveness of the educational plan, will be necessary to ensure compliance on both sides and to determine need for any modifications of the IEP or 504 Plan.

Case Revisited

Despite the current challenges James's parents are experiencing as detailed in the vignette at the beginning of this chapter, James's parents have done many things well:

1. *Early diagnosis and treatment*: James's parents pursued a diagnostic evaluation early when James first began exhibiting symptoms and obtained multimodal treatment, including parent training and medication management.
2. *School advocacy and intervention*: James had a 504 Plan in elementary and middle school with accommodations to address his executive functioning and behavioral challenges.

3. *Involvement with prosocial peers and activities*: James's parents worked hard when he was younger to arrange playdates with appropriate peers and fostered prosocial relationships. These relationships have persisted into adolescence and have protected James from affiliation with peers who may be a bad influence. In addition, they tried many extracurricular activities until finding one that he really enjoyed, which led to well-supervised interactions with prosocial peers.

4. *Monitoring and limit setting*: James is not permitted to drive himself to school (or anywhere else without an adult in the car) as he has not met the safety standards his parents set (e.g., driving at or under the speed limit without reminders). In addition, they have clear rules and expectations, as well as consequences related to his behavior, particularly on weekends when they are both traveling and James is home alone.

Nevertheless, James and his parents are struggling with circumstances common in families of teenagers with ADHD. Based on the existing literature, we recommend the following:

1. *Resumption of therapy*: Through the school-age years, James's parents grew increasingly competent in managing his behavior, and therapy appointments did not always fit into their increasingly busy schedule. However, as James's parents reflect on the unique challenges presented by the teenage years, they decide to resume treatment:

   (a) Key components of effective interventions include both *behavioral monitoring* and *medication management*:

      (i) James's parents resume working with a therapist trained in collaborative problem-solving and behavioral intervention to increase his independence in the morning, as well as other problem areas. Through setting clear expectations, rewards, and consequences, conflict is likely to decrease.

      (ii) James's parents also work with his prescribing physician to promote James's understanding about why he takes medication, how the medication works, his dosing, etc. The ultimate goal of increased adherence is addressed by transferring the responsibility of managing all aspects of his medication from his parents to James. Ongoing tracking of James's symptoms to ensure adequate medication management also is important as youth age.

   (b) James's therapist additionally monitors his social-emotional adjustment and identifies strategies for areas of difficulty as well as ways he can utilize his strengths to compensate for any areas of weakness.

   (c) To address the increasing parental discord and added stress on their marital relationship, James's parents may decide to pursue working with a couples' therapist as well.

2. *School advocacy*: James's parents recognize that he continues to require support to be successful in school. They partner with his teachers/school personnel to

reinstate his 504 Plan with accommodations related to James's impulsivity and executive functioning challenges. In addition, James's parents increase their monitoring in the area of academics, while James works explicitly on the development of his skills in the areas of executive functioning in which he most struggles. At the same time, his autonomy and self-advocacy skills are fostered as he participates in school team meetings.

3. *Monitoring and limit setting*: James's parents acknowledge that driving is not the only area of concern with regard to impulsivity and risk-taking. They engage in clear communication about expectations, rules, and consequences related to exploration of substances and sexual behavior. They leave him home alone as infrequently as their work schedules permit and rely upon their network of close friends, neighbors, and relatives to assist in supervision when they do have to be away for the entire weekend.

4. *Prioritize warm parent-child relationship*: Adolescents with ADHD often receive negative criticism from adults, teachers, and peers which can significantly impact their self-esteem. James's parents' belief in his ability to succeed is critical for his success. James and his parents are encouraged to engage in activities together that they all enjoy. In addition, maintaining warmth in the parent-child relationship is crucial.

5. *Opportunities for success*: James's parents continue to provide him with opportunities to succeed in extracurricular endeavors (e.g., flute). In addition, they continue to expose him to positive peer models and support friendships with desirable peers.

6. *Parental self-care*: James parents also take steps (e.g., exercise, hobbies, therapy, medication) to ensure their own physical and mental health needs are addressed. By prioritizing their own self-care, they recharge their parenting batteries, allowing for improved functioning across domains.

Conclusions

In this chapter, we have reviewed both vulnerabilities unique to adolescents with ADHD and promising interventions. Despite the complexity in studying youth with ADHD and their families, this area of inquiry is expanding as of late, with increasing research devoted to developing interventions specifically for adolescents. While it is never too late to intervene, intervention is recommended as *early* as challenges are detected.

Parenting a teenager with ADHD is understandably quite stressful and requires a combination of behavior planning, advocacy, therapy, medication management, and potentially other types of support and intervention. However, we hope that with increased knowledge comes confidence on the part of parents and providers working with parents. An understanding of increased risks and evidence-based interventions best equips parents to improve outcomes for adolescents with ADHD.

Tips
- Parenting an adolescent with ADHD can be frustrating, but parenting intentionally with warmth and involvement should pay off later.
- Teens with ADHD are high-risk drivers. This is a place for intense parent involvement and strict limit setting.
- Despite the drive for independence, expect greater involvement of parents whose adolescents have ADHD than those with unaffected adolescents.

References

1. Barkley RA, Fischer M, Smallish L, Fletcher K. Young adult outcome of hyperactive children: adaptive functioning in major life activities. J Am Acad Child Adolesc Psychiatry. 2006;45(2):192–202.
2. Kent KM, Pelham WE, Molina BSG, Sibley MH, Waschbusch DA, Yu J, et al. The academic experience of male high school students with ADHD. J Abnorm Child Psychol. 2011;39(3):451–62.
3. Barbaresi WJ, Katusic SK, Colligan RC, Weaver AL, Jacobsen SJ. Long-term school outcomes for children with attention-deficit/hyperactivity disorder: a population-based perspective. J Dev Behav Pediatr. 2007;28(4):265–73.
4. Langberg JM, Epstein JN, Becker SP, Girio-Herrera E, Vaughn AJ. Evaluation of the homework, organization, and planning skills (HOPS) intervention for middle school students with ADHD as implemented by school mental health providers. School Psych Rev. 2012;41(3):342–64.
5. Langberg JM, Epstein JN, Girio-Herrera E, Becker SP, Vaughn AJ, Altaye M. Materials organization, planning, and homework completion in middle-school students with ADHD: impact on academic performance. School Ment Health. 2011;3(2):93–101.
6. Miller M, Hinshaw SP. Does childhood executive function predict adolescent functional outcomes in girls with ADHD? J Abnorm Child Psychol. 2010;38(3):315–26.
7. Biederman J, Monuteaux MC, Doyle AE, Seidman LJ, Wilens TE, Ferrero F, et al. Impact of executive function deficits and attention-deficit/hyperactivity disorder (ADHD) on academic outcomes in children. 2004; Available from: http://www.ldchicago.com/efacoutcomes.pdf.
8. Sibley MH, Altszuler AR, Ross JM, Sanchez F, Pelham WE, Gnagy EM. A parent-teen collaborative treatment model for academically impaired high school students with ADHD. Cogn Behav Pract. 2014;21(1):32–42.
9. Sibley MH, Pelham WE, Derefinko KJ, Kuriyan AB, Sanchez F, Graziano PAA. Pilot trial of supporting teens' academic needs daily (STAND): a parent-adolescent collaborative intervention for ADHD. J Psychopathol Behav Assess. 2013;35(4):436–49.
10. Hoza B, Mrug S, Gerdes AC, et al. What aspects of peer relationships are impaired in children with attention-deficit/hyperactivity disorder? J Consult Clin Psychol. 2005;73(3):411–23.
11. Hoza B, Mrug S, Pelham WE, Greiner AR, Gnagy EM. A friendship intervention for children with attention-deficit/hyperactivity disorder: preliminary findings. J Atten Disord. 2003;6(3):87–98.
12. Zoromski AK, Owens JS, Evans SW, Brady CE. Identifying ADHD symptoms most associated with impairment in early childhood, middle childhood, and adolescence using teacher report. J Abnorm Child Psychol. 2015;43(7):1243–55.
13. Hoza B, Gerdes AC, Mrug S, Hinshaw SP, Bukowski WM, Gold JA, et al. Peer-assessed outcomes in the multimodal treatment study of children with attention deficit hyperactivity disorder. J Clin Child Adolesc Psychol. 2005;34(1):74–86.

14. Bagwell CL, Molina BSG, Pelham WE, Hoza B. Attention-deficit hyperactivity disorder and problems in peer relations: predictions from childhood to adolescence. J Am Acad Child Adolesc Psychiatry. 2001;40(11):1285–92.

15. Hoza B. Peer functioning in children with ADHD. J Pediatr Psychol. 2007;32(6):655–63.

16. Asher SR, Coie JD. Peer rejection in childhood. New York: Cambridge University Press; 1990.

17. Patterson GR, DeBaryshe BD, Ramsey E. A developmental perspective on antisocial behavior. Am Psychol. 1989;44(2):329–35.

18. Marshal MP, Molina BSG, Pelham WE Jr. Childhood ADHD and adolescent substance use: an examination of deviant peer group affiliation as a risk factor. Psychol Addict Behav. 2003;17(4):293–302.

19. Becker SP, Mehari KR, Langberg JM, Evans SW. Rates of peer victimization in young adolescents with ADHD and associations with internalizing symptoms and self-esteem. Eur Child Adolesc Psychiatry. 2017;26(2):201–14.

20. Keown LJ, Woodward LJ. Preschool boys with pervasive hyperactivity: early peer functioning and mother-child relationship influences. Soc Dev. 2006;15(1):23–45.

21. Hinshaw SP, Zupan BA, Simmel C, Nigg JT, Melnick S. Peer status in boys with and without attention-deficit hyperactivity disorder: predictions from overt and covert antisocial behavior, social isolation, and authoritative parenting beliefs. Child Dev. 1997;68(5):880–96.

22. Hurt EA, Hoza B, Pelham WE. Parenting, family loneliness, and peer functioning in boys with attention-deficit/hyperactivity disorder. J Abnorm Child Psychol. 2007;35(4):543–55.

23. Mikami AY, Jack A, Emeh CC, Stephens HF. Parental influence on children with attention-deficit/hyperactivity disorder: I. Relationships between parent behaviors and child peer status. J Abnorm Child Psychol. 2010;38(6):721–36.

24. Ray AR, Evans SW, Langberg JM. Factors associated with healthy and impaired social functioning in young adolescents with ADHD. J Abnorm Child Psychol. 2017;45(5):883–97.

25. Mikami AY, Lerner MD, Griggs MS, McGrath A, Calhoun CD. Parental influence on children with attention-deficit/hyperactivity disorder: II. Results of a pilot intervention training parents as friendship coaches for children. J Abnorm Child Psychol. 2010;38(6):737–49.

26. Centers for Disease Control and Prevention. WISQARS (Web-based Injury Statistics Query and Reporting System) Atlanta: US Department of Health and Human Services, CDC; 2015, 2019. https://www.cdc.gov/injury/wisqars/index.html#:~:text=WISQARS%E2%84%A2%20%E2%80%94%20Web%2Dbased%20Injury%20Statistics%20Query%20and%20Reporting%20System&text=CDC's%20WISQARS%E2%84%A2%20is%20an,and%20cost%20of%20injury%20data.

27. https://crashstats.nhtsa.dot.gov/Api/Public/ViewPublication/812498. NHTSA's National Center for Statistics and Analysis. 2018.

28. Chen L-H, Baker SP, Braver ER, Li G. Carrying passengers as a risk factor for crashes fatal to 16- and 17-year-old drivers. JAMA. 2000;283(12):1578.

29. Barkley RA, Guevremont DC, Anastopoulos AD, DuPaul GJ, Shelton TL. Driving-related risks and outcomes of attention deficit hyperactivity disorder in adolescents and young adults: a 3- to 5-year follow-up survey. Pediatrics. 1993;92(2):212–8.

30. Barkley RA, Cox D. A review of driving risks and impairments associated with attention-deficit/hyperactivity disorder and the effects of stimulant medication on driving performance. J Saf Res. 2007;38(1):113–28.

31. Ankem G, Klauer C, Ollendick T, Dingus T, Guo F. How risky are ADHD teen drivers? Analysis of ADHD teen drivers using naturalistic driving data. J Transp Heal. 2018;9:S13.

32. Woodward LJ, Fergusson DM, Horwood LJ. Driving outcomes of young people with attentional difficulties in adolescence. J Am Acad Child Adolesc Psychiatry. 2000;39(5):627–34.

33. Schatz NK, Fabiano GA, Morris KL, Shucard JM, Leo BA, Bieniek C. Parenting behaviors during risky driving by teens with attention-deficit/hyperactivity disorder. Behav Ther. 2014;45(2):168–76.

34. Beck KH, Shattuck T, Raleigh R. Parental predictors of teen driving risk. Am J Health Behav. 2001;25(1):10–20.

35. Knouse LE, Bagwell CL, Barkley RA, Murphy KR. Accuracy of self-evaluation in adults with ADHD. J Atten Disord. 2005;8(4):221–34.
36. Fabiano GA, Schatz NK, Hulme KF, Morris KL, Vujnovic RK, Willoughby MT, et al. Positive Bias in teenage drivers with ADHD within a simulated driving task. J Atten Disord. 2018;22(12):1150–7.
37. Fabiano GA, Schatz NK, Morris KL, Willoughby MT, Vujnovic RK, Hulme KF, et al. Efficacy of a family-focused intervention for young drivers with attention-deficit hyperactivity disorder. J Consult Clin Psychol. 2016;84(12):1078–93.
38. Molina BSG, Pelham WE. Childhood predictors of adolescent substance use in a longitudinal study of children with ADHD. J Abnorm Psychol. 2003;112(3):497–507.
39. Grant BF, Dawson DA. Age at onset of alcohol use and its association with DSM-IV alcohol abuse and dependence: results from the national longitudinal alcohol epidemiologic survey. J Subst Abus. 1997;9:103–10.
40. Sarver DE, McCart MR, Sheidow AJ, Letourneau EJ. ADHD and risky sexual behavior in adolescents: conduct problems and substance use as mediators of risk. J Child Psychol Psychiatry. 2014;55(12):1345–53.
41. Nigg JT. Attention-deficit/hyperactivity disorder and adverse health outcomes. Clin Psychol Rev. 2013;33(2):215–28.
42. Flory K, Molina BSG, Pelham WE Jr, Gnagy E, Smith B. Childhood ADHD predicts risky sexual behavior in young adulthood. J Clin Child Adolesc Psychol. 2006;35(4):571–7.
43. Rokeach A, Wiener J. The romantic relationships of adolescents with ADHD. J Atten Disord. 2018;22(1):35–45.
44. Walther CAP, Cheong J, Molina BSG, Pelham WE, Wymbs BT, Belendiuk KA, et al. Substance use and delinquency among adolescents with childhood ADHD: the protective role of parenting. Psychol Addict Behav. 2012;26(3):585–98.
45. Molina BSG, Marshal MP, Pelham WE, Wirth RJ. Coping skills and parent support mediate the association between childhood attention-deficit/hyperactivity disorder and adolescent cigarette use. J Pediatr Psychol. 2005;30(4):345–57.
46. Tandon M, Tillman R, Spitznagel E, Luby J. Parental warmth and risks of substance use in children with attention-deficit/hyperactivity disorder. Addict Res Theory. 2014;22(3):239–50.
47. Molina BSG, Flory K, Hinshaw SP, Greiner AR, Arnold LE, Swanson JM, et al. Delinquent behavior and emerging substance use in the MTA at 36 months: prevalence, course, and treatment effects. J Am Acad Child Adolesc Psychiatry. 2007;46(8):1028–40.
48. Huggins SP, Rooney ME, Chronis-Tuscano A. Risky sexual behavior among college students with ADHD: is the mother-child relationship protective? J Atten Disord. 2015;19(3):240–50.
49. Dittus PJ, Michael SL, Becasen JS, Gloppen KM, McCarthy K, Guilamo-Ramos V. Parental monitoring and its associations with adolescent sexual risk behavior: a meta-analysis. Pediatrics. 2015;136(6):e1587–99.
50. Dawson P, Guare R. Smart but scattered: the revolutionary "executive skills" approach to helping kids reach their potential. New York: Guilford Press; 2009.
51. Johnston C, Mash EJ. Families of children with attention-deficit/hyperactivity disorder: review and recommendations for future research. Clin Child Fam Psychol Rev. 2001;4(3):183–207.
52. Margari F, Craig F, Petruzzelli MG, Lamanna A, Matera E, Margari L. Parents psychopathology of children with attention deficit hyperactivity disorder. Res Dev Disabil. 2013;34(3):1036–43.
53. Chronis-Tuscano A, Stein MA. Pharmacotherapy for parents with attention-deficit hyperactivity disorder (ADHD). CNS Drugs. 2012;26(9):725–32.
54. American Psychiatric Association. Diagnostic and statistical manual of mental disorders. 5th ed. Arlington: American Psychiatric Association; 2013.
55. Johnston C, Mash EJ, Miller N, Ninowski JE. Parenting in adults with attention-deficit/hyperactivity disorder (ADHD). Clin Psychol Rev. 2012;32(4):215–28.
56. Chronis-Tuscano A, Wang CH, Woods KE, Strickland J, Stein MA. Parent ADHD and evidence-based treatment for their children: review and directions for future research. J Abnorm Child Psychol. 2017;45(3):501–17.

57. Babinski DE, Pelham WE, Molina BSG, Gnagy EM, Waschbusch DA, Wymbs BT, et al. Maternal ADHD, parenting, and psychopathology among mothers of adolescents with ADHD. J Atten Disord. 2016;20(5):458–68.
58. Griggs MS, Mikami AY. The role of maternal and child ADHD symptoms in shaping interpersonal relationships. J Abnorm Child Psychol. 2011;39(3):437–49.
59. Grimbos T, Wiener J. Testing the similarity fit/misfit hypothesis in adolescents and parents with ADHD. J Atten Disord. 2018;22(13):1224–34.
60. Wymbs BT, Pelham WE, Molina BSG, Gnagy EM, Wilson TK, Greenhouse JB, et al. Rate and predictors of divorce among parents of youths with ADHD. J Consult Clin Psychol. 2008;76(5):735–44.
61. Wymbs BT, Pelham WE Jr. Child effects on communication between parents of youth with and without attention-deficit/hyperactivity disorder. J Abnorm Psychol. 2010;119(2):366–75.
62. Barkley RA, Anastopoulos AD, Guevremont DC, Fletcher KE. Adolescents with attention deficit hyperactivity disorder: mother-adolescent interactions, family beliefs and conflicts, and maternal psychopathology. J Abnorm Child Psychol. 1992;20(3):263–88.
63. Wymbs BT, Pelham WE, Molina BSG, Gnagy EM. Mother and adolescent reports of Interparental discord among parents of adolescents with and without attention-deficit/hyperactivity disorder. J Emot Behav Disord. 2008;16(1):29–41.
64. Wiener J, Biondic D, Grimbos T, Herbert M. Parenting stress of parents of adolescents with attention-deficit hyperactivity disorder. J Abnorm Child Psychol. 2016;44(3):561–74.
65. Evans SW, Owens JS, Bunford N. Evidence-based psychosocial treatments for children and adolescents with attention-deficit/hyperactivity disorder. J Clin Child Adolesc Psychol. 2014;43(4):527–51.
66. Sibley MH, Swanson JM, Arnold LE, et al. Defining ADHD symptom persistence in adulthood: optimizing sensitivity and specificity. J Child Psychol Psychiatry. 2017;58(6):655–62.
67. Hodgkins P, Shaw M, Coghill D, Hechtman L. Amfetamine and methylphenidate medications for attention-deficit/hyperactivity disorder: complementary treatment options. Eur Child Adolesc Psychiatry. 2012;21(9):477–92.
68. Weisz JR, Hawley KM. Developmental factors in the treatment of adolescents. J Consult Clin Psychol. 2002;70(1):21–43.
69. Sibley MH, Graziano PA, Kuriyan AB, Coxe S, Pelham WE, Rodriguez L, et al. Parent-teen behavior therapy + motivational interviewing for adolescents with ADHD. J Consult Clin Psychol. 2016;84(8):699–712.
70. DosReis S, Mychailyszyn MP, Evans-Lacko SE, Beltran A, Riley AW, Myers MA. The meaning of attention-deficit/hyperactivity disorder medication and parents' initiation and continuity of treatment for their child. J Child Adolesc Psychopharmacol. 2009;19(4):377–83.
71. Brown TE. Smart but stuck: emotions in teens and adults with ADHD. 1st ed. San Francisco: John Wiley and Sons, Inc; 2014.
72. Miller WR, Rollnick S. Motivational interviewing: helping people change. New York: Guilford Press; 2013.
73. Greee R, Ablon JS. Treating explosive kids: the collaborative problem-solving approach. 1st ed. New York: Guilford Press; 2006.
74. Haydicky J, Shecter C, Wiener J, et al. Evaluation of MBCT for adolescents with ADHD and their parents: impact on individual and family functioning. J Child Fam Stud. 2015;24:76–94.
75. Sibley MH, Pelham WE, Evans SW, Gnagy EM, Ross JM, Greiner AR. An evaluation of a summer treatment program for adolescents with ADHD. Cogn Behav Pract. 2011;18(4):530–44.
76. Fabiano GA, Hulme K, Linke S, Nelson-Tuttle C, Pariseau M, Gangloff B, et al. The supporting a Teen's effective entry to the roadway (STEER) program: feasibility and preliminary support for a psychosocial intervention for teenage drivers with ADHD. Cogn Behav Pract. 2011;18(2):267–80.
77. Sibley MH, Pelham WE, Mazur A, Gnagy EM, Ross JM, Kuriyan AB. The effect of video feedback on the social behavior of an adolescent with ADHD. J Atten Disord. 2012;16(7):579–88.

78. Barkley R. Taking charge of ADHD third edition: the complete, authoritative guide for parents. New York: Guilford Press; 2013.
79. Chan E, Fogler JM, Hammerness PG. Treatment of attention-deficit/hyperactivity disorder in adolescents: a systematic review. JAMA. 2016;315(18):1997–2008.
80. McCarthy S, Asherson P, Coghill D, Hollis C, Murray M, Potts L, et al. Attention-deficit hyperactivity disorder: treatment discontinuation in adolescents and young adults. Br J Psychiatry. 2009;194(03):273–7.
81. Molina BSG, Hinshaw SP, Swanson JM, et al. The MTA at 8 years: prospective follow-up of children treated for combined-type ADHD in a multisite study. J Am Acad Child Adolesc Psychiatry. 2009;48(5):484–500.

Chapter 19
Living and Succeeding with ADHD in High School

Jonas Bromberg

Case Example

Jackson is a 14-year-old who will be starting ninth grade. He is attending a summer program (focused on environmental science) at the high school, in order to become familiar with the school grounds and meet peers. Jackson has ADHD and is treated with medication but has never received IEP support. In his summer program, he meets a group of 16-year-olds who will be entering 11th grade; Jackson starts spending time with them in the evenings and weekends. His parents are not sure if he is ready for this group.

Background

Each developmental transition brings a unique set of challenges for a student with ADHD. While the transition to high school is challenging for many teens, it can be particularly difficult for the student with ADHD, as the burden of managing projects, homework, and balancing academic and social activities increases significantly. Although many students with ADHD successfully make their way through their early school years, it is common for them to hit the well-known "ADHD wall" as they shift into high school.

Academic demands increase dramatically, and work becomes more complex. There is a greater emphasis on grades and significantly more homework. Teachers

J. Bromberg (✉)
Boston Children's Hospital, Boston, MA, USA

Pediatric Physicians' Organization at Children's, Wellesley, MA, USA

Harvard Medical School, Boston, MA, USA
e-mail: Jonas.bromberg@childrens.harvard.edu

© Springer Nature Switzerland AG 2020
A. Schonwald (ed.), *ADHD in Adolescents*,
https://doi.org/10.1007/978-3-030-62393-7_19

expect students to become more independent, work autonomously, organize themselves, initiate work, keep track of multiple assignments, and stay on top of long-term assignments. Socializing and extracurricular activities take on a greater level of importance during the teenage years.

High school is structured and organized in a way that seems especially unwelcoming for the student with ADHD. The day begins too early, before a student's natural rhythm tells them to be awake. It runs too long, with demands for attention and concentration that surpass the capacity of many students, even those without ADHD. Academic requirements force students to read and study topics that hold little or no interest to them (which, ironically, they are advised against doing once they graduate from high school). When you factor together the increase in academic and social pressures, the search for identity, and independence, along with burgeoning hormonal changes and emerging sexuality, it is easy to understand why so many adolescents with inattention, hyperactivity, and impulsivity struggle in high school. Not surprisingly, scholastic failure and dropout rates are higher among adolescents who have ADHD, than among adolescents who don't [1].

Though some high school students seem to "outgrow" their ADHD symptoms, the vast majority will do best with both treatment and academic support throughout high school. Here's a look at some of the challenges that high school students with ADHD face.

The Big Transition

The transition from middle school to high school is a big one and can be difficult for many teens. Academic work becomes more difficult; teachers who are working to foster increased independence may be less readily available, and expectations increase, especially in the later years as college approaches. On top of this, socializing and extracurricular activities become a more prominent part of life for most teens. These activities are often less of a struggle for teens and bring more pleasure than academic work, leading to a disproportionate interest and investment of energy, compared to academic activities. These changes introduce special challenges for teens with ADHD, as they adjust to the new cultural milieu that high school represents.

> At this age, many teens explicitly "forbid" their parents from coming too close to their new world.

In high school, the buildings are likely to be significantly bigger or even spread out between multiple buildings. The number of students in the school is typically greater, schedules may be more complex, and students may be in classes for the first time with peers who are in different grades. The rules and customs of high school are likely to be very different from those in earlier grades. Policies about being late, absences, the use of cell phones, and those for general conduct may be followed more strictly. In high school, parents typically have much less contact with school administrators, and teachers are less likely to get to know them.

During the high school years, students are expected to start playing a bigger role in their education and to take responsibility for getting the help and support they need. The daily preparation, organization, and planning required to navigate this new environment can be difficult, if not overwhelming, for many teens with ADHD. In high school, more responsibility is placed on the student for time management, being prepared, and balancing multiple class assignments (many of which may be larger projects, involving multiple steps, that are spread out over the course of a semester). Being in school with a larger number of peers experimenting with sex, substance use, and driving exposes young high schoolers to new risks and pressures. For teens who have difficulty with attention and learning, trouble making friends, difficulty navigating social life, and difficulty advocating for themselves, the transition to high school can be especially difficult.

Asking questions, obtaining support, and advocating for their own needs become gradually more important. High school students are expected to have greater self-awareness and be able to communicate about their academic needs and the accommodations that would be most helpful. In high school, many students with ADHD find that balancing afterschool activities or jobs gets complicated, especially when these activities are more enjoyable than the struggles and challenges of academic learning.

ADHD, Adolescent Risk Behavior, and Emotional Health

The combination of peer pressure and impulsivity leaves many high school students with ADHD more vulnerable than other teens to engage in risky behaviors, such as alcohol and other use, unprotected sex, and risky driving behavior. Many of these topics are explored in detail in other chapters of this book.

Adolescents with ADHD are more likely to engage in risky behaviors, such as substance abuse and unprotected sex [2]. Young adults who had ADHD in adolescence demonstrate earlier initiation of sexual activity and intercourse, have more sexual partners and more casual sex, and have more partner pregnancies [3].

Adolescents with ADHD demonstrate greater weekly marijuana use and daily cigarette smoking into young adulthood. This is often characterized by younger initiation of alcohol, cigarette, and marijuana use [4]. They are more likely to become daily smokers, initiate smoking at younger ages, and progress to regular smoking more quickly. Smokers with ADHD reported more intense withdrawal and cravings when trying to quit [5]. All of these factors may interfere with academic and social success.

To further complicate matters, other serious conditions may co-occur with ADHD. Approximately two out of three teens with ADHD have at least one other coexisting diagnosis, such as depression, anxiety, or behavioral problem [6]. Rates of depression, anxiety, and behavior issues are higher in teens with ADHD than in teens without the condition [7]. Students with multiple conditions are at higher risk than their peers for a multitude of academic difficulties, such as poor grades, being suspended or expelled, unexcused absences, not completing high school, and not going to college. For many high school students, the consequences of ADHD can diminish feelings of self-esteem and confidence.

> At a time of development when peer acceptance, friendships, and the pursuit of romance are at the center of a high school student's world, students with ADHD are at greatest risk of feeling as if they don't fit in.

Numerous strategies have been developed for caregivers to help their teens avoid risky behavior. More common recommendations include setting up consistent rules and applying them reliably and expecting one's teen to keep caregivers informed about who they are with, where they will be, and what they will be doing. Parents are advised to communicate frequently about strategies for better impulse control, to get to know their teen's friends and their parents, and to balance supervision with independence. They are further advised to resist too much close supervision yet to talk honestly with their teens about any need for additional supervision and support during high school while acknowledging their desire for independence. The goal of achieving greater self-reliance should be emphasized.

ADHD and Academic Achievement

High school can be especially challenging for a student with ADHD, and students with ADHD experience persistent academic underachievement, relative to their abilities.

High school students with ADHD experience greater levels of academic impairment, lower grade point averages, and placement in lower-level classes; fail more classes; and have significantly higher rates of dropout, in comparison to students without ADHD [8–10].

To make matters worse, high school students who have difficulty completing work and difficulty focusing in class are often seen as lacking in motivation and engagement, rather than as having a learning impairment. Underachievement in high school – and the self-doubt it creates – can have negative consequences that last well into adulthood.

But these negative outcomes are by no means certain. Many adolescents with ADHD do succeed in high school and complete college. Peer acceptance is one protective factor that promotes success [11]. Additional factors include higher IQ and fewer behavioral symptoms [12]. Establishing the right types of supports at home and at school, taking prescribed medication, and participating in behavioral treatment help many adolescents avoid these negative outcomes.

A research study by Mayes and Calhoun identified written expression as the most common learning problem among students with ADHD [13]. Consequently, writing assignments such as term papers, book reports, and even short essays can be very challenging for students with ADHD. For example, when writing a term paper, students with ADHD frequently have trouble remembering ideas, organizing the ideas, and consistently remembering punctuation, spelling, and grammar rules from long-term memory. Remembering multiple sources of information, organizing the bits and pieces into a meaningful and logical sequence, and reviewing and correcting errors can be problematic.

Strategies for Success

Fortunately, several approaches may assist teens and their families during the high school years. Each teen with ADHD has their own specific needs; we list specific strategies for those struggling with homework (Table 19.1), studying (Table 19.2), and self-management (Table 19.3).

High school students with ADHD and their families should work intentionally with schools. Think about the specific supports that will help the student succeed and that will address gaps proactively. Have in place systems to react quickly to problems that arise. Table 19.4 lists family-school interactions that promote these goals.

Table 19.1 Homework strategies for high schoolers with ADHD

Homework strategies
1. Institute a consistent "homework time" in your household
2. Turn off texting and social media alerts during this time
3. Set up a distraction-free workspace; avoid studying in the bedroom
4. Help your teen organize, prioritize, and check homework assignment
5. Establish daily and weekly timelines for assignments, and outline the steps that must be completed daily for each one
6. Break up long-term assignments into a set of small steps
7. Turn off cell phones, turn off email, turn off social media, and turn off instant messaging on personal computers
8. Turn off music and television
9. Keep your desk and workspace clear
10. Ask others not to disturb you while you are working

Table 19.2 Study strategies for high schoolers with ADHD

Study strategies
1. Help your student learn to break down complex assignments into manageable chunks
2. Use color-coded notebooks and files to identify each subject
3. Ask guidance staff and teachers for resources to help your student develop effective study habits
4. Connect with local ADHD support groups to find study skills training
5. Consider a tutor with special expertise working with adolescents with ADHD
6. Consider an ADHD coach or organizational coach
7. Use graphic organizers to provide visual prompts
8. Make the learning process as concrete and visual as possible

Table 19.3 Self-management strategies for high schoolers with ADHD

Self-management strategies
1. Begin teaching adolescents to advocate for themselves, to become active participants in getting their needs met
2. Encourage students to meet with their teachers to discuss their learning styles, what helps them learn best, and how to motivate them and help them stay focused and organized
3. Students should ask teachers to provide regular feedback and advice, to help them understand areas for improvement
4. Students and teachers should discuss strategies to maximize engagement and sustain attention
5. For long-term assignments, show intermediate work products to teachers along the way, to promote accountability and planning
6. Teach students to advocate for preferential seating to maximize focus on lectures and instruction and avoid being distracted by peers, windows, and noise from the hallway
7. If getting out of bed in the morning is a problem, set two alarms to go off in sequence, and put at least one alarm where you have to get out of bed to shut it off

Table 19.4 Family-school interaction strategies for high schoolers with ADHD

Family-school interaction strategies
1. Communicate with teachers regularly to stay informed about behavioral problems, difficulties understanding or completing homework assignments, poor test scores or grades, or other problems that may arise
2. Coordinate a consistent approach to teaching and supporting the development of study skills, time management, and organization strategies
3. Ask teachers to make special accommodations, such as simplifying and repeating instructions and providing written instructions for homework assignments
4. Get permission from teachers to record lectures if required
5. Get to know guidance and academic support staff at your child's school
6. Learn about the laws that pertain to academic support services for students with ADHD
7. Work with your child's school to determine if an academic evaluation is needed, to determine whether your student qualifies for specialized support services, or an individualized education plan (IEP)

Table 19.5 Organizational strategies for high schoolers with ADHD

Organizational strategies
1. Create a "launch pad" by the main entrance way, and put all of the things the student will need in the morning on the launch pad the night before (e.g., lunch, books, homework, backpack, keys)
2. Keep separate bags for books and schoolwork, sports equipment, and extra clothes or other personal items
3. Develop and use checklists to stay organized, stay on task, and complete work
4. Use the calendar, alarm, reminder, and note-keeping functions that are built into your adolescent's cell phone, to create to-do lists, track important information, and keep it all in one place
5. Use a visual representation of the day's schedule
6. Develop a clear strategy for prioritizing which tasks are most important, to make sure the most important tasks are completed first
7. Assign everything (cell phone, keys, medication, important documents) a place at home and at school
8. Create a plan (or "road map") for the week ahead on Sunday evening and for the weekend by no later than Friday afternoon
9. Closely monitor progress and establish rewards for homework completion
10. Establish a routine of reviewing your plan each morning (at a set time, like breakfast) to make sure you are aware of what's happening that day

ADHD and Organizational Challenges

Very few high school students with ADHD are well organized. Being disorganized can be one of the biggest problems for the high school student living with ADHD. Students with ADHD can toil for hours with an assignment and then not pass it in. They may forget where they left their backpacks. Being organized helps high schoolers spend less time looking for things, feel less overwhelmed, get more things accomplished with less stress, and even improve family relationships. Many strategies can help support better organization (Table 19.5).

ADHD and Demands on Working Memory

Working memory is the ability to keep information in your head and work with it mentally. High school students use working memory every day to complete a variety of tasks, such as following teacher's instructions and remembering what a teacher said so they can take accurate notes. This explains, in part, why students with ADHD and high IQs may still struggle in high school.

Educators and ADHD experts consider working memory to be one of the most important elements of functioning that can negatively impact high school student's academic success.

Most learning requires a combination of memorized facts and multiple steps to get to a solution. For example, with math word problems, a student must keep several numbers and questions in mind while figuring out how to solve a problem. They pull specific math rules and math facts from long-term memory while working toward a solution. Moving back and forth between working memory, long-term memory, and short-term memory can be a taxing effort for a student with ADHD [14]. Teachers may mistakenly attribute this challenge to laziness, yet the neurological deficits linked with ADHD make these tasks extremely difficult for students with ADHD.

In studying elementary school-aged students, researchers have found that working memory is a more powerful predictor of academic success than intelligence in the early years [14]. This research with young children is important when thinking about high school students, since working memory is a relatively stable construct over time. This means that a child with poor working memory at age ten is likely to have persistent deficits of working memory into their high school years. Fortunately, working memory can be improved (to a much greater degree than intelligence), if problems are identified early [15].

Many students with ADHD also have difficulty holding events in mind and using their sense of time to prepare for upcoming events and the future. As a result, they may inaccurately judge the passage of time and misjudge how much time it will take to finish a task, resulting in inadequate time to complete their assignments.

Deficits in working memory can negatively affect high school student behavior in numerous ways: at home, in the classroom, and socially. Memorizing math facts, spelling words, and dates requires working memory, as do performing mental computation, paraphrasing or summarizing, and organizing and writing essays. Because high school students with ADHD may have difficulty recalling the past, they may have limited insight and difficulty learning from past behavior. In part, this helps explain why they may repeat negative behaviors. Problems like difficulty in prioritizing, initiating, and completing work and being disorganized; forgetting homework; and difficulty in memorizing facts, organizing written work, carrying out long-term projects, arriving on time, and regulating and managing emotions are common academic problems linked to ADHD, working memory, and other executive function deficits.

ADHD and Social Skills

Impulsive comments, difficulty sustaining attention, the inability to sit still, forgetfulness, and misreading social cues are characteristics of ADHD that make it hard for some high school students with ADHD to make and keep friends. Research shows that children who have ADHD have fewer friends, are less likely to be accepted by their peers, and are more likely to experience social rejection during their teenage years [16].

Rules of society are not always taught explicitly; they are learned by paying attention to how other people behave. When other people are talking, you wait until they finish before responding. If you bump someone walking in the hallway, you say you're sorry. When there's a line at the movie theater, you wait your turn. Most teens do these things because they've naturally learned the social norms and social rules that guide how people interact with one another. However, teens with ADHD often have trouble learning and following these common social norms because they don't always notice these norms or they lack the impulse control to follow them. Students who have difficulty following social rules risk having others perceive them as self-centered, rude, or bad-mannered. Peers may find their behavior annoying and avoid them or leave them out of social groups and events. At its worst, this can lead some students with ADHD to be ostracized and bullied.

Concrete thinking, heightened sensitivity, and/or difficulty recognizing (or misreading) social cues can lead teens with ADHD to miss the nuances of humor (especially sarcasm and irony) and other abstract language, which increases the likelihood of emotional reactivity or impulsive outbursts. Your high schooler may think that others are mad at them, that nobody likes talking to them, or that others are being rude to them, even when that's not the case. Demonstrating or feeling empathy is difficult for some students who struggle with social cues. They may not know when to show empathy and when to let things go, causing them to overreact or underreact to their peers.

> Teens who experience difficulty reading social cues often don't understand how others experience and feel about them.

As a consequence of their diminished self-awareness, these students don't easily recognize when to modify their own behavior. These problems may lead teens to feel like friendships and participation in social activities may be too far out of reach, leading to isolation, feelings of frustration, and increase feelings of low self-confidence and self-esteem.

> Encourage attendance at social events, and help teens with ADHD learn to take a "nothing ventured, nothing gained" approach.

For many teens, the fear of rejection leads to avoidance of social opportunities. It is helpful to teens when parents validate their feelings and share their own experiences in high school. Point out examples of situations when your high schooler took risks socially and things ended up working out. Listen to your child's fears, and help them understand that it is normal to feel this way and that most kids (and adults) worry about being rejected socially.

For teens with ADHD, learning to understand these kinds of basic social conventions is the first step in knowing how to navigate the increasingly complex social world of high school. It is important for teens to learn appropriate social greetings, how to offer and receive compliments, and how to initiate and close conversations. With practice and consistent guidance from parents and teachers, students can learn to avoid distractions during social interactions, read body language and facial expressions, not violate other's personal space, avoid interrupting, how to maintain eye contact, and know the right time to end a brief interaction.

Adolescents with compromised listening skills, poor impulse control, and high emotional reactivity may benefit from anger management and conflict-resolution skills training. Parents, teachers, and coaches can offer observations and helpful advice about these and other behaviors that require improvement. Even a small social group may lessen the negative impact brought on by a broader lack of peer acceptance that many teens with ADHD experience. Parents can support their teen by asking them to invite friends to your home or on family outings, to help them promote close friendships. Gentle reminders to return phone calls, get to social events on time, and keep scheduled plans may help your teen succeed. Encouraging your teen to participate in extracurricular activities that offer social opportunities can help build social skills and nurture self-confidence. Help your teen identify activities they feel most confident about and where they are more likely to excel.

You can help your high schooler build social skills and feel prepared by role-playing common situations such as the following:

- Asking someone to go to the movies
- Refusing alcohol, drugs, or unwanted sex
- Starting a conversation in the cafeteria
- Greeting an unfamiliar adult, or classmate
- Going to a job interview
- Responding to something they don't understand
- Working on a group project
- Asking someone on a date
- Initiating conversation at a social event

ADHD and Driving

Driving represents one of the first steps toward independence in adolescents. Teenagers and driving are a perilous combination, especially when you consider that a leading cause of death in teens is automobile accidents [17]. When you have a teenager with ADHD, the driving risks increase significantly.

Driving is a set of interrelated, complex tasks that require many of the skills most affected by ADHD (such as planning ahead, following through, and staying on task). Variability in focus and attention, along with impulsivity, makes driving a risky proposition. Teen drivers with ADHD are up to four times more likely to have automobile accidents and incur injuries related to those accidents than teens without ADHD [18]. Does that mean that a teen ADHD should never drive and just keep getting rides from parents and friends? No, but parents should take a more planned and gradual approach to helping their teenagers become good drivers. Normal driving events, such as being distracted by things along the roadway, thoughts drifting while sitting in slow traffic or at a red light, talking to others in the car, listening to music, and incoming texts or phone calls, pose special risks to teenagers with ADHD.

> Helping teenagers with ADHD to become skilled and competent drivers requires a multifaceted approach that includes negotiation, training, and preparation.

Children and Adults with ADHD (CHADD) lists numerous helpful ideas [19].

Here is our list of ideas to help guide and support a teenager with ADHD, to become a skilled and safe driver:

1. Find a driving school that is designed specifically for teenagers with ADHD and other learning issues. Specialized driving programs may provide students with more time learning on interactive driving simulators, offer hazard prevention training to make the student more aware of potential hazards that can cause accidents, and provide significantly more "road hours" than what is normally included in a conventional driver-education program.
2. Take a more gradual approach, with multiple levels of supervised training and more frequent supervised practice driving sessions.
3. New drivers may benefit from training that emphasizes the use of safety checklists that include important tasks that easily become routine for non-ADHD drivers (e.g., buckling up, checking mirrors, setting climate controls before the trip starts).
4. Take a more participatory approach, regularly monitoring your teen's progress by riding along (during both the driver-education phase and after your teen has their driver's license). Parents should check in proactively, regularly, one-on-one, to see how comfortable (or uncomfortable) their teenager is feeling about their driving capabilities. Have them recount their experiences on the road, reporting any near accidents, missed turns, and other driving errors. Get into a routine of debriefing with them after they return from time out on the road. If your teenager is taking medication for ADHD, make sure it is taken when they will be driving.

Perhaps most important of all is helping your teenage driver minimize distractions while driving. Cell phones, the car stereo, eating and drinking, or carrying a group of friends can be seriously distracting for a skilled adult driver without ADHD but even more so to a teenage driver with ADHD [20]. Parents and teenagers should create clear rules, including turning off cell phones and other devices, tuning the car stereo before they begin to drive, and restricting the number of passengers in the car at a time. It is a parent's responsibility to create and implement rules and expectations for safe driving.

ADHD and Money Management

Functional problems like procrastination, disorganization, and impulsivity can have serious consequences on an adolescent's ability to manage money appropriately.

Managing money is a unique challenge for an adolescent with ADHD. ADHD-related difficulties with money include bouncing checks; losing or not paying bills; impulsive spending; being unable to save; losing money, bank cards, and checks; disorganized recordkeeping; getting in debt; and spending more than one's earnings.

Basic practices and principles of money management need to be reinforced with high school-aged adolescents with ADHD [21]. Help them clarify goals, identify problem areas with money, reduce impulsive spending, increase awareness of how money is spent, develop and use a spending plan, and get into the habit of saving. Helping adolescents with ADHD become aware of where their money is going (tracking purchases) helps them learn to account for their money. Recording purchases may help curb impulsivity and track where money is spent. Tracking spending into specific categories (such as food, movies, driving, clothing, cosmetics, music, hobbies) can help teach planning. This is also an opportunity to teach an adolescent to focus on saving and spending on things they love and value.

ADHD Students and a "Gap Year"

Typically, seniors who are college-bound have a summer break and transition immediately into college. In the 1970s, students, educators, and parents began questioning whether going straight into college was the best pathway for some students. The idea that taking a year to mature and decompress after twelve straight years of sitting in a classroom might be a better pathway for some high school graduates. The idea of pursuing special interests, traveling, and giving back to the world became known as a "gap year" [22].

Most research suggests positive benefits of a "gap year," such as increased maturity and self-confidence, higher motivation in college, improved communication skills, finding a sense of purpose, personal growth, greater interest and readiness for college [23, 24], and less "maladaptive behavior" as a result of their year off [25].

However, other studies show fewer differences in outcomes of students with and without gap years, and at least one found gap-year students were more likely to drop out of university [26].

ADHD and Dating

For the parent of an adolescent with ADHD, dating can be both exciting and worrisome.

Starting to date is a developmentally important experience. Impulsivity, poor problem-solving, and communications deficits can lead to uncomfortable, awkward, and even unsafe situations.

When it comes to dating, high schoolers with ADHD may need more support and direction from their parents than other students, so they can avoid problems and make the best choices for themselves. What most parents refer to as "dating" may be very different than what today's high school student's experience. Current teens may use phrases like "hanging-out" or "talking to" to refer to a peer they are romantically involved with, instead of the term "dating." Work to create a shared language with your teen, so you understand each other. Find out what language they use to refer to sexual behavior. Speaking openly about dating and sex can help teens feel comfortable talking about these topics. If you are uncomfortable talking with your teen about dating, begin by talking with other parents about how they approached the issues. It may take some work to find the right level of comfort, but avoiding the topic can have negative consequences, such as teens not having enough information to make good choices.

Many parents find talking with their high schooler about sex to be difficult or awkward, but avoiding the topic may lead to health risks, undesired pregnancy, or exploitation. Helping your teen understand your values, feelings, and expectations about sex is an important step in helping them clarify these things for themselves. Be as clear and direct as possible, so that their attention and language issues don't interfere with their understanding of what you're saying or come off as judgmental.

It can be helpful for many teens to begin their dating lives by going out in groups with other teens. This can be a safer place for many teens to practice dating skills, and friends can help each other stay safe, reduce feelings of pressure, and help each other make good choices.

Because structure and boundaries help adolescents with ADHD, set up clear rules and limits about dating. Just as you would with other friends, ask your high schooler to introduce you to the people they date, set clear time parameters and curfews, and insist on good communication about plans and where they will be. Encourage your teen to use their cell phone to set reminders, share location, and let you know if they are going to be late. Discuss specific ways that dating can put them at risk and how to minimize and avoid those risks. Help them think about situations that might make them feel uncomfortable and what they can do about it.

Case Revisited

Jackson's parents' concerns about his spending time with this older group are well-founded. High school peers may be driving, experimenting with substance use, and exploring sexual relationships. Beyond being younger than this crowd, Jackson's ADHD predisposes him to difficulty managing this more sophisticated social context and to making poor decisions with regard to his own safety and well-being. On the other hand, one goal of the program was to meet peers, and Jackson seems to have met that goal successfully. His parents might applaud this achievement and suggest Jackson invites his friends (and perhaps their families) to meet his parents. In clear and direct terms, parents can ask about sex, drugs, and other safety concerns, in support of Jackson's own values, confidence, and self-esteem. Together, they can agree on rules around who can drive a car with Jackson in it, that he shares his location on his phone with them, and that he lets his parents know explicitly where he is at all times. Further, his parents may use this opportunity of increasing independence to teach Jackson money management skills.

Conclusions

Despite our lists of strategies and suggestions to support adolescent success in high school, it may not be an easy time. Adolescence is traditionally filled with emotional angst, and parenting/educating teenagers can be hard, particularly those with ADHD. One way to look at it is this is the time when children and students are getting "ready to launch," when parents and teachers and clinicians are helping them prepare for the next steps with competence and confidence. There will always be some uncertainty and worry. Yet, knowing what to expect and how best to support the teen with ADHD can reduce the stress and increase the success.

> **Tips**
> - Gentle reminders to return phone calls, get to social events on time, and keep scheduled plans may help your teen succeed.
> - Find opportunities to teach teens with ADHD social conventions (greeting, waiting, personal space) explicitly.
> - Model productive anger management strategies in the course of daily life.
> - Get help! Assemble a team and use resources (such as www.CHADD.org); don't do it alone!

References

1. Trampush JW, Miller CJ, Newcorn JH, Halperin JM. The impact of childhood ADHD on dropping out of high school in urban adolescents/ young adults. J Atten Disord. 2009;13(2):127–36.
2. Huggins SP, Rooney ME, Chronis-Tuscano A. Risky sexual behavior among college students with ADHD: is the mother–child relationship protective? Journal of Attention Disorders. 2015;19(3):240–50.
3. Flory K, Brooke SG, Molina WE, et al. Childhood ADHD predicts risky sexual behavior in young adulthood. J Clin Child Adolesc Psychol. 2006;35(4):571–7.
4. Molina BS, Howard AL, Swanson JM, Stehli A, Mitchell JT, Kennedy TM, Epstein JN, Arnold LE, Hechtman L, Vitiello B, Hoza B. Substance use through adolescence into early adulthood after childhood-diagnosed ADHD: findings from the MTA longitudinal study. J Child Psychol Psychiatry. 2018;59:692–702.
5. Rhodes JD, Pelham WE, Gnagy EM, Shiffman S, Derefinko KJ, Molina BSG. Cigarette smoking and ADHD: an examination of prognostically relevant smoking behaviors among adolescents and young adults. Psychol Addict Behav. 2016;30(5):588–600.
6. Reale L, Bartoli B, Cartabia M, et al. Comorbidity prevalence and treatment outcome in children and adolescents with ADHD. Eur Child Adolesc Psychiatry. 2017;26(12):1443–57.
7. https://www.cdc.gov/ncbddd/adhd/data.html#another.
8. DuPaul GJ, Volpe RJ, Jitendra AK, Lutz JG, Lorah KS, Gruber R. Elementary school students with AD/HD: predictors of academic achievement. J Sch Psychol. 2004;42:285–301.
9. Barkley RA, Fischer M, Edelbrock CS, Smallish L. The adolescent outcome of hyperactive children diagnosed by research criteria: I. An 8-year prospective follow-up study. J Am Acad Child Adolesc Psychiatry. 1990;29(4):546–57.
10. Mannuzza S, Klein RG, Moulton JL 3rd. Young adult outcome of children with "situational" hyperactivity: a prospective, controlled follow-up study. J Abnorm Child Psychol. 2002;30(2):191–8.
11. Dvorsky MR, Langberg JM, Evans SW, Becker SP. The protective effects of social factors on the academic functioning of adolescents with ADHD. J Clin Child Adolesc Psychol. 2018;47(5):713–26.
12. Modesto-Lowe V, Yelunina L, Hanjan K. Attention-deficit/hyperactivity disorder: a shift toward resilience? Clin Pediatr (Phila). 2011;50(6):518–24.
13. Mayes SD, Calhoun SL. Learning, attention, writing, and processing speed in typical children and children with ADHD, autism, anxiety, depression, and oppositional-defiant disorder. Child Neuropsychol. 2007;13(6):469–93.
14. Kofler MJ, Sarver DE, Harmon SL, et al. Working memory and organizational skills problems in ADHD. J Child Psychol Psychiatry. 2018;59(1):57–67.
15. Dehn MJ. Supporting and strengthening working memory in the classroom to enhance executive functioning. In: Goldstein S, Naglieri JA, editors. Handbook of executive functioning. New York: Springer Science + Business Media; 2014. p. 495–507.
16. Bagwell C, et al. Attention-deficit hyperactivity disorder and problems in peer relations: predictions from childhood to adolescence. J Am Acad Child Adolesc Psychiatry. 2001;40(11):1285–92.
17. Heron M. Deaths: leading causes for 2016. National Vital Statistics Reports; 67(6). Hyattsville: National Center for Health Statistics; 2016.
18. https://behindthewheelwithadhd.com/the-statistics/.
19. https://chadd.org/for-parents/teens-with-adhd-and-driving/#:~:text=Compared%20with%20his%20peers%2C%20your,there%20has%20been%20a%20problem.
20. Jerome L, Segal A, Habinski L. What we know about ADHD and driving risk: a literature review, meta-analysis and critique. J Can Acad Child Adolesc Psychiatry. 2006;15(3):105–25.
21. https://www.understood.org/en/school-learning/choosing-starting-school/leaving-high-school/how-various-learning-and-thinking-differences-can-cause-trouble-with-money-management.

22. https://gapyearassociation.org/blog/a-short-history-of-the-gap-year/#:~:text=In%20 modern%20times%20the%20roots,education%20and%20enlisted%20after%20graduation.
23. Coetzee M, Bester S. The possible value of a gap-year: a case study. S Afr J High Educ. 2009;23:609–23.
24. King A. Minding the gap? Young people's accounts of taking a gap-year as a form of identity work in higher education. J Youth Stud. 2011;14:341–57.
25. Hoe N. American Gap Association Alumni Survey. Philadelphia: Institute for Survey Research at Temple University; 2015.
26. Parker PD, Thoemmes F, Duineveld JJ, Salmela-Aro K. I wish I had (not) taken a gap-year? The psychological and attainment outcomes of different post-school pathways. Dev Psychol. 2015;51(3):323–33.

Chapter 20
Assembling a Team

Alison Rosenberg Mostyn

Case Example

Clark is a 14-year-old ninth grader with ADHD. He takes stimulant medication with good effect, prescribed by his pediatrician. He saw a counselor at school when he was younger to help with anger management. Now in high school, Clark's grades are dropping from B's to C's. He has trouble getting all of his work done and retreats into his bedroom to listen to music. He has friends, and there are no concerns for substance or alcohol use. His parents are not sure how to support him.

Background

It is important to assemble a team so that an adolescent with ADHD can be supported by a group of caring adults and peers to help them through the maze of the teenage years. The team should work collaboratively to ensure the adolescent's success now and into the future. An adolescent who has a support team has the advantage of having a variety of perspectives to help them. A doctor may only see a patient in their office for a 30-minute appointment; a parent does not see how their son or daughter is interacting with peers in the school cafeteria on a day-to-day basis. A psychologist does not have the privilege of seeing their patient score the winning soccer goal. Therefore, it is essential that parents work diligently to assemble a team so that their child's strengths and challenges can be appreciated across settings (Table 20.1). The Committee on Children with Disabilities of the American Academy of Pediatrics notes that collaboration between parents and medical and

A. R. Mostyn (✉)
Boston Children's Hospital, Boston, MA, USA
e-mail: Alison.Rosenberg-Mostyn@childrens.harvard.edu

© Springer Nature Switzerland AG 2020
A. Schonwald (ed.), *ADHD in Adolescents*,
https://doi.org/10.1007/978-3-030-62393-7_20

Table 20.1 Possible members of the team for the teen with ADHD

Possible members of the team	
Adolescent	Parents/guardians
Case manager	Peers
College counselor	Primary care provider
Developmental-behavioral pediatrician	Professional advocate or attorney
Evaluator/psychologist	Psychiatrist
Extracurricular activity instructor/coach	School guidance counselor or therapist
General education and/or special education teacher	Siblings
Mental health clinician (psychologist, social worker)	Supervisor at a job
Mentor	Tutor

educational providers leads to better outcomes for children and adolescents with disabilities [1]. Indeed, having a team to support success is critical in the life of an adolescent with ADHD.

Ideally, the adolescent should feel supported by an array of adults in their life, as well as peers. It may be useful to talk to the adolescent directly about this "team" approach so that they have an understanding of why certain professionals are involved in their lives. A teen may feel frustrated that they have to go to weekly tutoring or therapy sessions. These supportive services may make them feel different from their peers. Emphasize that the tutor or therapist is part of their "team" and that there are many adults who want to see them do well. Some adolescents need a few more team members to meet their full potential. Applying a strengths-based approach, a team for an adolescent with ADHD should not be viewed as a deficit but rather as tool that is key for optimal performance at home, in school, and in the community.

Parents/Guardians

Parents are likely going to be the organizers of the adolescent's team. They will be looking for the medical, mental health, and educational professionals who can treat and meet the needs of their child. Parents may find it useful to research and prepare questions for these professionals prior to meeting them. Professionals in these fields have different approaches. Parents know their children best and will likely have an intuitive sense of which professionals will be a good match for them and their child. Parents will also need to decide when more supports are needed or when particular team members may no longer be necessary.

Parents not only assemble the team but also will need to manage and synthesize the information and recommendations that team members bring to the table and turn these into realities for their child.

Team members may not agree on all treatment recommendations, and it will be up to the parent with input from the adolescent to select treatment modalities that make the most sense and will be the most effective.

Though parents are putting together a team for their child, they are in reality also assembling this team for themselves. Parenting a teenager with ADHD has unique challenges. Therefore, parents are seeking support not only for the child but also for themselves as part of this process. The team can at times support the adolescent and at other times the entire family.

The Medical Home and the Adolescent's Medical Team

Medical professionals are a critical part of the adolescent's team. A medical professional may make the ADHD diagnosis and help inform not only medical treatments but can also assist in recommending accommodations in school and effective strategies for a successful home environment.

Ideally, the adolescent's medical care should begin in a primary care medical home (PCMH). The American Academy of Pediatrics defines the medical home as having the following attributes: accessible, family-centered, continuous, comprehensive, coordinated, compassionate, and culturally effective. They state that a medical home works to build collaborations between medical providers, families, and the community [2].

When possible, parents should seek care that is delivered in this medical home model in order to access the most supports. The PCMH recognizes that communication between a child's "team" members, such as a therapist, school guidance counselor, and pediatrician, is essential in making sure that medical care is well informed and appropriate. If a child is very inattentive in the school setting but nowhere else, the primary care provider should have a good sense of this. If this is the case, it would be prudent to investigate comorbid learning difficulties if inattention in the classroom is not seen in other settings. Therefore, coordination between the medical and school team, such as the coordinated care referenced in the medical home model, is crucial in making an ADHD diagnosis.

If an adolescent receives care in a PCMH, there are often professionals, such as a case manager, working in the PCMH who are tasked with helping families coordinate care for their child. This can be extremely helpful to parents who are trying to navigate care for their child with ADHD. One study even found that parents of children with ADHD diagnoses receiving care in the medical home model were "significantly less likely to report financial or employment burden than families whose children received primary care in practices not meeting all criteria for a PCMH. In fact, exposure to a complete PCMH accounted for a nearly 50% reduction in the risk of financial or employment burden" [3]. If there are professionals who are helping families navigate the medical and school systems, parents will not have to carry as much of the burden and can rely on these team members with expertise in these matters.

> In addition, the medical home model reflects the notion that parents are experts on their children and takes a less "top down" approach than traditional Western medicine has taken in the past in working with children with ADHD.

This model also recognizes how critical culturally appropriate medical care is when treating adolescents with ADHD. As mentioned in earlier chapters, the culture of the family must be considered when developing a treatment plan for an adolescent with ADHD. The medical home model recognizes that culture impacts a family's understanding of a diagnosis, as well as a family's selection of treatment options [2].

A primary care provider may be sufficient for managing the treatment needs of a teenager with ADHD. However, some adolescents may be referred to a developmental-behavioral pediatrician and/or a psychiatrist for more specialized care. Start with the adolescent's current medical provider (ideally a clinician in a practice that meets the standards for a medical home model), and inquire whether specialty care is warranted. More specialized care is typically needed when there are ongoing concerns that have not been resolved or if there are comorbid diagnoses in addition to ADHD. More than 50% of children with ADHD have another medical diagnosis, and 35% have a psychiatric diagnosis [4]. Therefore, specialty care beyond the primary care team is often needed, given the comorbid diagnoses typically seen in children with ADHD.

If the adolescent is referred to a specialist, when they have their first appointment with the medical professional, it may be helpful to think of it as an interview. Some questions a parent/caregiver may want to consider asking a new medical professional include the following:

- What is your experience working with adolescents with ADHD?
- What types of treatment do you typically recommend for ADHD?
- How will I/we (the parents or caregivers) be involved in treatment decisions, and how will the adolescent be involved?
- What is the easiest way to communicate with you?
- Until what age can my child remain your patient?
- Is telehealth an option for our visits?

Medical professionals partner with families to determine whether medication is the most appropriate course of action to treat the adolescent's ADHD symptoms. The medical team will monitor the efficacy of the medical interventions and will work with parents and adolescents to make adjustments to the treatment plan as needed.

The medical team can also provide recommendations that can help inform the school team about what accommodations the adolescent will need to optimize academic and social success. They can provide school teams and parents with advice around whether the adolescent will need an individualized education plan (IEP) or a 504 plan to provide the supports they need at school. The Committee on Children with Disabilities recommends that the primary care pediatrician participates in the writing of an IEP. Most pediatricians will not be available to attend an IEP or 504 plan meeting in person. Some will be able to participate by telephone or virtually. If a pediatrician cannot participate in a meeting, parents can ask them to document their recommendations in a letter [1]. Parents can also ask members of their child's medical team to review an IEP or 504 plan prior to signing it.

Mental Health Team

Depending upon the current needs and comorbid diagnoses of the adolescent, they may also need a mental health provider (psychologist, social worker, or other licensed mental health professional) who provides therapeutic support. Adolescents may have a mental health provider who is affiliated with their primary care provider, practicing independently in the community, and/or based at their school. If an adolescent is supported by mental health clinicians both at school and elsewhere, it is essential that these providers consistently communicate to ensure seamless care. These professionals will provide guidance in terms of behavioral interventions that can be put into place at school, at home, and in the community to help the adolescent be successful. The mental health provider can also provide consultation to schools.

If an adolescent has a comorbid mental health condition, such as anxiety or depression, mental health treatment for both ADHD and the other diagnosis is vital. These conditions must be co-treated with ADHD, as it can be hard to tease out which difficulties are impacting the adolescent the most. Both conditions are likely impacting the other, and comprehensive mental health treatment is warranted.

> Another role of the mental health provider is to assist with school advocacy.

Some clinicians will have more expertise in this area than others. Parents can ask a mental health provider to attend a school meeting or, if that is not possible, to put their recommendations in writing. The mental health provider can also coach parents about how to advocate for school services they recommend.

School Team

The demands of middle school and high school can create many challenges for adolescents with ADHD. Arthur L. Robin notes that often times, academic difficulties for children with ADHD do not arise until high school when demands change. This is particularly true for children who did not have hyperactive or challenging behaviors that impacted school success at a younger age [5]. It is important for parents to be aware that as a child transitions to a new school (middle or high school) or a new academic structure (different teachers for all subjects), problems may arise that were not present in the past.

Every school district varies in terms of the supports and staff available to work with students with disabilities. Parents and students should be proactive as early in the school year as possible to inform school staff of needs related to ADHD. It may be helpful to think of every new school year as a fresh start. While there may be some staff who work with a student throughout their middle school and high school career, generally, it will vary from year to year. It is the responsibility of the parents (and the adolescent) to educate teachers and other support staff about the diagnosis of ADHD and what supports are needed.

> Ask at the beginning of the school year for school staff's email addresses and telephone numbers, and inquire how to best communicate with them to ensure a timely response.

School supports may be formal, through an individualized education program (IEP) or 504 plan, or there may be informal strategies that work well that can be implemented as long as school staff is aware of them. It is important to discuss these with school staff and to determine the best way to ensure ongoing communication with them. Some school districts offer parents access to their child's grades and assignments through online applications. This can be useful to parents who are monitoring their child's academic progress closely. If a parent has access to their child's assignments and grades, they can better determine when it is appropriate to step in versus letting the adolescent navigate a particular class on their own. If an adolescent receives treatment from a mental health professional at school, parents should be proactive in reaching out to this person to inquire directly how they can support the child's attentional difficulties.

Parents should not assume that members of an adolescent's school team are communicating with one another. Parents should request in person meetings with all professionals working with their child to make sure everyone has a good understanding about what strategies are effective in supporting their child's attentional needs.

Many adolescents have difficulty completing their homework, particularly adolescents with ADHD. A school professional or a therapist can help parents and the adolescent establish processes around homework. Solely being responsible for their own homework is not effective for teenagers with ADHD [5]. A useful intervention is a homework contract that details how homework will be done and outlines how long-term assignments will be broken into smaller chunks. Assistance with backpack organization can also be instrumental in helping with school success [6].

Table 20.2

Class/teacher:	
Homework completed for today:	Yes/no
Homework assignment for tonight:	
Long-term project/assignment and due date(s):	
Overdue assignments:	
Additional comments:	
Parent signature:	
Teacher signature:	

A home/school communication system can be a useful tool to assist adolescents with assignment completion and test preparation. Parents can help keep track of homework and grades if they are in regular communication with education professionals. Arthur L. Robin recommends written home and school communication on a weekly basis and notes that a guidance counselor should get involved if weekly communication is not sufficient in monitoring academic progress. A strengths-based system is also helpful in having the adolescent focus on positive behaviors (completing tasks) as opposed to focusing on negative behaviors [5].

Here is a sample home/school communication log that can be modified to fit a specific student's needs (Table 20.2).

Special Education/504 Plan Team

If parents, school personnel, or medical professionals are concerned about an adolescent's school progress, parents can consider obtaining an individualized education program (IEP) evaluation or requesting a 504 plan in order for their child to receive a higher level of support. According to a study conducted by Murray et al., high school students with ADHD without an IEP or 504 plan were not provided with many accommodations [7]. Therefore, it is important that if needed, supports are formalized.

In the United States, parents can request an individualized education program (IEP) evaluation to ensure access to a free appropriate public education, in accordance with the Individuals with Disabilities Education Act (IDEA) of 1990, reauthorized in 2004 [8]. To initiate this process, parents need to put a request for an IEP evaluation in writing in the area of the suspected disability. If the adolescent's ADHD is impacting their learning, it is appropriate to request a cognitive and educational evaluation to determine if they need specialized instruction. According to an update in IDEA in 2004, initial evaluations for students must be conducted within 60 days of a school receiving written parental consent, though this can vary from state to state [9].

The initial IEP meeting held after an evaluation should include everyone who evaluated the student, in addition to parents. The adolescent, when appropriate, should be present at their IEP meeting as well. Parents are able to bring an attorney, advocate, therapist, family member, or any other supportive person in the adolescent's life. These additional team members may provide useful insight to the IEP team about what services the adolescent needs. Parents also have the right to request an interpreter for these meetings.

> Parents often feel that the evaluators are speaking another language and using jargon that is not understandable in IEP meetings.

Parents should ask professionals as many questions as they need to so that they have a good understanding of the findings of the evaluations and the team's proposal or denial of specialized instruction.

Some students with ADHD will need an individualized education program (IEP) in order to make progress in an academic setting, while others will not [8]. Some students who do not qualify for an IEP still may benefit from a 504 plan. Section 504 of the Rehabilitation Act ensures that schools make accommodations for students with disabilities [8]. Students with ADHD generally benefit from preferential seating, extra time on examinations, and frequent breaks. These are the types of accommodations that can be included in a 504 plan.

If an adolescent has an IEP or 504 plan, the team working with the student at school must have a formal meeting annually to review progress [9]. The team should also determine whether the special education supports in the IEP or the accommodations provided as part of the 504 plan are appropriate or need to be enhanced.

Psychologists/Evaluators

If the adolescent has ongoing difficulties or if a family is not in agreement with the IEP evaluation, parents should consult with the members of their child's "ADHD team" to determine if a psychological or neuropsychological evaluation is warranted. This can include cognitive testing, academic testing, and assessments of executive functioning, social communication, and social-emotional functioning. The psychologist/neuropsychologist who conducts this testing will become part of the adolescent's team. They will write a report with diagnoses and recommendations based on the testing. If specific interventions are requested, parents can ask if the evaluator is available to attend a school meeting so that they can speak to their recommendations. An adolescents' health insurance may or may not cover the cost of this evaluation. If a parent disagrees with the school system about the provision of special education services, they can also request that the school pays for this evaluation.

Attorney/Advocate

When parents are concerned that their child is not making adequate progress in their public school, it may be appropriate to hire an advocate or an attorney who focuses on special education issues. This is a professional who has expert knowledge in special education and disability policies and can help negotiate school services and accommodations on behalf of the child with the school district.

Tutors

Families can consider hiring a tutor if the adolescent is experiencing ongoing academic struggles, either at the middle school, high school, or college level. If all professionals that a family has consulted believe that the adolescent's school is offering optimal supports, either through general education, special education, or accommodations through a 504 plan, and the adolescent is still struggling, then finding a tutor may be useful. A tutor can focus upon executive functioning skills or can provide support in a specific subject area, depending on the adolescent's needs. Parents should interview tutors to make sure they understand ADHD and inquire what experience the tutor has in working with children with attentional challenges. Tutors can be costly, but many local agencies provide reduced cost or free support. Peer-to-peer tutoring is often available in high schools, and local colleges and universities may offer additional tutoring options.

Mentors

For adolescents with ADHD, mentors can serve as role models and offer guidance in a supportive manner. According to a study conducted by Miranda-Chan et al., "Having a naturally occurring mentor in adolescence was associated with better psychological well-being, greater overall satisfaction with a romantic partner, greater education attainment, and less criminal activity in young adulthood" [10]. There are formal mentorship programs, or perhaps the adolescent has a more informal mentor, such as an athletic coach, who is willing to spend more time with them and provide some additional guidance to help prepare the adolescent for the future. Michael Sandler specifically recommends a mentor for college students with ADHD; this can be someone in the office of disabilities or a professor who has a good understanding of the challenges a student with ADHD may encounter [11].

College Team

Prior to applying to college, it is important for students with ADHD to work with their high school's college counselor to seek input about the optimal environment for higher education. If the adolescent's high school does not have a college counselor, some families hire a private college counselor with expertise in finding programs for students with ADHD or other learning differences.

For those adolescents who move out of their family's home and live at their college, parents will not be present to assist with work completion as they were in high school. It is important to consider this when determining if an adolescent is prepared to handle the work load of college on their own. Getting the "team's" input regarding this choice is essential. A therapist or college counselor can help facilitate a conversation with the adolescent and family around this topic.

> When considering colleges, families should contact the office of disability services to obtain information regarding the college's resources for a student with ADHD.

Michael Sandler recommends asking if there is a staff member who specializes in working with students with ADHD as opposed to staff who work with disabilities in general. He also suggests asking about what services/accommodations can be provided, and families should compare and contrast options at different colleges [11]. There may be extra services available at some colleges for additional fees, but families should be aware of what is included with tuition.

Once in college, if a student is struggling, they should work to get professors on their team by meeting with them and explaining their attentional challenges. Professors can help provide guidance and accommodations to help with successful academic outcomes. Edward Filo notes that while the disability services staff can be helpful, professors in particular subject areas can be better equipped to determine accommodations in their specific academic domain [12]. Being proactive at the beginning of a semester can be key to ensuring that professors understand a student's motivation and desire to succeed [12].

Most colleges have health centers, and if ongoing medical care for ADHD or mental health care is warranted, the campus health center likely has medical professionals who can provide these services. Some will help find local care accessible to their college students. Again, it can be useful to research this information when making a decision about college. Families can compare and contrast college options and help determine the best fit if they know the resources available.

Peer Supports

As adolescence is a time during which peers and fitting in are of utmost importance, it can be helpful for teenagers with ADHD to connect to peers who are dealing with similar struggles. If medical providers have recommended that an adolescent takes medication to help with attention or hyperactivity, it can be useful to connect the adolescent with other teenagers who have taken ADHD medication so that they can have a better understanding of how this treatment option may have helped others [6]. A peer support group for college students with ADHD can provide another layer of support in addition to a disability services office [12]. In addition, it can be useful to connect an adolescent with ADHD with a successful peer role model who does not have ADHD. School guidance counselors and college disability offices may be able to recommend informal or more formalized peer supports to families and adolescents.

Support Groups for Parents

Parents of children with ADHD face unique challenges, and it may be helpful for parents to join a support group specific to parenting a child with attention difficulties. As part of a support group, parents may feel less isolated and may learn new strategies to help their child by listening to the success and struggles of other parents in a similar situation. These can be in-person groups or groups that exist on the internet [13].

Employment

If the adolescent has a job, another member of their team is their employer. The adolescent will need to decide if it would be helpful to disclose their ADHD diagnosis to their supervisor. If a disclosure is made, the adolescent is entitled to reasonable accommodations, in accordance with the Americans with Disabilities Act and Rehabilitation Act of 1973 [14]. The adolescent should consider, in consultation with their team, which accommodations have been helpful in the academic setting. They should then brainstorm how those accommodations will translate into a workplace setting. A supervisor can also become a valuable member of the adolescent's team, helping them discern how their strengths can shine and their attentional challenges can be accommodated to optimize workplace performance [14].

Other Supports

An adolescent probably has people in their lives who are supporting them but do not have any expertise in ADHD. These adults may include athletic coaches, family members, a youth group advisor, or another member of the adolescent's community. It is important to consider these more informal supports as part of the adolescent's team, as they can offer insight into more of the adolescent's strengths and successes in a way that a therapist or educator may not appreciate or understand. Sometimes, it is helpful for these people to participate in IEP or 504 plan meetings.

The Adolescent as Part of the Team

It cannot be overstated that the adolescent themselves must be a member of their team to ensure that their voice is heard in the decisions that are made about them and in establishing the supports they need to be successful. It can be useful for an adolescent to attend IEP or 504 plan meetings so that they can provide the team with information about how supports are helping them and if there are additional services that they think may be of benefit to them. An adolescent should prepare for the meeting beforehand by either writing down or thinking about the following:

> Starting at age fourteen, children can be invited to their IEP or 504 plan annual meetings.

- What should your school team know about you?
- What would you like your school team to know about how your ADHD impacts your school work?
- What is the team already doing that is helping you? What can they do to help you more?

Even if an adolescent does not have formalized supports through an IEP or 504 plan, their team should help empower them to advocate for themselves by setting up meetings with teachers and supportive professionals as needed.

Case Revisited

Clark's situation is not unusual. Often academic difficulties for children with ADHD do not arise until high school when demands change. He and his parents may start brainstorming the reasons that he is struggling to get his work done; executive function demands, social stressors, medication nonadherence, new-onset anxiety, or depression all come to mind as possible explanations. A meeting with his primary care provider may help identify the next steps to take, which may include requesting an IEP evaluation, supporting executive function with school supports or tutoring, and a referral for counseling to address social-emotional struggles. Reviewing medication adherence should be part of these conversations. Clark and his family should start to build his team, considering this a proactive step in supporting his success as he moves into more challenging situations and setting him up to thrive in high school and thereafter.

Conclusions

The most important role that the team can play is helping the adolescent stay positive and future oriented. Adolescence can be a trying time for anyone, and those with ADHD face additional challenges. Therefore, building a multidisciplinary support system for an adolescent with ADHD is critical. A team of family members, medical professionals, educators, professionals specializing in ADHD, mentors, peer supports, and other relevant supportive adults can help navigate the unique obstacles that adolescents with ADHD encounter, launching them into successful early adulthood. The team should also support their family in their journey as well.

Tips
- Include your teen when you put a team together. Talk about why specific people will be important to their success.
- Keep a list of your team, with contact phone numbers and emails.
- A bigger team does not mean a more problematic situation.

References

1. Committee on Children with Disabilities. The pediatrician's role in development of an individual education plan (IEP) and/or an individual service plan (IFSP). Pediatrics. 1999;104(1):124–7.
2. "What is a Medical Home?" In American Academy of Pediatrics. https://medicalhomeinfo. aap.org/overview/Pages/Whatisthemedicalhome.aspx. Accessed 10 Dec 2018.
3. Ronis DD, Baldwin CD, Blumkin A, Kuhlthau K, Szilagyi PG. Patient-centered medical home and family burden in attention-deficit hyperactivity disorder. J Dev Behav Pediatr. 2015;36(6):417–25.
4. Knapp CA, Hinojosa M, Baron-Lee J, Fernandez-Baca D, Hinojosa R, Thompson L. Factors associated with a medical home among children with attention-deficit hyperactivity disorder. Matern Child Health J. 2012;16(9):1171–8.
5. Robin AL. ADHD in adolescents. New York: Guilford Press; 1998.
6. Robin AL. ADHD in adolescents. In: Brown TE, editor. ADHD comorbidities. Washington, D.C: American Psychiatric Publishing; 2009. p. 69–81.

7. Murray, et al. Prevalence and characteristics of school services for high school students with attention-deficit/hyperactivity disorder. School Ment Health. 2014;6(4):264–78.
8. Engel M, Mariko Favini P, Sindelar T. Legal issues in the education of children with special health care needs. In: Porter SM, Branowicki PA, Palfrey JS, editors. Supporting students with special health care needs. Baltimore: Paul H. Brookes Publishing; 2014. p. 37–64.
9. Wright PW, Wright PD. Special education law. 2nd ed. Virginia: Harbor House Law Press, Inc.; 2011.
10. Miranda-Chan T, Fruiht V, Dubon V, Wray-Lake L. The functions and longitudinal outcomes of adolescents' naturally occurring mentorships. Am J Community Psychol. 2016;57:47–59.
11. Sander M. College confidence with ADD. Illinois: Sourcebooks, Inc.; 2008.
12. Filo E. From ADHD to Tourette syndrome: supporting students with social disorders in higher education. Pennsylvania: LRP Publications; 2005.
13. Northen H, Kurland R. Social work with groups. 3rd ed. New York: Columbia Press; 2001.
14. Sarkis E. Addressing attention-deficit/hyperactivity disorder in the workplace. Postgrad Med. 2014;126:25–30.

Index

© Springer Nature Switzerland AG 2020
A. Schonwald (ed.), *ADHD in Adolescents*,
https://doi.org/10.1007/978-3-030-62393-7

Printed in the United States
by Baker & Taylor Publisher Services